Neuropsychology of Sports-Related Concussion

Neuropsychology of Sports-Related Concussion

EDITED BY **PETER A. ARNETT**

AMERICAN PSYCHOLOGICAL ASSOCIATION
Washington, DC

The opinions and statements published are the responsibility of the authors, and such opinions and statements do not necessarily represent the policies of the American Psychological Association.

Published by
American Psychological Association
750 First Street, NE
Washington, DC 20002
www.apa.org

APA Order Department
P.O. Box 92984
Washington, DC 20090-2984
Phone: (800) 374-2721; Direct: (202) 336-5510
Fax: (202) 336-5502; TDD/TTY: (202) 336-6123
Online: http://www.apa.org/pubs/books
E-mail: order@apa.org

In the U.K., Europe, Africa, and the Middle East, copies may be ordered from
Eurospan Group
c/o Turpin Distribution
Pegasus Drive
Stratton Business Park
Biggleswade, Bedfordshire
SG18 8TQ United Kingdom
Phone: +44 (0) 1767 604972
Fax: +44 (0) 1767 601640
Online: https://www.eurospanbookstore.com/apa
E-mail: eurospan@turpin-distribution.com

Typeset in Goudy by Circle Graphics, Inc., Columbia, MD

Printer: Thomson-Shore, Dexter, MI
Cover Designer: Beth Schlenoff Design, Bethesda, MD

Library of Congress Cataloging-in-Publication Data

Names: Arnett, Peter A., editor. | American Psychological Association, publisher.
Title: Neuropsychology of sports-related concussion / edited by Peter A. Arnett.
Description: First edition. | Washington, DC : American Psychological Association,
   [2019] | Includes bibliographical references and index.
Identifiers: LCCN 2018016364 (print) | LCCN 2018017007 (ebook) |
   ISBN 9781433829826 (eBook) | ISBN 1433829827 (eBook) | ISBN 9781433829796
   (hardcover) | ISBN 1433829797 (hardcover)
Subjects: | MESH: Brain Concussion—physiopathology | Brain Concussion—
   complications | Athletic Injuries | Neuropsychology—methods |
   Post-Concussion Syndrome
Classification: LCC RC394.C7 (ebook) | LCC RC394.C7 (print) | NLM WL 354 |
   DDC 617.4/81044—dc23
LC record available at https://lccn.loc.gov/2018016364

British Library Cataloguing-in-Publication Data
A CIP record is available from the British Library.

Printed in the United States of America

http://dx.doi.org/10.1037/0000114-000

10 9 8 7 6 5 4 3 2 1

CONTENTS

CONTRIBUTORS

Michael L. Alosco, PhD, Boston University Alzheimer's Disease Center, Boston University CTE Center, Department of Neurology, Boston University School of Medicine, Boston, MA

Peter A. Arnett, PhD, Psychology Department, Neuropsychology of Sports Concussion & MS Programs, Pennsylvania State University, University Park

Breton M. Asken, MS, ATC, Department of Clinical and Health Psychology, University of Florida, Gainesville

William B. Barr, PhD, Department of Neurology, New York University School of Medicine, New York

Megan Bradson, BS, Psychology Department, Pennsylvania State University, University Park

Abigail C. Bretzin, MS, ATC, Department of Kinesiology, Sport Related Concussion Laboratory, Michigan State University, East Lansing

Jared M. Bruce, PhD, Department of Psychology, Department of Biomedical and Health Informatics, University of Missouri, Kansas City

Michael W. Collins, PhD, Department of Orthopaedic Surgery, University of Pittsburgh Medical Center, Sports Medicine Concussion Program, Pittsburgh, PA

Tracey Covassin, PhD, ATC, FNATA, Department of Kinesiology, Sport Related Concussion Laboratory, Michigan State University, East Lansing

Ruben J. Echemendia, PhD, University Orthopedics Center, Concussion Clinic, State College, PA

Sheri A. Fedor, PT, DPT, NCS, Centers for Rehab Services, Inova Physical Therapy Center, Fairfax, VA

Meghan E. Fox, PhD, ATC, Movement Science Department, Grand Valley State University, Allendale, MI

Morgan Glusman, MS, Department of Psychology, University of Missouri, Kansas City

Emily C. Grossner, MS, Department of Psychology, Pennsylvania State University, University Park

Neha Gupta, BS, Eberly College of Science, Schreyer Honors College, Pennsylvania State University, University Park

Erin Guty, MS, Department of Psychology, Pennsylvania State University, University Park

Rose C. Healy, BA, Boston University Alzheimer's Disease Center, Boston University CTE Center, Department of Neurology, Boston University School of Medicine, Boston, MA

Jill R. Henley, PsyD, Integrated Center for Child Development, Sports Psychology Department, Newton, MA

Frank G. Hillary, PhD, Department of Psychology, Pennsylvania State University, University Park

Arthur Maerlender, PhD, ABPP-CN, Center for Brain, Biology and Behavior, University of Nebraska, Lincoln

Andrew R. Mayer, PhD, Mind Research Network; Department of Neurology, University of New Mexico, Albuquerque

Michael A. McCrea, PhD, Department of Neurosurgery, Medical College of Wisconsin, Milwaukee

Victoria C. Merritt, PhD, VA San Diego Healthcare System, San Diego, CA

Jessica Meyer, PhD, Psychology Department, Pennsylvania State University, University Park, PA

Lindsay D. Nelson, PhD, Department of Neurosurgery, Medical College of Wisconsin, Milwaukee

Amanda R. Rabinowitz, PhD, Moss Rehabilitation Research Institute, Elkins Park, PA

Wayne J. Sebastianelli, MD, Pennsylvania State College of Medicine, Pennsylvania State Sports Medicine, State College, PA

Semyon M. Slobounov, PhD, Department of Kinesiology, Pennsylvania State University, University Park

Robert A. Stern, PhD, Boston University Alzheimer's Disease Center, Boston University CTE Center, Departments of Neurology, Neurosurgery, and Anatomy and Neurobiology, Boston University School of Medicine, Boston, MA

Denise S. Vagt, PsyD, Florida Institute of Technology, Melbourne

Alexa E. Walter, MS, Department of Kinesiology, Pennsylvania State University, University Park

Frank M. Webbe, PhD, Director of Concussion Management, Florida Institute of Technology, Melbourne

Melissa N. Womble, PhD, Inova Medical Group Orthopaedics & Sports Medicine, Inova Sports Medicine Concussion Program, Fairfax, VA

ACKNOWLEDGMENTS

This book is dedicated to my loving wife, Melissa, and my children, Nathan and Raina. Thank you so much for your inspiration and support over the years. I want to thank my brother, Jeffrey, who has been an inspiration to me throughout my career as a scholar and scientist, as well as a true friend. I also want to thank my other siblings: Steve, for his initial intellectual inspiration for me to pursue a career in academia; Mike, whose career in medicine helped fuel my interest in combining medical and psychiatric issues in my career; and Claudia, whose dedication to addressing mental health issues with her work helped encourage me to do the same. I am also grateful to all of the graduate students with whom I have been privileged to work during my academic and clinical career. Your creativity, dedication, and hard work have truly made my career worthwhile. Special thanks to those students who have served as concussion program coordinators for me at Penn State, including Chris Bailey, Aaron Rosenbaum, Fiona Barwick, Amanda Rabinowitz, Gray Vargas, Victoria Merritt, Jessica Meyer, and Erin Guty. This research and clinical program could not have been done without you, and I am forever grateful for the time and talent you have dedicated to this! Finally, I thank all of the athletes whom I have seen over the years as part of the Penn State Concussion Program. It has been a privilege providing clinical care to you to help ensure your safe return-to-play. I hope this book will help provide even better care to concussed athletes in the future.

Neuropsychology of Sports-Related Concussion

INTRODUCTION

PETER A. ARNETT

The Penn State Sports Concussion Program was initially developed by Drs. Ruben J. Echemendia and Margot Putukian in the 1990s. After both left Penn State in the early 2000s, I was asked to assume responsibility for the part of the program focusing on neuropsychology and gladly took it on. Since that time, during about the past 15 years, sports concussion has received increasingly intense research and media attention. In the past, concussions in sports were often disregarded as "dings," or "getting your bell rung." Currently, no one with even relatively casual knowledge of concussion would say these things. With Ann McKee's Boston University group recently publishing their chronic traumatic encephalopathy (CTE) study on former National Football League (NFL) players, the potential long-term impact of repeated concussions has been brought into vivid relief. Her Boston University group found that 110 of the 111 former NFL players' brains were consistent with CTE (Mez et al., 2017). With that said, acute sports concussions, although serious neurological events, if approached with knowledge and care, can often be managed well.

http://dx.doi.org/10.1037/0000114-001
Neuropsychology of Sports-Related Concussion, P. A. Arnett (Editor)

AUDIENCE AND SCOPE FOR THE BOOK

In this book, the focus is on concussions that occur through participation in sport. There are certainly other mechanisms of concussion that could lead to similar outcomes (e.g., blast injury as a result of combat injuries, motor vehicle accidents), but treatment of concussions that occur outside of the context of sports goes beyond the scope of this book. Although the various chapters sometimes provide slightly different definitions of sports concussion, all are consistent with McCrory and colleagues' (2017) recent consensus statement indicating that "sport related concussion is a traumatic brain injury induced by biomechanical forces" (p. 839).

With this in mind, I think readers will find much to round out their knowledge of sports concussion in this book, with chapters written by some of the leading experts in this field. Even if you have relatively little understanding of sports concussion, you will find this book to be accessible and easy to follow. If you already have more specialized knowledge, the chapters will expand your understanding with cutting-edge researchers in the field providing an up-to-date accounting of particular areas. Almost all chapters end with a section titled "Key Questions to Be Addressed in the Next 5 Years" that details suggested directions for research moving forward.

If you are involved in the management of sports-related concussions, this book will also meet your needs. Nearly every chapter includes a case study that illustrates its main theme. Of note, all cases included have been de-identified to protect the confidentiality of the individuals discussed. Additionally, most chapters have a section at the end titled "Key Clinical Take-Home Points" that includes fundamental knowledge that all health care providers involved in the care of sports concussion can use immediately. Finally, as a didactic teaching tool, this book can be used as core reading for a class on sports-related concussion that is at the upper undergraduate or beginning graduate level course.

ORGANIZATION OF THE BOOK

In terms of its organization, the book is divided into four topical sections that are essential for understanding neuropsychological aspects of sports concussion. The first section, Symptom Outcomes and Management, includes chapters by Michael A. McCrea and colleagues on persistent postconcussive symptoms; Melissa N. Womble, Michael (Micky) W. Collins, and colleagues from the University of Pittsburgh group on posttraumatic headache and migraine assessment; and a final chapter, by Erin Guty, Megan Bradson, and me, at Penn State on depression and anxiety in sports concussion management.

The second section, Biological Underpinnings and Consequences, includes three informative chapters. The initial chapter, by Victoria C. Merritt and me, focuses on genetic factors, with the next chapter by Emily C. Grossner, Andrew R. Mayer, and Frank G. Hillary, providing an informative review of the use of neuroimaging in sports concussion. The final chapter of this section is on CTE by Michael L. Alosco, Rose C. Healy, and Robert A. Stern from the Boston University group. The third section, Factors Affecting the Validity of Neuropsychological Results, addresses a range of important measurement issues that can affect the validity of neuropsychological results in the sports concussion context. Tracey Covassin and her collaborators at Michigan State provide an authoritative review on sex differences in sports concussion, followed by a chapter by Amanda R. Rabinowitz on issues relating to the assessment of effort on testing based on some of her seminal work in this area. The next chapter, by Arthur (Art) Maerlender, provides a wide-ranging review of a host of validity issues in neuropsychological assessment in this context, followed by a final chapter by Jessica Meyer and me that presents some empirical data comparing the sensitivity of the ImPACT test with traditional neuropsychological measures. The final section, Specialty Contributions to Sports Concussion, begins with an excellent chapter by Ruben J. Echemendia and colleagues focusing on neuropsychology in professional sports, taking advantage of his many years of experiences consulting with Major League Soccer, the NFL, and the National Hockey League, among other professional sports leagues. A chapter by my colleagues at Penn State, Alexa E. Walter and Semyon (Sam) M. Slobounov, then presents a fascinating presentation of virtual-reality paradigms as applied to sports concussion, followed by a chapter by one of the central players in developing the field of pediatric concussion, Frank M. Webbe and his colleague Denise S. Vagt. The final substantive chapter of the book is written by Neha Gupta and Wayne J. Sebastianelli; the latter is medical director of Penn State Sports Medicine and has had long-term involvement working with that institution's athletes. This chapter focuses on how the paradigm for management of concussions in orthopedic settings has changed dramatically in recent years.

QUESTIONS ADDRESSED BY THE BOOK

With this overview in mind, you will be able to address a number of important questions upon reading this book:

1. How are persistent postconcussion symptoms (including headache, depression, and anxiety, among others) best managed, and what do we still need to learn about such symptoms to improve our care of concussed athletes?

2. Why is it important to understand genetic and other biological factors that may alter risk for persisting symptomatology post-concussion, and what do we do with this information?
3. When taking into consideration all the factors that can influence the validity of neuropsychological tests in the sports concussion context, what approach will allow us to provide the most accurate assessment of cognitive functioning postconcussion?
4. Finally, how should we alter our approach to managing sports concussion in different contexts and populations to provide the most accurate assessment and treatment?

To conclude, I hope you will enjoy this book. It provides authoritative accounts of some central areas of interest in the neuropsychology of sports concussion. Each chapter can be digested and considered on its own, but by reading the entire book, you will appreciate the significance of the broader themes covered. Happy reading!

REFERENCES

McCrory, P., Meeuwisse, W., Dvořák, J., Aubry, M., Bailes, J., Broglio, S., . . . Vos, P. E. (2017). Consensus statement on concussion in sport—The 5th international conference on concussion in sport held in Berlin, October 2016. *British Journal of Sports Medicine, 51*, 838–847.

Mez, J., Daneshvar, D. H., Kiernan, P. T., Abdolmohammadi, B., Alvarez, V. E., Huber, B. R., . . . McKee, A. C. (2017). Clinicopathological evaluation of chronic traumatic encephalopathy in players of American football. *JAMA, 318*, 360–370.

I

SYMPTOM OUTCOMES AND MANAGEMENT

1

PERSISTENT POSTCONCUSSIVE SYMPTOMS AFTER SPORT-RELATED CONCUSSION

MICHAEL A. McCREA, BRETON M. ASKEN,
LINDSAY D. NELSON, AND WILLIAM B. BARR

Sport-related concussion (SRC) is widely recognized as a major international public health issue that has become a focus of increasing concern from clinicians, researchers, sporting organizations, and athletes themselves over the past 20 years (Barr & McCrea, 2001; DeKosky, Ikonomovic, & Gandy, 2010; Langlois, Rutland-Brown, & Wald, 2006; McCrory et al., 2017). The annual incidence of nonfatal traumatic brain injuries (TBIs) from sports and recreation activities in persons aged 19 years or younger is estimated to be more than 2.6 million per year in the United States (Centers for Disease Control and Prevention, 2011). Concussion is now among the most frequent sports injuries at all participation levels, including youth sports (Guskiewicz, Weaver, Padua, & Garrett, 2000; Halstead, Walter, & The Council on Sports Medicine and Fitness, 2010). From 1997 to 2007, emergency department visits for 8- to 13-year-olds affected by concussion in organized sports doubled and increased by more than 200% in the 14- to 19-year-old group (Bakhos, Lockhart, Myers, & Linakis, 2010).

http://dx.doi.org/10.1037/0000114-002
Neuropsychology of Sports-Related Concussion, P. A. Arnett (Editor)

Elevated incidence and reporting rates likely reflect improved SRC awareness and recognition and do not necessarily indicate that sports have become more dangerous over time (LaRoche, Nelson, Connelly, Walter, & McCrea, 2016).

Increases in the reported incidence of SRC over the past several years also drive concerns about potential long-term effects of injury on neurologic, cognitive, psychological, and social functioning (DeKosky et al., 2010; McCrory et al., 2017). These reemerging concerns that exposure to multiple concussions and repetitive subclinical brain trauma in collision sports may increase an athlete's long-term risk for neurodegenerative pathology were originally raised almost 100 years ago (Martland, 1928; McKee et al., 2013). In the interim and continuing to the present day, the risk of persistent symptoms (e.g., headaches, cognitive dysfunction), often referred to as *postconcussion syndrome* (PCS), has been another primary concern with respect to the chronic effects of concussion.

This chapter focuses on the latter, including a broad overview of best practice approaches to diagnosis, assessment, and management of athletes with persistent symptoms after SRC. In doing so, we review existing evidence from studies specifically of SRC, while also noting findings from the wealth of literature on persistent symptoms and PCS in the context of civilian mild TBI (mTBI). Given the nature of this text and its likely readership, special attention is paid to the valuable role of the neuropsychologist in the evaluation and treatment of athletes who experience persistent SRC symptoms. This book dedicates other sections to the discussion of more chronic effects of repetitive concussion or head impact exposure, including chronic traumatic encephalopathy.

NATURAL HISTORY OF RECOVERY AFTER SRC

Extensive research over the past 2 decades has significantly advanced our scientific understanding of the true natural history of clinical recovery following SRC. A 2003 report was the first to plot the continuous time course of recovery immediately following and within several days after SRC, indicating that more than 90% of athletes reported symptom recovery within 1 week. Figure 1.1 displays the recovery curves for symptoms, cognitive performance, and postural stability from this study (McCrea et al., 2003). Several other prospective studies have since demonstrated that the overwhelming majority of athletes achieve a complete recovery in symptoms, cognitive functioning, postural stability, and other functional impairments over a period of approximately 1 to 2 weeks after SRC (Belanger & Vanderploeg, 2005; Broglio & Puetz, 2008; Collins et al., 1999; Guskiewicz et al., 2003; Macciocchi, Barth, Alves, Rimel, & Jane, 1996).

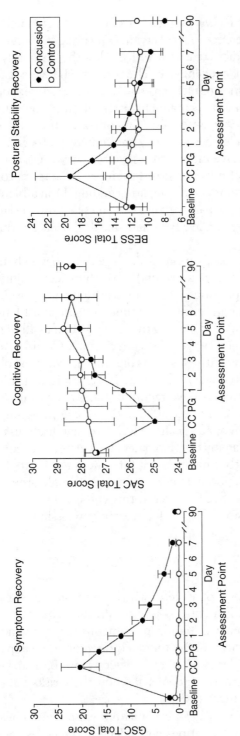

Figure 1.1. Recovery curves from the National Collegiate Athletic Association Concussion Study. Symptom, cognitive, and postural stability recovery in concussion and control participants. Higher scores on the Graded Symptom Checklist (GSC) indicate more severe symptoms; lower scores on the Standardized Assessment of Concussion (SAC) indicate poorer cognitive performance; higher scores on the Balance Error Scoring System (BESS) indicate poorer postural stability. Error bars reflect 95% confidence intervals. CC = time of concussion; PG = postgame or postpractice. From "Acute Effects and Recovery Time Following Concussion in Collegiate Football Players: The NCAA Concussion Study," by M. McCrea, K. M. Guskiewicz, S. W. Marshall, W. Barr, C. Randolph, R. C. Cantu, . . . J. P. Kelly, 2003, *JAMA, 290*, p. 2559. Copyright 2003 by the American Medical Association. Adapted with permission.

Recovery times after SRC vary significantly by recruitment methods. That is, there is a significant difference in recovery times reported from truly prospective, population-based studies compared with studies that primarily enrolled clinic patients or samples of convenience. The core issue here is a major ascertainment bias that confounds results across studies. Prospective, population-based studies provide the most accurate characterization of the acute effects and natural history of recovery after SRC. In contrast, clinic-based studies are systematically confounded because they are limited to observed recovery times in patients who (a) have inherently longer recovery times and (b) seek consultation in specialty clinics because of their persistent symptoms. This consideration is also important when comparing findings from athlete-focused SRC literature to emergency department mTBI studies because the latter often reflects more serious injuries and less systematic medical oversight throughout the recovery process.

Select studies have focused on clarifying the extent to which individual factors (e.g., age, sex, psychological factors) other than acute injury characteristics may be related to prolonged recovery in athletes after SRC. Limited research has suggested a lengthier recovery time in younger athletes (Field, Collins, Lovell, & Maroon, 2003), citing that roughly half of all high school athletes required more than 14 days to recover (Lau, Collins, & Lovell, 2012). Unfortunately, many of these studies did not include control subjects and applied criteria for "recovery" that may have resulted in high false-positive rates. Other researchers have reported that female athletes experience increased symptoms (Colvin et al., 2009) and cognitive impairment (Dougan, Horswill, & Geffen, 2014) after SRC, although findings regarding sex differences in recovery are mixed (Frommer et al., 2011; Zuckerman et al., 2012), and many studies that have found differences are limited by small samples of female athletes, poorly matched male and female groups, or lack of preinjury baseline data. (See Chapter 7, this volume, by Covassin et al. for a more detailed discussion of sex differences in concussion.)

PROLONGED RECOVERY AFTER SRC

There is a sizable subset of athletes whose symptoms persist past this typical window of recovery. Few data exist on the precise frequency of athletes who do not follow this course of rapid, spontaneous recovery and instead exhibit prolonged postconcussive symptoms or other functional impairments. Furthermore, empirical evidence on what risk factors may be associated with prolonged recovery time or poor outcome, and how these risks can be modified in a clinical setting, is inconsistent.

McCrea and colleagues (2013) used data from a multicenter prospective study from 1999 to 2008 investigating acute effects and recovery after SRC.

In total, 18,531 player seasons (i.e., total sport seasons of participation by all athletes) were analyzed. All athletes enrolled in the study had baseline data collected on the Graded Symptom Checklist, Balance Error Scoring System, Standardized Assessment of Concussion, and a brief battery of neuropsychological tests. During the study period, 570 athletes sustained an SRC. Of those, 57 (10%) were classified as having a prolonged recovery, although not necessarily PCS, based on the study definition of SRC symptoms lasting more than 7 days.

In addition to having longer lasting symptoms, the prolonged recovery group performed worse on several cognitive measures during the acute period compared with the typical recovery group (Figure 1.2 describes symptom, cognitive, and postural stability recovery for the prolonged recovery, typical recovery, and control groups). Nearly a quarter (25%, or 2.5% of total injured sample) of the prolonged recovery group's symptoms persisted until the long-term follow-up date of the study (either day 45 or 90 postinjury) without evidence of persisting differences on cognitive functioning or balance measures. Injury-related factors associated with prolonged recovery included the occurrence of unconsciousness, posttraumatic amnesia, and higher symptom severity within 24 hours of injury. In particular, athletes who suffered loss of consciousness had 4.15 times higher odds of experiencing symptoms beyond 7 days compared with those who did not lose consciousness.

These findings and additional literature raise suspicion that a more severe biomechanical injury causes greater disruption of normal brain function, ultimately requiring a longer recovery time. On the basis of the collection of prospective studies across sports, prolonged symptoms (e.g., greater than 7–10 days) are believed to occur in 10% to 25% of athletes (Makdissi, Cantu, Johnston, McCrory, & Meeuwisse, 2013; McCrea et al., 2003; Morgan et al., 2015). Similar to what is estimated from studies of mTBI in nonathlete samples, the prevalence estimate and factors responsible for the presence of persistent symptoms following SRC remains a topic of contention and further investigation in brain injury research (Iverson et al., 2017).

PCS: DEFINITIONAL AND DIAGNOSTIC CHALLENGES

Postconcussive disorder (PCD) or *postconcussion syndrome* are commonly referenced in clinical settings but are poorly defined and often misunderstood terms. Throughout this chapter, we use the term *postconcussion syndrome*, or PCS, when describing persistent symptomatology lasting weeks to months after SRC (depending on the preferred definition). We differentiate PCS from "prolonged" or "protracted" symptoms, which some studies use to describe symptom resolution taking longer than the typical 7 to 10 days.

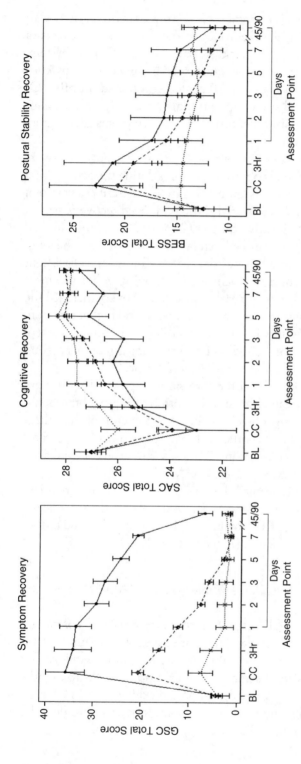

Figure 1.2. Patterns of recovery in symptoms, cognitive function, and postural stability after sport-related concussion in athletes with typical versus prolonged recovery compared with noninjured control subjects. Symptom, cognitive, and postural stability recovery in two groups of concussed participants (prolonged recovery vs. typical recovery; defined by persistence of symptoms) and control participants. Higher scores on the Graded Symptom Checklist (GSC) indicate more severe symptoms; lower scores on the Standardized Assessment of Concussion (SAC) indicate poorer cognitive performance; higher scores on the Balance Error Scoring System (BESS) indicate poorer postural stability. Error bars reflect 95% confidence intervals. CC = time of concussion; PG = postgame/postpractice. Acute injury characteristics (loss of consciousness, posttraumatic amnesia, retrograde amnesia) and postinjury symptom severity were predictive of prolonged recovery, with no relationship found between prolonged recovery and other personal characteristics (e.g., gender, sport, mechanism of injury, neuropsychological impairment). Typical recovery group (open circles); prolonged recovery group (filled circles); and normal control group (Xs). From "Incidence, Clinical Course, and Predictors of Prolonged Recovery Time Following Sport-Related Concussion in High School and College Athletes," by M. McCrea, K. Guskiewicz, C. Randolph, W. B. Barr, T. A. Hammeke, S. W. Marshall, . . . J. P. Kelly, 2013, *Journal of the International Neuropsychological Society, 19,* p. 26. Copyright 2013 by The International Neuropsychological Society. Adapted with permission.

PCS has been proposed for diagnostic use when concussion symptoms, such as neurologic, cognitive, behavioral, or somatic complaints, persist beyond the acute and subacute periods and become chronic, with *chronic* often operationalized as beyond 1 or 3 months (American Psychiatric Association, 1994; World Health Organization, 1992a, 1992b). Figure 1.3 lists the diagnostic guidelines in a research and clinical setting for PCS, according to the *International Classification of Diseases* (10th rev.; ICD–10). The confusion and ambiguity of these terms in the clinical setting undoubtedly reflects the lack of consensus terminology used in the research. The inconsistent definitions and measures used for PCS classification significantly limit our understanding of incidence, prevalence, and risk factors. Currently, studies rely on subjective symptom checklists (e.g., the Rivermead Post-Concussion Symptoms Questionnaire [King, Crawford, Wenden, Moss, & Wade, 1995], Post-Concussion Scale [Lovell et al., 2006], Sport Concussion Assessment Tool—3: Symptom Evaluation [McCrory et al., 2013]) and somewhat arbitrary symptom duration cutoffs. For example, minimum symptom durations have been reported as brief as 14 days and as long as 3 months, and symptom requirements range from presence of any symptoms to a minimum of three symptoms (Babcock et al., 2013; Heitger, Jones, & Anderson, 2008; Lau, Kontos, Collins, Mucha, & Lovell, 2011). Recognizing some individuals may have a protracted recovery relative to expected timelines without being diagnosed with a post-concussion *syndrome* is important in both a clinical and a research setting.

The cause of PCS is unclear because research has yet to yield a reliable or validated diagnostic biomarker of either PCS risk or presence with adequate sensitivity and specificity. Lishman (1988) proposed the idea that the physiological effects of brain injury contribute most strongly during the acute stage, but psychosocial influences primarily drive symptom expression in more chronic stages. As such, accurate symptom attribution in the weeks to months following mTBI is difficult because the symptoms commonly associated with PCS, such as chronic headache or decreased concentration, may be secondary to non-mTBI factors, such as musculoskeletal injury, chronic pain, or psychological factors. Regardless, it has been reasonably well established that PCS, in lieu of other explanatory factors, is not a unidimensional condition but rather an outcome influenced by cognitive, emotional, medical, psychosocial, and motivational factors (Iverson, Zasler, & Lange, 2007; McCrea, 2007). Treatment must incorporate a broad biopsychosocial framework, which emphasizes the critical role of the neuropsychologist.

Inconsistent definitions, factors beyond mTBI affecting symptoms, and attributional biases make PCS one of the more controversial and challenging conditions in the neurosciences to diagnose and treat. Contributing to the controversy is a limited understanding of mTBI among many primary care and specialty professionals who do not routinely provide care to individuals after

General F07	"Personality and Behavioral Disorders due to Brain Disease, Damage, and Dysfunction"
G1	Objective evidence (from physical and neurological examination and laboratory tests) and/or history, of cerebral disease, damage, or dysfunction
G2	Absence of clouding of consciousness and of significant memory deficit
G3	Absence of sufficient or suggestive evidence for an alternative causation of the personality or behavior disorder that would justify placement in section F6 ("Other Mental Disorders due to Brain Damage and Dysfunction and to Physical Disease")

F07.2 (Research Criteria)	"Postconcussional Syndrome"
A	The general criteria of F07 must be met
B	History of head trauma with loss of consciousness, preceding the onset of symptoms by a period of up to four weeks (objective EEG, brain imaging, or oculonystagmographic evidence of brain damage may be lacking)
C	At least three of the following:
(1)	Complaints of unpleasant sensations and pains, such as headache, dizziness (usually lacking the features of true vertigo), general malaise and excessive fatigue, or noise intolerance
(2)	Emotional changes, such as irritability, emotional lability, both easily provoked or exacerbated by emotional excitement or stress, or some degree of depression and/or anxiety
(3)	Subjective complaints of difficulty in concentration and in performing mental tasks, and of memory complaints, without clear objective evidence (e.g., psychological tests) of marked impairment
(4)	Insomnia
(5)	Reduced tolerance to alcohol
(6)	Preoccupation with the above symptoms and fear of permanent brain damage, to the extent of hypochondriacal over-valued ideas and adoption of the sick role
General	The syndrome occurs following head trauma (usually sufficiently severe to result in loss of consciousness) and includes a number of disparate symptoms such as headache, dizziness (usually lacking the features of true vertigo), fatigue, irritability, difficulty in concentrating and performing mental tasks, impairment of memory, insomnia, and reduced tolerance to stress, emotional excitement, or alcohol. These symptoms may be accompanied by feelings of depression or anxiety, resulting from some loss of self-esteem and fear of permanent brain damage. Such feelings enhance the original symptoms and a vicious circle results. Some patients become hypochondriacal, embark on a search for diagnosis and cure, and may adopt a permanent sick role. The etiology of these symptoms is not always clear, and both organic and psychological factors have been proposed to account for them. The nosological status of this condition is thus somewhat uncertain. There is little doubt, however, that this syndrome is common and distressing to the patient.
Diagnostic Guidelines	At least three of the features described above should be present for a definite diagnosis. Careful evaluation with laboratory techniques (electroencephalography, brain stem evoked potentials, brain imaging, oculonystagmography) may yield objective evidence to substantiate the symptoms but results are often negative. The complaints are not necessarily associated with compensation motives.

Figure 1.3. Diagnostic guidelines in the research and clinical settings for "Postconcussional Syndrome" according to the World Health Organization (1992a). EEG = electroencephalogram.

brain injury or recognize the nonspecific nature of the postconcussion symptoms. Such factors can lead to misdiagnosis and misattribution of symptoms. For example, while acute headache after concussion is common and often related to the physiological effects of brain injury, chronic headaches after concussion can be related to musculoskeletal injuries (e.g., cervical muscle strain) that may have occurred at the time of the concussive event but are not from the brain concussion per se. Leddy et al. (2015) found that symptom reporting alone did not differentiate subjects considered physiologically recovered based on a validated exertional protocol from those with normal treadmill performance but abnormal cervical–vestibular examination findings. They emphasized the need to perform specific exertional versus orthopedic–vestibular examinations when attempting to determine etiology of persistent symptoms. Chronic headaches, regardless of underlying cause, may precipitate a PCS diagnosis when etiology may be unrelated to mTBI effects.

Similarly, attention and concentration problems directly related to the early pathophysiology after mTBI can persist after the brain dysfunction has resolved due to the indirect contributions of ancillary symptoms (e.g., chronic pain, dizziness, or sleep disturbance). Formal diagnosis of PCS requires not only that symptoms persist beyond a stipulated time frame but also that other differential diagnoses and confounds that may explain the patient's symptoms (e.g., somatic symptom disorders, factitious disorder, posttraumatic stress disorder [PTSD], malingering) have been ruled out. This is often extremely challenging when multiple etiologies for concussion-like symptoms exist.

There are also population-specific risk considerations when managing a patient's recovery. The main goal for most civilian mTBI patients involves returning to work or school where, depending on the nature of one's job, there is likely minimal risk for exacerbating the injury or sustaining another injury. For athletes, however, there is often significant motivation to return to athletic activity with high likelihood of exposure to reinjury. The sports medicine clinician is tasked with the difficult responsibility of balancing the neurobiological risks of returning the chronically symptomatic athlete to sports participation with the negative psychosocial effects associated with prolonged removal from their sport which, in turn, can mimic or exacerbate ongoing symptoms in the postconcussion period (Mainwaring, Hutchison, Bisschop, Comper, & Richards, 2010). Neuropsychologists are uniquely trained in recognizing and appreciating the interplay of these symptom sources.

PCS AFTER SRC

Athletes warrant separate consideration from civilian populations, particularly in more elite samples, such as collegiate and professional athletes. From a research interpretation standpoint, it is important for clinicians to recognize that most athletes undergo consistent medical oversight and are often a far less biased sample than relying on emergency department visits. Perhaps even more important, in the event an athlete sustains an SRC, he or she often has daily access to medical personnel (typically a certified athletic trainer). This allows for constant modifications and adjustments to the rehabilitation process by clinicians with specific training in managing concussion relative to many emergency department or primary care physicians.

Athletes, on average, are likely to be in better health than nonathletes when they sustain a concussion and exhibit a lower rate of preexisting risk factors, such as psychiatric diagnoses. These reasons, among others, may explain the different recovery trajectories seen in civilian versus athlete-specific literature, as well as differences in what is considered "normal" recovery. Patients visiting an emergency department or primary care physician might commonly be told that a 3- to 4-week recovery is normal, whereas sports medicine clinicians typically expect symptoms to last only 1 to 2 weeks. Therefore, "protracted recovery" and symptom duration indicating a "postconcussion syndrome" might be very different constructs for athletes versus civilians. With that in mind, we discuss the understanding of PCS in athlete populations specifically, while referencing concepts from civilian literature that likely also apply to athletes.

There is comparatively little information regarding the rates and predictors of PCS in athlete samples. Although injury factors such as loss of consciousness, posttraumatic amnesia, and more severe acute symptoms are found to predict prolonged recovery time (i.e., symptoms lasting greater than 7 days) in a minority of athletes (McCrea et al., 2013), findings are inconsistent (Iverson et al., 2017; Tator & Davis, 2014; Zuckerman et al., 2016). Risk factors identified in civilian mTBI literature may be differentially prevalent in athlete-specific samples, but considering their effects is equally essential.

Researchers involved in studies of SRC only recently began appreciating the complexity of interacting factors potentially helpful in predicting or explaining prolonged recovery and PCS (Morgan et al., 2015). Attempts to apply concepts from civilian mTBI literature include a focus on psychological factors (e.g., misattribution, nocebo effect, "good-old-days" phenomena) underlying risk for PCS (Gunstad & Suhr, 2001). As a group, athletes have been found to underestimate the level of baseline symptoms present before the injury and to overestimate changes in symptoms occurring after the injury, consistent with a model of expectation as etiology (Mittenberg, DiGiulio, Perrin, & Bass, 1992). Another study found that athletes have a general expectation for a healthy recovery from concussion, which differs from the types of expectations observed in other groups (Gunstad & Suhr, 2001).

Preparticipation examinations and the development of formalized concussion management protocols provide readily available medical history, demographic, and injury-specific data for clinicians that is relevant for informing symptom attribution and prolonged recovery risk following SRC. However, evaluating and determining symptom etiology of an athlete's symptoms remains challenging the further removed from the injury. Examining base rates of concussion-like symptoms provides incremental evidence of what might be considered normal symptom expression, ultimately exposing the non-specificity of the symptoms that make up the formal diagnostic criteria for PCS.

Along those lines, Iverson and colleagues described the prevalence of subjects meeting ICD–10 PCS symptom criterion in the absence of a diagnosed concussion (i.e., during baseline assessment) in more than 30,000 adolescent student athletes. This diagnosis requires presence of symptoms in three of six domains, four of which are directly examined by most standard concussion symptom checklists (cognitive, somatic/physical, emotional/mood, and sleep/insomnia). They found 20.4% of male subjects and 28.0% of female subjects reported such symptoms at baseline, and the most robust predictors of these symptoms included history of migraines, learning disability and attention-deficit/hyperactivity disorder (ADHD), and previous psychiatric diagnoses (Iverson et al., 2015). Asken, Snyder, Smith, Zaremski, and Bauer (2017) described similar rates of adolescent athletes reporting PCS-like symptoms at baseline, and found only 36% of their sample were completely "asymptomatic" at baseline (i.e., a symptom score of 0), highlighting the high prevalence of concussion-like symptoms in the absence of concussion. Male and female college athletes also report PCS-like symptoms at a clinically significant rate (12.8% and 21.7%, respectively), with sleep-related and physical symptoms being by far the most common and only 40.1% of athletes reporting completely asymptomatic profiles (Asken, Snyder, Clugston, et al., 2017). Taken together, the high rate of concussion-like symptoms in healthy individuals raises the question of whether someone with minor residual symptoms weeks to months after a concussion is still suffering direct effects of the injury or is simply experiencing the normal ("base rate") degree of nonspecific symptomatology. These findings emphasize the potential benefit of the neuropsychologist in differential diagnosis and intervention with consideration of preexisting and concomitant risks for symptom manifestation.

Preinjury risk factors identified within the adult civilian mTBI literature for development of PCS include a number of personality variables and a prior history of psychiatric disturbance (Broshek, De Marco, & Freeman, 2015; Silverberg & Iverson, 2011). Predictive factors for PCS in children include learning difficulties, behavioral problems, and a previous history of head injury (Zemek, Farion, Sampson, & McGahern, 2013). Thus far, similar findings have been reported among the few studies examining PCS in athlete samples. Zuckerman et al. (2016) found previous history of concussion doubled the risk of a PCS diagnosis in a large data set of collegiate athletes, but, unfortunately, the authors were unable to account for many relevant medical history factors in their multivariate prediction model (Zuckerman et al., 2016). One study of youth athletes found personal or family history of mood disorder, other psychiatric illness, life stressors, and migraine increased PCS risk (Morgan et al., 2015). This study also found the rate of PCS to be increased in association with delayed symptom onset. This is interesting in the context of recent data suggesting that athletes who delay reporting their concussion symptoms experience a longer recovery than those who are immediately removed from athletic participation (Asken et al., 2016; Elbin et al., 2016). Conceivably, athletes with a delayed symptom onset likely continued participating in their sport during the immediate postconcussion phase and may have exposed their brain to further subclinical impacts or potentially detrimental effects of acute high-intensity physical exertion. Another study reported that more than 80% of their PCS cases in athletes had a history of at least one prior concussion (Tator & Davis, 2014). A high percentage of these cases also reported a history of premorbid psychiatric condition, ADHD, learning disability, and migraine.

Across civilian mTBI and athlete SRC studies, preexisting psychiatric conditions or psychiatric symptom reporting are among the most consistent and robust predictors of protracted recovery. This is not altogether surprising when considering both the neurobiological and psychosocial outcomes associated with a concussion. Preexisting depression and/or anxiety may be exacerbated by the neurometabolic cascade resulting from acute concussion (Giza & Hovda, 2014). More broadly, individuals with poor coping mechanisms or maladaptive reactions to adverse events will be at significant risk of persistent symptoms from a psychosocial standpoint. In a diathesis–stress model, a concussion represents a substantial "stress" threat when considering the abrupt lifestyle changes. For example, many student athletes define much of their self-worth by their athletic identity as well as academic or extracurricular involvements. Acute concussion management often dictates immediate removal from these activities and creates a stressful and frustrating environment for the athlete. Preexisting abilities and strategies adapting to such adverse events (i.e., "resilience"), social support networks, recovery trajectories relative to personal expectations, and real or perceived pressure to resume normal activities quickly all represent significant modifiers to the recovery process irrespective of the direct neurobiological effects of concussion. Importantly, these risks exist even in the absence of a formally diagnosed psychiatric condition and may be represented by ancillary factors such as a family history of psychiatric disorders or subjective symptom reporting within psychiatric domains during baseline assessments. Nelson and colleagues found baseline self-reported somatic symptoms to be the strongest premorbid predictor of symptom duration after SRC (Nelson et al., 2016). As such, clinicians must identify individuals at high risk for maladaptive reactions to their injury so that they can be educated or possibly referred for early psychological intervention.

NEUROBIOLOGICAL HYPOTHESES OF PERSISTENT SRC SYMPTOMATOLOGY

Advances in neuroimaging and more direct measurement of physiological outcomes following SRC have led to interesting but often inconsistent findings. The contradictory results reflect the heterogeneity of SRC but nonetheless provide important considerations for treatment and monitoring of persistent symptoms. Research focusing on autonomic functioning considers outcomes such as heart rate variability and cerebral blood flow (CBF) and the effects of physical exertion both as a diagnostic tool and treatment intervention. Diffusion tensor imaging (DTI) purportedly measures microstructural white matter changes, and a handful of studies have examined DTI outcomes as a diagnostic and prognostic tool for PCS. Similarly, blood biomarker research offers some promise as a means of measuring residual central nervous system pathophysiological processes. We briefly discuss the state of this literature and the clinical utility of considering these neurobiological factors.

Leddy and colleagues postulated that SRC involves multiple physiological systems throughout the body. Their review identified heart rate variability as a potentially useful measure of disturbed autonomic nervous system functioning, as evidenced by imbalanced parasympathetic–sympathetic nervous system activation. CBF alterations are also observed after concussion and are believed to underlie symptom exacerbation during physical exertion. Using arterial spin labeling magnetic resonance imaging, Meier and colleagues found persistently reduced CBF in a subgroup of collegiate athletes with protracted recovery (Meier et al., 2015). Reduced CBF was also noted in small groups of pediatric SRC subjects (Bartnik-Olson et al., 2014), and evidence suggests reduced CBF may outlast observable or reported clinical symptoms (Wang et al., 2016). Specifically related to exercise, an integral component of the athlete's return to activity protocol, two studies reported evidence of autonomic dysfunction in a sample of PCS patients based on CBF response to exertion and a more symptom-limited intolerance to exercise (Clausen, Pendergast, Willer, & Leddy, 2016; Kozlowski, Graham, Leddy, Devinney-Boymel, & Willer, 2013). Leddy et al. (2010) described a reliable method for differentiating physiologically versus autonomically based PCS symptoms using exertional test performance. Specifically, they contended that the ability to exercise to voluntary exhaustion (85%–90% of maximum heart rate) for 20 minutes without significant symptom exacerbation indicates physiological resolution of PCS symptoms. In other words, persistent symptoms not exacerbated by the exertional test are not due to autonomic dysfunction and therefore may necessitate different treatment courses. The role of subthreshold exercise intervention as a rehabilitative tool for PCS is described in more detail later in the chapter.

DTI outcomes after mTBI inconsistently differentiate PCS patients. In civilian studies, "poor outcome patients" with symptoms at least 3 months postinjury demonstrated more severe white matter abnormalities than "good-outcome patients," and the "good-outcome" group did not differ from healthy control participants on DTI outcomes (Messé et al., 2011). However, Lange et al. (2015) found no DTI differences between mTBI subjects meeting ICD–10 PCS criteria (symptoms for at least 1 month) and those not meeting criteria. Similarly, Waljas and colleagues reported DTI measures differentiating mTBI patients from healthy control participants, but not between mTBI patients based on ICD–10 PCS status. Few studies have specifically examined athlete PCS samples using DTI. Findings indicate DTI outcomes differed between adolescent PCS athletes with and without cognitive symptoms (Bartnik-Olson et al., 2014) and inconsistent regional white matter differences between athletes with PCS compared with control participants, but no correlation of DTI measures and symptom changes (Polak, Leddy, Dwyer, Willer, & Zivadinov, 2015). To date, there is insufficient evidence supporting the use of DTI as diagnostic or prognostic of PCS (Asken, DeKosky, Clugston, Jaffee, & Bauer, 2018).

Blood biomarkers contribute to our understanding of prognosis and outcomes after more severe forms of TBI and are recently being studied more rigorously in mTBI and SRC populations. Kawata et al. (2016) provided an excellent review of commonly studied blood biomarkers and how they relate to the effects of brain injury. Shahim and colleagues (2016) recently identified elevated neurofilament light protein and reduced beta-amyloid burden as potential markers of risk for persistent PCS symptoms lasting more than 1 year in a sample of Swedish hockey players, but no association with levels of total tau, glial fibrillary acidic protein, or neurogranin. In a similar cohort, Siman et al. (2015) reported serum alpha-2-spectrin N-terminal fragment and serum tau levels differentiated athletes with normal versus prolonged (although not necessarily PCS-like) recoveries. Current blood biomarker research in SRC predominantly focuses on diagnostic sensitivity and specificity. To date, no reliable or validated blood-based biomarker has been identified. Papa, Ramia, Edwards, Johnson, and Slobounov (2015) described the generally small sample sizes and highly variable postinjury assessment points across most SRC blood biomarker studies and inconsistent correlations of biomarker concentrations with concussion-like symptoms. The authors concluded that current literature does not yet support a validated biomarker for the effects of SRC. The application of this research in measuring residual physiological dysfunction decoupled from clinical recovery is interesting but in its infancy. Detailed reviews of the application and findings of blood-based biomarkers in SRC research have previously been published (Papa, 2016; Papa et al., 2015; Zetterberg & Blennow, 2016).

NEUROPSYCHOLOGICAL EVALUATION OF PERSISTENT SYMPTOMS AFTER SRC

Clinicians involved in the diagnosis and treatment of SRC will undoubtedly encounter cases of complicated recovery, characterized by symptoms persisting beyond the period associated with a "normal" resolution of symptoms (Makdissi et al., 2013). Defining a patient's condition as "prolonged recovery" versus PCS likely matters only for insurance billing purposes or if education and treatment planning will differ, and it is important to remember the highly variable required symptom durations that currently exist for classifying PCS. In some cases, one might attribute prolonged recovery to underlying neurophysiological causes, including histories of recent or multiple concussions, or persisting autonomic dysfunction, which may be elucidated through previously referenced exertional testing protocols (Leddy & Willer, 2013). In other cases, there will be no obvious neurobiological or physiological causes, raising concerns about the presence of a more psychosocial-based persistent PCS.

Neuropsychologists have been leaders in the effort to develop evidenced-based guidelines for evaluation and management of SRC. Many neuropsychologists have made major contributions to advance scientific understanding of SRC, participated in the clinical treatment of athletes who have sustained a concussion, and disseminated information critical to injury prevention. Neuropsychologists benefit from a sophisticated understanding of the current literature in this field and the complexities of symptom etiology, which enables provision of the highest level of care to patients. Clinically, the role of the neuropsychologist in SRC is perhaps most appreciated in the case of persistent symptomatology.

In many cases, athletes will have been symptomatic for weeks to months before obtaining neuropsychological services. Evaluating the appropriateness of the patient's treatment to that point is essential given the wealth of misinformation on concussion management and the unfortunate reality that many physicians are unaware of the most current treatment recommendations. One of the most commonly observed mismanagement practices involves restricting athletes to complete physical and cognitive rest past the point of acute recovery and until they report being completely asymptomatic.

For student athletes, this often includes absolute removal from sport participation (including attending practices and other team events) as well as partial or complete academic withdrawal.

Similar to most sport-related injuries (e.g., ligament sprains, muscle strains), an initial period of rest is important for allowing initiation of proper recovery and inflammatory processes. However, the goal should be reintegration to physical and cognitive activity as soon as tolerated, while avoiding situations in which the athlete may experience further head impacts if concerns of incomplete recovery remain. Recent evidence, albeit limited, and modern expert opinion suggest that prolonged rest may be as detrimental as no rest period at all, and active rehabilitation strategies should be explored (Buckley, Munkasy, & Clouse, 2016; Collins et al., 2016; DiFazio, Silverberg, Kirkwood, Bernier, & Iverson, 2016; Leddy, Baker, & Willer, 2016; Sawyer, Vesci, & McLeod, 2016; Thomas, Apps, Hoffmann, McCrea, & Hammeke, 2015; K. J. Schneider et al., 2017). Specific recommendations for guiding return to physical and cognitive activity, and the importance of a multidisciplinary management approach, are described in more detail later in the chapter. Anecdotally, allowing athletes previously on complete restriction to begin even light physical and cognitive activity can have a substantial positive effect on their mood and attitude about recovery that, altogether, has neurobiological and psychosocial benefits.

Athletes experiencing prolonged symptomatology after SRC represent a heterogeneous and complicated patient population. This *miserable minority*, a term originally applied to nonathlete, civilian mTBI patients (Ruff, Camenzuli, & Mueller, 1996), now includes athletes who have returned to baseline or normative expectations on functional testing but continue reporting symptoms, athletes who report being asymptomatic but continually fail to achieve adequate performance on functional tests, or both report symptoms and exhibit poor performance on neurocognitive testing. When the symptoms-only patient presents, a neuropsychology referral can be beneficial for refining etiological attribution of symptoms. In instances where an athlete reports being asymptomatic but fails to return to baseline or normative standards on cognitive test performance, more comprehensive neuropsychological testing (e.g., traditional assessments) may be warranted to more conclusively define the source of underlying impairment and better understand the patient's strengths and weaknesses across a broad range of neurocognitive domains. Comprehensive neuropsychological evaluations are rarely indicated but are occasionally invaluable for either identifying lingering problems or providing reassurance of cognitive normalcy to the patient.

Arguably, the most important aspect of a neuropsychological evaluation of persistent PCS is the clinical interview. In addition to gaining a better understanding of the patient's treatment to that point, a detailed history of symptom course and timing is essential. The expectation after "typical" SRC is that symptoms peak shortly after the injury and then progressively resolve over time. Instances of symptom plateauing or worsening after a period of improvement should trigger the clinician to investigate both neurobiological and psychosocial sources of the abnormal symptom progression, as well as consideration of concussion-like symptom base rates to assist in determining whether current symptomatology is indeed abnormal for the patient or if a "good-old-days" bias may play a role. Other important influences include, but are not limited to, preexisting psychiatric symptoms, sleep disturbances, neurodevelopmental disorders (e.g., learning disability, ADHD), substance use, and general adjustment to their current situation. It is likely that persistent cognitive complaints or observed deficits (via computerized neurocognitive testing or decreased performance in school) prompted the referral to neuropsychology, and the patient may expect definitive answers regarding the connection between residual brain damage from their SRC and his or her cognitive symptoms. The degree to which such patients appreciate other biopsychosocial influences will be highly variable and important for the clinician to address during the evaluation because these factors frequently represent important treatment targets.

A focused approach to neuropsychological assessment can be helpful to guide interventions aimed at athletes reporting persistent symptoms after SRC (Barr & McCrea, 2010; Nelson, Janecek, & McCrea, 2013). Not faced with time constraints found in the setting of acute diagnosis and recovery, testing of cognitive functioning in patients with prolonged effects of SRC can be accomplished effectively with a 1- to 2-hour neuropsychological test battery assessing a combination of cognitive and aforementioned psychosocial symptom influences. Although athletes might end up reporting a wide range of symptoms after SRC, findings from the evidence-based literature indicate that attention, processing speed, and memory are the functions commonly affected and should receive the most attention through neuropsychological testing (Belanger, Curtiss, Demery, Lebowitz, & Vanderploeg, 2005). Because access to a baseline evaluation with formal neuropsychological tests is unlikely, appropriate normative referencing relative to some combination of similar age, sex, education, and sociodemographic samples is essential for interpreting performance relative to "expected" scores. (For more discussion of this issue, see Chapter 10, this volume, by Meyer and Arnett on evidence-based approaches to neuropsychological assessment.) There is minimal utility of commercially available computerized neurocognitive assessments this far out from injury, particularly if the athlete has already taken such assessments multiple times. At most, a neuropsychologist may wish to use a computerized assessment as a screening measure for determining whether more formal neuropsychological assessment is warranted.

Often in cases of SRC, the neuropsychologist is in a position of providing assurance and communicating that the results of testing indicate no residual cognitive consequences of brain injury, contrary to what might be reported by other health care professionals or the subjective complaints of the patient. The goal would be to provide the patient with evidence-based information on recovery that will help him or her return to school, sports, and other activities as soon as possible, as well as education regarding other symptom etiologies. The goal of the neuropsychological evaluation will be to provide the athlete, family, and others an explanation of factors other than the physiological effects of "brain damage" that are likely to be playing a role in the maintenance of persisting symptoms and how those factors can be addressed through appropriate cognitive, physical, or psychological intervention, or other forms of rehabilitation (e.g., vestibular therapy, pharmacological intervention).

MULTIDISCIPLINARY MANAGEMENT AND REHABILITATION OF PERSISTENT SYMPTOMS AFTER SRC

Active treatment and rehabilitation of SRC is currently the focus of substantial research efforts. For student athletes, outcome targets include returning to physical or athletic activity (i.e., "return to play"), returning to academics (i.e., "return to learn"), and managing ancillary symptomatology via psychotherapeutic or pharmacological intervention. These diverse but overlapping treatment avenues ideally use a multidisciplinary clinical approach that might involve neuropsychology, neurology, physical–vestibular therapy, and coordinated care with team clinicians (athletic trainers and physicians) as well as school officials important for implementing academic accommodations when indicated. In the absence of a clinical setting that provides "one-stop-shop" access to all of these specialties, findings from a comprehensive neuropsychological evaluation and clinical interview can serve the essential role of making appropriate referral recommendations.

Athletes restricted from physical activity for an extended period of time because of persistent symptomatology should be strongly considered for initiating subthreshold exertional activity (Leddy, Hinds, Sirica, & Willer, 2016). A referral to physical therapy or their athletic trainer to oversee the protocol is preferred. The recommended protocol is the Buffalo Concussion Treadmill Test, described in detail Leddy and Willer (2013). Importantly, this protocol has been demonstrated to be safe for patients who are currently symptomatic and may differentiate the source of symptomatology. Whereas acute concussion management focuses on symptom *presence* as a limiting activity factor, clinicians managing persistent cases often successfully use symptom *exacerbation* and perceived exertion. Allowing an athlete to reengage in physical activity can have profound impacts on their mood, as well as enhance their recovery. Griesbach and colleagues demonstrated benefits of aerobic exercise in preclinical models performed 2 to 3 weeks after concussion, as well as upregulation of brain-derived neurotrophic factor (a protein important for neuron repair and functional restoration) after voluntary exercise approximately 1 month after injury (Griesbach, Hovda, Molteni, Wu, & Gomez-Pinilla, 2004; Griesbach, Tio, Nair, & Hovda, 2014).

Conversely, extending the restricted activity period may lead to secondary negative neurobiological and psychosocial effects of SRC (Berlin, Kop, & Deuster, 2006; Leddy, Baker, & Willer, 2016). If concerns about exercise intensity remain beyond the acute recovery period, it is recommended, at a minimum, that athletes engage in some form of light activity each day (e.g., going for a walk)—progressing as tolerated—and avoid being sedentary. Situations in which the athletes may be exposed to head impacts should continue to be avoided until high-intensity physical activity and sport-specific, noncontact activities are achieved in combination with minimal to no residual symptoms (McCrory, Meeuwisse, Aubry, et al., 2013; McCrory, Meeuwisse, Dvořák, et al., 2017). For more comprehensive reviews of physical activity and rest following concussion see Broglio et al. (2015); DiFazio et al. (2016); Leddy, Hinds, et al. (2016); Sawyer et al. (2016); K. J. Schneider et al. (2013, 2017); and Silverberg and Iverson (2013).

Recently, researchers and clinicians began focusing more direct efforts and emphases on returning to cognitive activity, typically in the context of academic reintegration. The same principles and negative effects associated with extended removal from sport and athletic activity apply to removal from school and extracurricular activities. Additionally, recommendations for reintegration are similar and should be initiated as soon as possible. For many student athletes in high school and collegiate settings, extended or even brief removal from academics is a significant source of stress and anxiety. A recent review by Johnson and colleagues indicated that cognitive rest is almost universally recommended as an early intervention after concussion, yet only one study found that doing so reduced symptom duration, and academic adjustments in school are relatively infrequent (Brown et al., 2014; Johnson, Provenzano, Shumaker, Valovich-McLeod, & Bacon, 2016).

Findings from a neuropsychological evaluation should inform recommendations for academic accommodations, implementation of which requires establishing relationships with and monitoring compliance by appropriate school officials. In a collegiate setting, this might entail developing a plan with the school's disabilities resource center. A survey study from Olympia and colleagues identified common accommodations that included extended assignment deadlines, rest periods during the school day, postponed or staggered test dates, reduced workload, and accommodations for light and noise sensitivity (Olympia, Ritter, Brady, & Bramley, 2016). If neuropsychological testing reveals difficulties with concentration or working memory, an additional accommodation may be use of a notetaker, which would allow the student athlete to sit in the classroom and simply listen. Many of the academic accommodations are not unlike those that might be implemented for a student with ADHD, with the main difference being that the ultimate goal is rescinding the accommodations as soon as possible and progressing the student athlete's independence as symptoms allow. Return-to-learn recommendations for persistent PCS patients specifically have not been described. However, a progression of activities similar to return-to-play are recommended and may include partial attendance initially, breaks during the school day, breaks when studying or completing homework, and gradual progression to a full school day and workload (Master, Gioia, Leddy, & Grady, 2012). Supervised symptom monitoring when performing cognitive activities is also important for tracking tolerance and determining the aggressiveness with which the student can resume normal cognitive activities (Gioia et al., 2010). Several recent reviews have been published on the topic of cognitive rest and return to learn protocols (Arbogast et al., 2013; DiFazio et al., 2016; Eastman & Chang, 2015; Iverson & Gioia, 2016; McAbee, 2015; K. H. Schneider, 2016).

Physical and cognitive activities as rehabilitative approaches are relatively new in the mTBI literature and have focused mostly on athletes. Previous interventions targeting persistent PCS cases used traditional psychotherapeutic approaches such as cognitive behavior therapy (CBT) for treatment of PCS (Al Sayegh, Sandford, & Carson, 2010), although no controlled trials of this treatment modality have been attempted in a sports setting. Similarly, sleep is frequently affected by SRC, and poor sleep can mimic or exacerbate many of the symptoms associated with SRC. Identifying potentially poor sleep habits is essential to minimizing this complicating factor. In addition to basic sleep hygiene recommendations, a more formal or abbreviated course of CBT for insomnia (CBTi) may be appropriate for athletes exhibiting symptoms of insomnia or excessive daytime fatigue. If sleep problems accompany symptoms of depression, stress, and anxiety, CBTi is likely an appropriate treatment option (Stepanski & Wyatt, 2003; Taylor & Pruiksma, 2014). Of note, although it makes intuitive sense that treatments effective in civilian studies would be effective for athletes as well, there may potentially be barriers to accessing or seeking treatment considering the often-unique demographic and socioeconomic makeup of certain sports and athletic organizations.

As we have discussed, even in the absence of identifiable preinjury risk factors, an SRC may trigger psychiatric difficulties such as anxiety and depression. Determining the "chicken and the egg" in these scenarios becomes increasingly challenging over time. Regardless, such ancillary interactions are important targets for treatment in cases of prolonged recovery. Cognitive behavioral health treatments that focus on *cognitive restructuring* may be effective for athletes who remain symptomatic beyond the window of normal recovery following SRC. Athletes with well-established PCS frequently develop inaccurate or distorted perceptions of their injury, their recovery, their preserved abilities, and their outcome (Iverson et al., 2007). Psychotherapies focusing on cognitive restructuring work toward dismantling the distorted self-perceptions that frequently accompany PCS and replace them with *accurate beliefs and appraisals* related to one's injury, recovery, preserved ability, and outcome postinjury (Miller & Mittenberg, 1998). Ferguson and Mittenberg (1996) developed a six-session structured CBT program that helps patients understand how psychological factors can intensify and maintain PCS-related symptoms and teach PCS patients cognitive-behavioral techniques to manage stress and cope more effectively with symptoms. Iverson et al. (2007) reviewed cognitive errors or biases exhibited by patients with PCS that can complicate recovery and promote disability.

Proactive, preventative interventions also demonstrated effectiveness in mitigating onset of persistent PCS. Because psychological and social factors of disease (and PCS) are clearly modifiable variables (e.g., the patient, the provider, and the patient's environment can influence outcome), it should not be surprising that mTBI patients who receive brief behavioral health treatments very early postinjury (hours or days) report fewer and less severe PCS-related symptoms months later, relative to control patients with mTBI who do not receive brief behavioral interventions (Borg et al., 2004; Comper, Bisschop, Carnide, & Tricco, 2005; Paniak, Toller-Lobe, Reynolds, Melnyk, & Nagy, 2000; Ponsford et al., 2002).

PCS treatment clearly requires and benefits most from integrated, multidisciplinary assessment and management. A more detailed description of incorporating other medical specialties is outside the purview of this chapter, but recent consensus statements and expert meetings outline this concept (Collins et al., 2016; Ellis et al., 2017). Vestibular and physical therapy interventions are becoming increasingly popular for patients experiencing persistent dizziness or oculomotor dysfunction, or who may have sustained a concomitant orthopedic injury (frequently cervical). A referral to a physical therapist with specialized training in vestibular therapy can be an effective means of promoting symptom resolution in patients presenting with these symptoms (Broglio et al., 2015; Grabowski, Wilson, Walker, Enz, & Wang, 2017; K. J. Schneider et al., 2014). Many clinicians prefer not to use medications in the acute SRC recovery period but explore such options in persistent PCS cases. Referral to a neurologist for pharmacological considerations may incrementally benefit the patient suffering from migraines, debilitating headaches, significant sleep problems, or severe psychiatric symptoms. The goal for persistent PCS patients is reintegration into their normal physical and cognitive activities and resumption of medical care by their certified athletic trainer or primary care physician (whom many state laws require dictate the ultimate clearance for return to sport). This often necessitates more aggressive and multimodal treatment than the typical SRC case. The neuropsychologist is uniquely positioned to recognize sources of persistent problems and can recommend the most appropriate referrals because many of these treatment approaches fall outside the direct expertise of neuropsychologists.

CASE STUDY

Patient AB is a 17-year-old female athlete who sustained a concussion during a high school soccer game. She was evaluated by her athletic trainer after she reported headaches and dizziness after a play in which she challenged an opponent for a header and subsequently landed with the back of her head striking the ground. She was immediately removed from play and restricted from returning that game.

AB reported to the athletic training room daily over the following week for serial assessment. She exhibited persistent headaches, dizziness, difficulty concentrating, worsening sleep latency, and cognitive test scores below baseline performance. Medical history was negative for prior concussion, diagnosed psychiatric disorder, ADHD, or learning disability. Her athletic trainer referred her to her primary care physician, who recommended continued strict physical and cognitive rest, including removal from school and restriction from attending or participating in team-related and other extracurricular activities until asymptomatic. Her symptoms were managed conservatively. AB continued reporting symptoms 4 weeks postinjury, at which point her physician diagnosed her with PCS and referred her for a more formal neuropsychological evaluation.

Neuropsychological testing indicated lower than expected performance on measures of verbal fluency, processing speed, and working memory. Clinical interview revealed AB to be a high-achieving student involved in multiple clubs and extracurricular activities. She described significant symptoms of anxiety and frustration due to persistent dizziness, sleep problems, and falling behind in school. She reported feeling irritable and depressed over not being able to be around her teammates, socialize with friends, or participate in other extracurricular activities. The neuropsychologist concluded that cognitive difficulties were likely driven by these worsening mood symptoms, which were also significantly interfering with sleep. Primary recommendations included low-level physical activity, limited return to academic activities with temporary accommodations, allowing attendance at team practices and games, initiation of CBT with emphases on cognitive restructuring and sleep problems, and a referral to a physical therapist with specialized training in vestibular therapy.

The physical therapist diagnosed AB with benign positional paroxysmal vertigo and performed canalith repositioning procedures, which resulted in significant reductions in dizziness symptoms. AB then completed the Buffalo Concussion Treadmill Test under supervision of the physical therapist, who concluded that the physiological effects of AB's concussions had resolved on the basis of minimal symptom exacerbation with higher intensity activity. She was cleared for initiation of the return-to-play protocol without exposure to further head impacts until other symptoms improved. Concurrently, AB's psychotherapist elected to begin a course of CBT for insomnia, which uses behavioral approaches reversing poor sleep habits that had developed since the injury, relaxation techniques, and cognitive restructuring strategies targeting maladaptive thought patterns and frustrations over AB's recovery.

AB reported rapid improvement in anxiety, depression, and sleep symptoms after clearance for participation in team-related activities, increased physical activity, and catching up with academic work. Following 4 weeks of physical and vestibular therapy and CBT, AB reported complete symptom resolution, performed all noncontact steps of the return to play protocol, and returned to school full time without accommodations. She returned to baseline performance on all concussion tests and was then cleared by her physician for contact practice. After achieving full return to play and academics, AB continued at-home vestibular exercises prescribed by the physical therapist and completed two additional sessions of cognitive behavioral therapy focusing on concerns of reinjury and symptom reemergence.

CLINICAL TAKE-HOME POINTS

1. *Persistent PCS may arise from multiple etiologies beyond the residual effects of SRC, necessitating the need for skilled differential diagnosis and multidisciplinary treatment and management.*
2. *Preexisting psychiatric symptomatology is among the strongest and most consistent predictors of prolonged recovery after SRC.*
3. *Strict physical and cognitive rest for several weeks after SRC is not recommended.* Emerging research and international consensus guidelines now indicate that reintegration of activity may promote neurobiological recovery processes and mitigate the negative psychosocial effects of extended removal from sport and school.

KEY QUESTIONS TO BE ADDRESSED IN THE NEXT 5 YEARS

1. *What is the optimal timing to introduce physical and cognitive activity despite incomplete symptom resolution?*
2. *What is the clinical utility of neurobiological markers (advanced imaging, blood biomarkers, etc.) in tracking recovery processes and identifying patients at risk of persistent PCS?*
3. *What are the risks of premature return to sport (i.e., exposure to potential SRC mechanisms) and academics in the presence of subjective symptoms but absence of objective neurobiological dysfunction?*

REFERENCES

Al Sayegh, A., Sandford, D., & Carson, A. J. (2010). Psychological approaches to treatment of postconcussion syndrome: A systematic review. *Journal of Neurology, Neurosurgery, & Psychiatry, 81,* 1128–1134. http://dx.doi.org/10.1136/jnnp.2008.170092

American Psychiatric Association. (1994). *Diagnostic and statistical manual of mental disorders* (4th ed.). Washington, DC: Author.

Arbogast, K. B., McGinley, A. D., Master, C. L., Grady, M. F., Robinson, R. L., & Zonfrillo, M. R. (2013). Cognitive rest and school-based recommendations following pediatric concussion: The need for primary care support tools. *Clinical Pediatrics, 52,* 397–402. http://dx.doi.org/10.1177/0009922813478160

Asken, B. M., DeKosky, S. T., Clugston, J. R., Jaffee, M. S., & Bauer, R. M. (2018). Diffusion tensor imaging (DTI) findings in adult civilian, military, and sport-related mild traumatic brain injury (mTBI): A systematic critical review. *Brain Imaging and Behavior, 12,* 585–612. http://dx.doi.org/10.1007/s11682-017-9708-9

Asken, B. M., McCrea, M. A., Clugston, J. R., Snyder, A. R., Houck, Z. M., & Bauer, R. M. (2016). "Playing through it": Delayed reporting and removal from athletic activity after concussion predicts prolonged recovery. *Journal of Athletic Training, 51,* 329–335. http://dx.doi.org/10.4085/1062-6050-51.5.02

Asken, B. M., Snyder, A. R., Clugston, J. R., Gaynor, L. S., Sullan, M. J., & Bauer, R. M. (2017). Concussion-like symptom reporting in non-concussed collegiate athletes. *Archives of Clinical Neuropsychology, 32,* 963–971.

Asken, B. M., Snyder, A. R., Smith, M. S., Zaremski, J. L., & Bauer, R. M. (2017). Concussion-like symptom reporting in non-concussed adolescent athletes. *The Clinical Neuropsychologist, 31,* 138–153. http://dx.doi.org/10.1080/13854046.2016.1246672

Babcock, L., Byczkowski, T., Wade, S. L., Ho, M., Mookerjee, S., & Bazarian, J. J. (2013). Predicting postconcussion syndrome after mild traumatic brain injury in children and adolescents who present to the emergency department. *JAMA Pediatrics, 167,* 156–161. http://dx.doi.org/10.1001/jamapediatrics.2013.434

Bakhos, L. L., Lockhart, G. R., Myers, R., & Linakis, J. G. (2010). Emergency department visits for concussion in young child athletes. *Pediatrics, 126,* e550–e556. http://dx.doi.org/10.1542/peds.2009-3101

Barr, W. B., & McCrea, M. (2001). Sensitivity and specificity of standardized neurocognitive testing immediately following sports concussion. *Journal of the International Neuropsychological Society, 7,* 693–702. http://dx.doi.org/10.1017/S1355617701766052

Barr, W. B., & McCrea, M. (2010). Diagnosis and assessment of concussion. In F. M. Webbe (Ed.), *The handbook of sport neuropsychology* (pp. 91–112). New York, NY: Springer.

Bartnik-Olson, B. L., Holshouser, B., Wang, H., Grube, M., Tong, K., Wong, V., & Ashwal, S. (2014). Impaired neurovascular unit function contributes to persistent symptoms after concussion: A pilot study. *Journal of Neurotrauma, 31,* 1497–1506. http://dx.doi.org/10.1089/neu.2013.3213

Belanger, H. G., Curtiss, G., Demery, J. A., Lebowitz, B. K., & Vanderploeg, R. D. (2005). Factors moderating neuropsychological outcomes following mild traumatic brain injury: A meta-analysis. *Journal of the International Neuropsychological Society, 11,* 215–227. http://dx.doi.org/10.1017/S1355617705050277

Belanger, H. G., & Vanderploeg, R. D. (2005). The neuropsychological impact of sports-related concussion: A meta-analysis. *Journal of the International Neuropsychological Society, 11,* 345–357. http://dx.doi.org/10.1017/S1355617705050411

Berlin, A. A., Kop, W. J., & Deuster, P. A. (2006). Depressive mood symptoms and fatigue after exercise withdrawal: The potential role of decreased fitness. *Psychosomatic Medicine, 68,* 224–230. http://dx.doi.org/10.1097/01.psy.0000204628.73273.23

Borg, J., Holm, L., Peloso, P. M., Cassidy, J. D., Carroll, L. J., von Holst, H., . . . Yates, D. (2004). Non-surgical intervention and cost for mild traumatic brain injury: Results of the WHO Collaborating Centre Task Force on Mild Traumatic Brain Injury. *Journal of Rehabilitation Medicine, 36,* 76–83. http://dx.doi.org/10.1080/16501960410023840

Broglio, S. P., Collins, M. W., Williams, R. M., Mucha, A., & Kontos, A. P. (2015). Current and emerging rehabilitation for concussion: A review of the evidence. *Clinics in Sports Medicine, 34,* 213–231. http://dx.doi.org/10.1016/j.csm.2014.12.005

Broglio, S. P., & Puetz, T. W. (2008). The effect of sport concussion on neurocognitive function, self-report symptoms and postural control: A meta-analysis. *Sports Medicine, 38,* 53–67. http://dx.doi.org/10.2165/00007256-200838010-00005

Broshek, D. K., De Marco, A. P., & Freeman, J. R. (2015). A review of postconcussion syndrome and psychological factors associated with concussion. *Brain Injury, 29,* 228–237. http://dx.doi.org/10.3109/02699052.2014.974674

Brown, N. J., Mannix, R. C., O'Brien, M. J., Gostine, D., Collins, M. W., & Meehan, W. P., III. (2014). Effect of cognitive activity level on duration of post-concussion symptoms. *Pediatrics, 133*, e299–e304. http://dx.doi.org/10.1542/peds.2013-2125

Buckley, T. A., Munkasy, B. A., & Clouse, B. P. (2016). Acute cognitive and physical rest may not improve concussion recovery time. *The Journal of Head Trauma Rehabilitation, 31*, 233–241. http://dx.doi.org/10.1097/HTR.0000000000000165

Centers for Disease Control and Prevention. (2011, October 7). Nonfatal traumatic brain injuries related to sports and recreation activities among persons aged ≤19 years—United States, 2001–2009. *Morbidity and Mortality Weekly Report, 60*, 1337–1342.

Clausen, M., Pendergast, D. R., Willer, B., & Leddy, J. (2016). Cerebral blood flow during treadmill exercise is a marker of physiological postconcussion syndrome in female athletes. *The Journal of Head Trauma Rehabilitation, 31*, 215–224. http://dx.doi.org/10.1097/HTR.0000000000000145

Collins, M. W., Grindel, S. H., Lovell, M. R., Dede, D. E., Moser, D. J., Phalin, B. R., . . . McKeag, D. B. (1999). Relationship between concussion and neuropsychological performance in college football players. *JAMA, 282*, 964–970. http://dx.doi.org/10.1001/jama.282.10.964

Collins, M. W., Kontos, A. P., Okonkwo, D. O., Almquist, J., Bailes, J., Barisa, M., . . . Zafonte, R. (2016). Statements of agreement from the Targeted Evaluation and Active Management (TEAM) Approaches to Treating Concussion Meeting held in Pittsburgh, October 15–16, 2015. *Neurosurgery, 79*, 912–929. http://dx.doi.org/10.1227/NEU.0000000000001447

Colvin, A. C., Mullen, J., Lovell, M. R., West, R. V., Collins, M. W., & Groh, M. (2009). The role of concussion history and gender in recovery from soccer-related concussion. *The American Journal of Sports Medicine, 37*, 1699–1704. http://dx.doi.org/10.1177/0363546509332497

Comper, P., Bisschop, S. M., Carnide, N., & Tricco, A. (2005). A systematic review of treatments for mild traumatic brain injury. *Brain Injury, 19*, 863–880. http://dx.doi.org/10.1080/02699050400025042

DeKosky, S. T., Ikonomovic, M. D., & Gandy, S. (2010). Traumatic brain injury—Football, warfare, and long-term effects. *The New England Journal of Medicine, 363*, 1293–1296. http://dx.doi.org/10.1056/NEJMp1007051

DiFazio, M., Silverberg, N. D., Kirkwood, M. W., Bernier, R., & Iverson, G. L. (2016). Prolonged activity restriction after concussion: Are we worsening outcomes? *Clinical Pediatrics, 55*, 443–451. http://dx.doi.org/10.1177/0009922815589914

Dougan, B. K., Horswill, M. S., & Geffen, G. M. (2014). Athletes' age, sex, and years of education moderate the acute neuropsychological impact of sports-related concussion: A meta-analysis. *Journal of the International Neuropsychological Society, 20*, 64–80.

Eastman, A., & Chang, D. G. (2015). Return to learn: A review of cognitive rest versus rehabilitation after sports concussion. *NeuroRehabilitation, 37,* 235–244. http://dx.doi.org/10.3233/NRE-151256

Elbin, R. J., Sufrinko, A., Schatz, P., French, J., Henry, L., Burkhart, S., . . . Kontos, A. P. (2016). Removal from play after concussion and recovery time. *Pediatrics, 138,* e20160910. http://dx.doi.org/10.1542/peds.2016-0910

Ellis, M. J., Ritchie, L. J., McDonald, P. J., Cordingley, D., Reimer, K., Nijjar, S., . . . Russell, K. (2017). Multidisciplinary management of pediatric sports-related concussion. *The Canadian Journal of Neurological Sciences, 44,* 24–34.

Ferguson, R. J., & Mittenberg, W. (1996). Cognitive–behavioral treatment of postconcussion syndrome: A therapist's manual. In V. B. Van Hasselt & M. Hersen (Eds.), *Sourcebook of psychological treatment manuals for adult disorders* (pp. 615–655). New York, NY: Plenum Press. http://dx.doi.org/10.1007/978-1-4899-1528-3_16

Field, M., Collins, M. W., Lovell, M. R., & Maroon, J. (2003). Does age play a role in recovery from sports-related concussion? A comparison of high school and collegiate athletes. *The Journal of Pediatrics, 142,* 546–553. http://dx.doi.org/10.1067/mpd.2003.190

Frommer, L. J., Gurka, K. K., Cross, K. M., Ingersoll, C. D., Comstock, R. D., & Saliba, S. A. (2011). Sex differences in concussion symptoms of high school athletes. *Journal of Athletic Training, 46,* 76–84. http://dx.doi.org/10.4085/1062-6050-46.1.76

Gioia, G., Vaughan, C., Reesman, J., McGuire, E., Gathercole, L., Padia, H., . . . Wells, C. (2010). Characterizing post-concussion exertional effects in the child and adolescent. *Journal of the International Neuropsychological Society, 16*(Suppl. 1), 178.

Giza, C. C., & Hovda, D. A. (2014). The new neurometabolic cascade of concussion. *Neurosurgery, 75*(Suppl. 4), S24–S33. http://dx.doi.org/10.1227/NEU.0000000000000505

Grabowski, P., Wilson, J., Walker, A., Enz, D., & Wang, S. (2017). Multimodal impairment-based physical therapy for the treatment of patients with postconcussion syndrome: A retrospective analysis on safety and feasibility. *Physical Therapy in Sport, 23,* 22–30. http://dx.doi.org/10.1016/j.ptsp.2016.06.001

Griesbach, G. S., Hovda, D. A., Molteni, R., Wu, A., & Gomez-Pinilla, F. (2004). Voluntary exercise following traumatic brain injury: Brain-derived neurotrophic factor upregulation and recovery of function. *Neuroscience, 125,* 129–139. http://dx.doi.org/10.1016/j.neuroscience.2004.01.030

Griesbach, G. S., Tio, D. L., Nair, S., & Hovda, D. A. (2014). Recovery of stress response coincides with responsiveness to voluntary exercise after traumatic brain injury. *Journal of Neurotrauma, 31,* 674–682. http://dx.doi.org/10.1089/neu.2013.3151

Gunstad, J., & Suhr, J. A. (2001). "Expectation as etiology" versus "the good old days": Postconcussion syndrome symptom reporting in athletes, headache sufferers, and depressed individuals. *Journal of the International Neuropsychological Society, 7,* 323–333. http://dx.doi.org/10.1017/S1355617701733061

Guskiewicz, K. M., McCrea, M., Marshall, S. W., Cantu, R. C., Randolph, C., Barr, W., . . . Kelly, J. P. (2003). Cumulative effects associated with recurrent concussion in collegiate football players: The NCAA Concussion Study. *JAMA, 290,* 2549–2555. http://dx.doi.org/10.1001/jama.290.19.2549

Guskiewicz, K. M., Weaver, N. L., Padua, D. A., & Garrett, W. E., Jr. (2000). Epidemiology of concussion in collegiate and high school football players. *The American Journal of Sports Medicine, 28,* 643–650. http://dx.doi.org/10.1177/03635465000280050401

Halstead, M. E., Walter, K. D., & The Council on Sports Medicine and Fitness. (2010). Clinical report—Sport-related concussion in children and adolescents. *Pediatrics, 126,* 597–615. http://dx.doi.org/10.1542/peds.2010-2005

Heitger, M. H., Jones, R. D., & Anderson, T. J. (2008, August). *A new approach to predicting postconcussion syndrome after mild traumatic brain injury based upon eye movement function.* Paper presented at the 2008 30th Annual International Conference of the IEEE Engineering in Medicine and Biology Society, Vancouver, Canada.

Iverson, G. L., Gardner, A. J., Terry, D. P., Ponsford, J. L., Sills, A. K., Broshek, D. K., & Solomon, G. S. (2017). Predictors of clinical recovery from concussion: A systematic review. *British Journal of Sports Medicine, 51,* 941–948. http://dx.doi.org/10.1136/bjsports-2017-097729

Iverson, G. L., & Gioia, G. A. (2016). Returning to school following sport-related concussion. *Physical Medicine and Rehabilitation Clinics of North America, 27,* 429–436. http://dx.doi.org/10.1016/j.pmr.2015.12.002

Iverson, G. L., Silverberg, N. D., Mannix, R., Maxwell, B. A., Atkins, J. E., Zafonte, R., & Berkner, P. D. (2015). Factors associated with concussion-like symptom reporting in high school athletes. *JAMA Pediatrics, 169,* 1132–1140. http://dx.doi.org/10.1001/jamapediatrics.2015.2374

Iverson, G. L., Zasler, N. D., & Lange, R. T. (2007). Post-concussive disorder. In N. D. Zasler, D. I. Katz, & R. D. Zafonte (Eds.), *Brain injury medicine: Principles and practice* (pp. 373–405). New York, NY: Demos Medical.

Johnson, R. S., Provenzano, M. K., Shumaker, L. M., Valovich-McLeod, T. C., & Bacon, C. E. (2016). The effect of cognitive rest as part of post-concussion management for adolescent athletes: A critically appraised topic. *Journal of Sport Rehabilitation, 26,* 437–446.

Kawata, K., Liu, C. Y., Merkel, S. F., Ramirez, S. H., Tierney, R. T., & Langford, D. (2016). Blood biomarkers for brain injury: What are we measuring? *Neuroscience and Biobehavioral Reviews, 68,* 460–473. http://dx.doi.org/10.1016/j.neubiorev.2016.05.009

King, N. S., Crawford, S., Wenden, F. J., Moss, N. E. G., & Wade, D. T. (1995). The Rivermead Post Concussion Symptoms Questionnaire: A measure of symptoms commonly experienced after head injury and its reliability. *Journal of Neurology, 242,* 587–592. http://dx.doi.org/10.1007/BF00868811

Kozlowski, K. F., Graham, J., Leddy, J. J., Devinney-Boymel, L., & Willer, B. S. (2013). Exercise intolerance in individuals with postconcussion syndrome. *Journal of Athletic Training, 48,* 627–635. http://dx.doi.org/10.4085/1062-6050-48.5.02

Lange, R. T., Panenka, W. J., Shewchuk, J. R., Heran, M. K., Brubacher, J. R., Bioux, S., . . . Iverson, G. L. (2015). Diffusion tensor imaging findings and postconcussion symptom reporting six weeks following mild traumatic brain injury. *Archives of Clinical Neuropsychology, 30,* 7–25. http://dx.doi.org/10.1093/arclin/acu060

Langlois, J. A., Rutland-Brown, W., & Wald, M. M. (2006). The epidemiology and impact of traumatic brain injury: A brief overview. *The Journal of Head Trauma Rehabilitation, 21,* 375–378. http://dx.doi.org/10.1097/00001199-200609000-00001

LaRoche, A. A., Nelson, L. D., Connelly, P. K., Walter, K. D., & McCrea, M. A. (2016). Sport-related concussion reporting and state legislative effects. *Clinical Journal of Sport Medicine, 26,* 33–39. http://dx.doi.org/10.1097/JSM.0000000000000192

Lau, B. C., Collins, M. W., & Lovell, M. R. (2012). Cutoff scores in neurocognitive testing and symptom clusters that predict protracted recovery from concussions in high school athletes. *Neurosurgery, 70,* 371–379. http://dx.doi.org/10.1227/NEU.0b013e31823150f0

Lau, B. C., Kontos, A. P., Collins, M. W., Mucha, A., & Lovell, M. R. (2011). Which on-field signs/symptoms predict protracted recovery from sport-related concussion among high school football players? *The American Journal of Sports Medicine, 39,* 2311–2318. http://dx.doi.org/10.1177/0363546511410655

Leddy, J. J., Baker, J. G., Merchant, A., Picano, J., Gaile, D., Matuszak, J., & Willer, B. (2015). Brain or strain? Symptoms alone do not distinguish physiologic concussion from cervical/vestibular injury. *Clinical Journal of Sport Medicine, 25,* 237–242. http://dx.doi.org/10.1097/JSM.0000000000000128

Leddy, J. J., Baker, J. G., & Willer, B. (2016). Active rehabilitation of concussion and post-concussion syndrome. *Physical Medicine and Rehabilitation Clinics of North America, 27,* 437–454. http://dx.doi.org/10.1016/j.pmr.2015.12.003

Leddy, J. J., Hinds, A., Sirica, D., & Willer, B. (2016). The role of controlled exercise in concussion management. *PM&R, 8*(Suppl. 3), S91–S100. http://dx.doi.org/10.1016/j.pmrj.2015.10.017

Leddy, J. J., Kozlowski, K., Donnelly, J. P., Pendergast, D. R., Epstein, L. H., & Willer, B. (2010). A preliminary study of subsymptom threshold exercise training for refractory post-concussion syndrome. *Clinical Journal of Sport Medicine, 20,* 21–27. http://dx.doi.org/10.1097/JSM.0b013e3181c6c22c

Leddy, J. J., & Willer, B. (2013). Use of graded exercise testing in concussion and return-to-activity management. *Current Sports Medicine Reports, 12,* 370–376. http://dx.doi.org/10.1249/JSR.0000000000000008

Lishman, W. A. (1988). Physiogenesis and psychogenesis in the "post-concussional syndrome." *The British Journal of Psychiatry, 153,* 460–469. http://dx.doi.org/10.1192/bjp.153.4.460

Lovell, M. R., Iverson, G. L., Collins, M. W., Podell, K., Johnston, K. M., Pardini, D., . . . Maroon, J. C. (2006). Measurement of symptoms following sports-related concussion: Reliability and normative data for the post-concussion scale. *Applied Neuropsychology, 13,* 166–174. http://dx.doi.org/10.1207/s15324826an1303_4

Macciocchi, S. N., Barth, J. T., Alves, W., Rimel, R. W., & Jane, J. A. (1996). Neuropsychological functioning and recovery after mild head injury in collegiate athletes. *Neurosurgery, 39,* 510–514. http://dx.doi.org/10.1227/00006123-199609000-00014

Mainwaring, L. M., Hutchison, M., Bisschop, S. M., Comper, P., & Richards, D. W. (2010). Emotional response to sport concussion compared to ACL injury. *Brain Injury, 24,* 589–597. http://dx.doi.org/10.3109/02699051003610508

Makdissi, M., Cantu, R. C., Johnston, K. M., McCrory, P., & Meeuwisse, W. H. (2013). The difficult concussion patient: What is the best approach to investigation and management of persistent (>10 days) postconcussive symptoms? *British Journal of Sports Medicine, 47,* 308–313. http://dx.doi.org/10.1136/bjsports-2013-092255

Martland, H. S. (1928). Punch drunk. *JAMA, 91,* 1103–1107. http://dx.doi.org/10.1001/jama.1928.02700150029009

Master, C. L., Gioia, G. A., Leddy, J. J., & Grady, M. F. (2012). Importance of "return-to-learn" in pediatric and adolescent concussion. *Pediatric Annals, 41,* 1–6. http://dx.doi.org/10.3928/00904481-20120827-09

McAbee, G. N. (2015). Pediatric concussion, cognitive rest and position statements, practice parameters, and clinical practice guidelines. *Journal of Child Neurology, 30,* 1378–1380. http://dx.doi.org/10.1177/0883073814551794

McCrea, M. (2007). *Mild traumatic brain injury and post-concussion syndrome: The new evidence base for diagnosis and treatment.* New York, NY: Oxford University Press.

McCrea, M., Guskiewicz, K. M., Marshall, S. W., Barr, W., Randolph, C., Cantu, R. C., . . . Kelly, J. P. (2003). Acute effects and recovery time following concussion in collegiate football players: The NCAA Concussion Study. *JAMA, 290,* 2556–2563. http://dx.doi.org/10.1001/jama.290.19.2556

McCrea, M., Guskiewicz, K., Randolph, C., Barr, W. B., Hammeke, T. A., Marshall, S. W., . . . Kelly, J. P. (2013). Incidence, clinical course, and predictors of prolonged recovery time following sport-related concussion in high school and college athletes. *Journal of the International Neuropsychological Society, 19,* 22–33. http://dx.doi.org/10.1017/S1355617712000872

McCrory, P., Meeuwisse, W. H., Aubry, M., Cantu, B., Dvorák, J., Echemendia, R. J., . . . Turner, M. (2013). Consensus statement on concussion in sport: The 4th International Conference on Concussion in Sport held in Zurich, November 2012. *British Journal of Sports Medicine, 47,* 250–258. http://dx.doi.org/10.1136/bjsports-2013-092313

McCrory, P., Meeuwisse, W., Dvořák, J., Aubry, M., Bailes, J., Broglio, S., . . . Vos, P. E. (2017). Consensus statement on concussion in sport—The 5th international conference on concussion in sport held in Berlin, October 2016. *British Journal of Sports Medicine, 51*, 838–847. http://dx.doi.org/10.1136/bjsports-2017-097699

McKee, A. C., Stein, T. D., Nowinski, C. J., Stern, R. A., Daneshvar, D. H., Alvarez, V. E., . . . Baugh, C. M. (2013). The spectrum of disease in chronic traumatic encephalopathy. *Brain, 136*, 43–64.

Meier, T. B., Bellgowan, P. S., Singh, R., Kuplicki, R., Polanski, D. W., & Mayer, A. R. (2015). Recovery of cerebral blood flow following sports-related concussion. *JAMA Neurology, 72*, 530–538. http://dx.doi.org/10.1001/jamaneurol.2014.4778

Messé, A., Caplain, S., Paradot, G., Garrigue, D., Mineo, J. F., Soto Ares, G., . . . Lehéricy, S. (2011). Diffusion tensor imaging and white matter lesions at the subacute stage in mild traumatic brain injury with persistent neurobehavioral impairment. *Human Brain Mapping, 32*, 999–1011. http://dx.doi.org/10.1002/hbm.21092

Miller, L. J., & Mittenberg, W. (1998). Brief cognitive behavioral interventions in mild traumatic brain injury. *Applied Neuropsychology, 5*, 172–183. http://dx.doi.org/10.1207/s15324826an0504_2

Mittenberg, W., DiGiulio, D. V., Perrin, S., & Bass, A. E. (1992). Symptoms following mild head injury: Expectation as aetiology. *Journal of Neurology, Neurosurgery & Psychiatry, 55*, 200–204. http://dx.doi.org/10.1136/jnnp.55.3.200

Morgan, C. D., Zuckerman, S. L., Lee, Y. M., King, L., Beaird, S., Sills, A. K., & Solomon, G. S. (2015). Predictors of postconcussion syndrome after sports-related concussion in young athletes: A matched case-control study. *Journal of Neurosurgery. Pediatrics, 15*, 589–598. http://dx.doi.org/10.3171/2014.10.PEDS14356

Nelson, L. D., Janecek, J. K., & McCrea, M. A. (2013). Acute clinical recovery from sport-related concussion. *Neuropsychology Review, 23*, 285–299. http://dx.doi.org/10.1007/s11065-013-9240-7

Nelson, L. D., Tarima, S., LaRoche, A. A., Hammeke, T. A., Barr, W. B., Guskiewicz, K., . . . McCrea, M. A. (2016). Preinjury somatization symptoms contribute to clinical recovery after sport-related concussion. *Neurology, 86*, 1856–1863. http://dx.doi.org/10.1212/WNL.0000000000002679

Olympia, R. P., Ritter, J. T., Brady, J., & Bramley, H. (2016). Return to learning after a concussion and compliance with recommendations for cognitive rest. *Clinical Journal of Sport Medicine, 26*, 115–119. http://dx.doi.org/10.1097/JSM.0000000000000208

Paniak, C., Toller-Lobe, G., Reynolds, S., Melnyk, A., & Nagy, J., (2000). A randomized trial of two treatments for mild traumatic brain injury: 1 year follow-up. *Brain Injury, 14*, 219–226. http://dx.doi.org/10.1080/026990500120691

Papa, L. (2016). Potential blood-based biomarkers for concussion. *Sports Medicine and Arthroscopy Review, 24*, 108–115. http://dx.doi.org/10.1097/JSA.0000000000000117

Papa, L., Ramia, M. M., Edwards, D., Johnson, B. D., & Slobounov, S. M. (2015). Systematic review of clinical studies examining biomarkers of brain injury in athletes after sports-related concussion. *Journal of Neurotrauma, 32*, 661–673. http://dx.doi.org/10.1089/neu.2014.3655

Polak, P., Leddy, J. J., Dwyer, M. G., Willer, B., & Zivadinov, R. (2015). Diffusion tensor imaging alterations in patients with postconcussion syndrome undergoing exercise treatment: A pilot longitudinal study. *The Journal of Head Trauma Rehabilitation, 30*, E32–E42. http://dx.doi.org/10.1097/HTR.0000000000000037

Ponsford, J., Willmott, C., Rothwell, A., Cameron, P., Kelly, A. M., Nelms, R., & Curran, C. (2002). Impact of early intervention on outcome following mild head injury in adults. *Journal of Neurology, Neurosurgery & Psychiatry, 73*, 330–332. http://dx.doi.org/10.1136/jnnp.73.3.330

Ruff, R. M., Camenzuli, L., & Mueller, J. (1996). Miserable minority: Emotional risk factors that influence the outcome of a mild traumatic brain injury. *Brain Injury, 10*, 551–565. http://dx.doi.org/10.1080/026990596124124

Sawyer, Q., Vesci, B., & McLeod, T. C. (2016). Physical activity and intermittent postconcussion symptoms after a period of symptom-limited physical and cognitive rest. *Journal of Athletic Training, 51*, 739–742. http://dx.doi.org/10.4085/1062-6050-51.12.01

Schneider, K. H. (2016). Cognitive rest: An integrated literature review. *The Journal of School Nursing, 32*, 234–240. http://dx.doi.org/10.1177/1059840515607344

Schneider, K. J., Iverson, G. L., Emery, C. A., McCrory, P., Herring, S. A., & Mccuwisse, W. H. (2013). The effects of rest and treatment following sport-related concussion: A systematic review of the literature. *British Journal of Sports Medicine, 47*, 304–307. http://dx.doi.org/10.1136/bjsports-2013-092190

Schneider, K. J., Leddy, J. J., Guskiewicz, K. M., Seifert, T., McCrea, M., Silverberg, N. D., . . . Makdissi, M. (2017). Rest and treatment/rehabilitation following sport-related concussion: A systematic review. *British Journal of Sports Medicine, 51*(12). http://dx.doi.org/10.1136/bjsports-2016-097475

Schneider, K. J., Meeuwisse, W. H., Nettel-Aguirre, A., Barlow, K., Boyd, L., Kang, J., & Emery, C. A. (2014). Cervicovestibular rehabilitation in sport-related concussion: A randomised controlled trial. *British Journal of Sports Medicine, 48*, 1294–1298. http://dx.doi.org/10.1136/bjsports-2013-093267

Shahim, P., Tegner, Y., Gustafsson, B., Gren, M., Ärlig, J., Olsson, M., . . . Blennow, K. (2016). Neurochemical aftermath of repetitive mild traumatic brain injury. *JAMA Neurology, 73*, 1308–1315. http://dx.doi.org/10.1001/jamaneurol.2016.2038

Silverberg, N. D., & Iverson, G. L. (2011). Etiology of the post-concussion syndrome: Physiogenesis and psychogenesis revisited. *NeuroRehabilitation, 29*, 317–329.

Silverberg, N. D., & Iverson, G. L. (2013). Is rest after concussion "the best medicine?": Recommendations for activity resumption following concussion in athletes, civilians, and military service members. *The Journal of Head Trauma Rehabilitation, 28*, 250–259. http://dx.doi.org/10.1097/HTR.0b013e31825ad658

Siman, R., Shahim, P., Tegner, Y., Blennow, K., Zetterberg, H., & Smith, D. H. (2015). Serum SNTF increases in concussed professional ice hockey players and relates to the severity of postconcussion symptoms. *Journal of Neurotrauma, 32*, 1294–1300. http://dx.doi.org/10.1089/neu.2014.3698

Stepanski, E. J., & Wyatt, J. K. (2003). Use of sleep hygiene in the treatment of insomnia. *Sleep Medicine Reviews, 7*, 215–225. http://dx.doi.org/10.1053/smrv.2001.0246

Tator, C. H., & Davis, H. (2014). The postconcussion syndrome in sports and recreation: Clinical features and demography in 138 athletes. *Neurosurgery, 75*(Suppl. 4), S106–S112. http://dx.doi.org/10.1227/NEU.0000000000000484

Taylor, D. J., & Pruiksma, K. E. (2014). Cognitive and behavioural therapy for insomnia (CBT-I) in psychiatric populations: A systematic review. *International Review of Psychiatry, 26*, 205–213. http://dx.doi.org/10.3109/09540261.2014.902808

Thomas, D. G., Apps, J. N., Hoffmann, R. G., McCrea, M., & Hammeke, T. (2015). Benefits of strict rest after acute concussion: A randomized controlled trial. *Pediatrics, 135*, 213–223. http://dx.doi.org/10.1542/peds.2014-0966

Wang, Y., Nelson, L. D., LaRoche, A. A., Pfaller, A. Y., Nencka, A. S., Koch, K. M., & McCrea, M. A. (2016). Cerebral blood flow alterations in acute sport-related concussion. *Journal of Neurotrauma, 33*, 1227–1236. http://dx.doi.org/10.1089/neu.2015.4072

World Health Organization. (1992a). *The ICD–10 classification of mental and behavioural disorders—Clinical descriptions and diagnostic guidelines.* Retrieved from http://www.who.int/classifications/icd/en/bluebook.pdf

World Health Organization. (1992b). *The ICD–10 classification of mental and behavioural disorders—Diagnostic criteria for research.* Retrieved from http://www.who.int/classifications/icd/en/GRNBOOK.pdf

Zemek, R. L., Farion, K. J., Sampson, M., & McGahern, C. (2013). Prognosticators of persistent symptoms following pediatric concussion: A systematic review. *JAMA Pediatrics, 167*, 259–265. http://dx.doi.org/10.1001/2013.jamapediatrics.216

Zetterberg, H., & Blennow, K. (2016). Fluid biomarkers for mild traumatic brain injury and related conditions. *Nature Reviews Neurology, 12*, 563–574. http://dx.doi.org/10.1038/nrneurol.2016.127

Zuckerman, S. L., Solomon, G. S., Forbes, J. A., Haase, R. F., Sills, A. K., & Lovell, M. R. (2012). Response to acute concussive injury in soccer players: Is gender a modifying factor? *Journal of Neurosurgery: Pediatrics, 10*, 504–510. http://dx.doi.org/10.3171/2012.8.PEDS12139

Zuckerman, S. L., Totten, D. J., Rubel, K. E., Kuhn, A. W., Yengo-Kahn, A. M., & Solomon, G. S. (2016). Mechanisms of injury as a diagnostic predictor of sport-related concussion severity in football, basketball, and soccer: Results from a regional concussion registry. *Neurosurgery, 63*(Suppl. 1), 102–112. http://dx.doi.org/10.1227/NEU.0000000000001280

2

POSTTRAUMATIC HEADACHE AND MIGRAINE ASSESSMENT AND MANAGEMENT AFTER SPORT-RELATED CONCUSSION

MELISSA N. WOMBLE, JILL R. HENLEY,
SHERI A. FEDOR, AND MICHAEL W. COLLINS

This chapter discusses the similarities in pathophysiology between concussion and migraine, which may be responsible for the high rates of posttraumatic headaches and migraines after sport-related concussion (SRC). We also describe proper management and treatment when headaches and migraines are present after injury.

HEADACHE AND MIGRAINE IN THE GENERAL POPULATION

Within the general population, headache is a common somatic complaint (Zasler, 2015). Specifically, headaches are estimated as affecting approximately half of the global population at least once each year (Patel et al., 2016; Wöber-Bingöl, 2013). It is estimated that up to 4% of the world's

Michael W. Collins is cofounder, shareholder, and board member of ImPACT Applications, Inc. However, ImPACT was not the focus of the current chapter. No other authors have competing interests to report.

http://dx.doi.org/10.1037/0000114-003
Neuropsychology of Sports-Related Concussion, P. A. Arnett (Editor)

adult population experience chronic headaches, which occur 15 or more days per month (Patel et al., 2016). Many types of headaches exist, although the primary headache disorders include tension-type and migraine headaches. The International Headache Society (2013) has defined a tension-type headache as an episodic, typically bilateral, pressing or tightening-type headache that does not worsen with regular physical activity and is not associated with nausea, although photophobia or phonophobia may be present. Current estimates predict a lifetime prevalence of tension-type headaches at 30% to 78% (International Headache Society [IHS], 2013; Wöber-Bingöl, 2013). Headaches can also be caused by a number of other medical conditions, such as injury to the head or neck or medication overuse (IHS, 2013). Although increased headache frequencies have been observed in certain regions of the world, headaches are a pandemic worldwide and affect individuals of all genders, ages, and ethnicities. Frequent or severe headaches can negatively affect daily life in terms of occupational and academic performance as well as quality of life (IHS, 2013; Kacperski, Hung, & Blume, 2016; Patel et al., 2016).

Migraine has been identified as the third most prevalent disorder worldwide and seventh largest cause of disability (Burstein, Noseda, & Borsook, 2015; IHS, 2013). Migraine is suspected to involve cortical, subcortical, and brainstem areas responsible for the regulation of autonomic, affective, cognitive, and sensory functions (Burstein et al., 2015). The IHS (2013) has defined migraine as an episodic, unilateral, pulsating-type headache that worsens with regular physical activity and is associated with symptoms including nausea, phonophobia, and photophobia, or a combination of these. Current estimates predict a mean prevalence of migraine at approximately 10% for pediatric populations and 15% for adult populations (Burstein et al., 2015; Wöber-Bingöl, 2013).

Migraine is a complex neurological process involving multiple clinical phases, including the preheadache (comprising the prodrome and possible aura), early headache, advanced headache, and postdrome (Linde, Mellberg, & Dahlöf, 2006). Within the preheadache phase, the prodrome signals an impending migraine with premonitory symptoms such as changes in cognition, mood, sensations, and bodily functions (e.g., gastrointestinal complaints) that occur on average 9.42 hours before pain (Kelman & Rains, 2005). Questionnaire studies have revealed that more than 80% of adults and 70% of children can identify the prodrome and therefore are sometimes able to take precautionary measures, such as using abortive migraine medications (Cuvellier, Mars, & Vallée, 2009). Aura, also a component of the preheadache phase, represents a cluster of focal neurological symptoms developing gradually in 5 to 20 minutes to include visual, somatosensory, dysphasic symptoms, or a combination of these (IHS, 2013; Linde et al., 2006). Aura has a clear onset and termination that is fully reversible; however, aura does not occur with each attack or in all patients. Intervention during aura may successfully abort the headache process (IHS, 2013). The early and advanced headache phases of migraine are generally similar for those with and without aura. Specifically, migraine attacks can last anywhere from 4 to 72 hours for adult populations and 1 to 72 hours for pediatric populations, with full remission between attacks (IHS, 2013). The postdrome phase is not well understood, but it is known to represent a period of increased vulnerability within the central nervous system (IHS, 2013; Linde et al., 2006).

With regard to the pathophysiology of migraine with aura, there is evidence of regional cerebral blood flow and cortical spreading depression in the brainstem and cortical regions (Burstein et al., 2015; Silberstein, 2004). Specifically, reduction of blood flow begins in the primary visual cortex and spreads anteriorly, in a wave of cortical neuronal and glial depolarization at a rate of 2 to 5 mm per second to the primary somatosensory and motor cortices (IHS, 2013; Lashley, 1941; Silberstein, 2004). These structures lie in close proximity to the trigeminal vascular system, which innervates the parenchyma as well as the meninges (Silberstein, 2004). Interestingly, blood flow changes and spreading depression do not seem to occur in migraine without aura (IHS, 2013). As discussed, migraine can be associated with a prodrome in a majority of migraine patients, which is associated with diffuse cerebral dysfunction beginning in the hypothalamus (Blau, 1980). This diffuse cerebral dysfunction provokes changes in the brainstem and cortex, affecting meningeal vasculature associated with typical migraine symptoms, including headache. Nociception in the dural and meningeal vasculature have been found responsible for the pain sensation during migraine (IHS, 2013).

CONCUSSION

Concussion has been defined as a complex pathophysiological process caused by biomechanical force, resulting in transient neurological dysfunction (Giza & Hovda, 2014; McCrory et al., 2017; Mild Traumatic Brain Injury Committee of the Head Injury Interdisciplinary Special Interest Group of the American Congress of Rehabilitation Medicine, 1993). A concussion may be caused by a direct or indirect blow to the head, face, neck, or elsewhere on the body if the force of the impact is transmitted to the head (e.g., whiplash injury; McCrory et al., 2017). Concussion is viewed as a functional rather than structural injury due to underlying ionic shifts, metabolic changes, and alterations in neurotransmission (Giza & Hovda, 2014; McCrory et al., 2017). Concussion is undetectable with traditional imaging methods. However, advanced imaging techniques, such as diffusion tensor imaging, show promise, especially in the adolescent population, in detecting associated microstructural damage (Echemendia, 2012; Giza & Hovda, 2014). After concussion, patients experience a constellation of physical, cognitive, and emotional symptoms that are transient in nature. These symptoms are reflective of a temporary neuronal disturbance rather than cell death (Giza & Hovda, 2014). It has generally been thought that 80% to 90% of athletes recover from an SRC within 7 to 14 days (McCrory et al., 2013); however, new research has shown that recovery can last up to 4 weeks for symptoms, 3 to 4 weeks for memory, and 3 weeks for vestibular and oculomotor dysfunction (Henry, Elbin, Collins, Marchetti, & Kontos, 2016). Demographic (e.g., sex) and postinjury factors (e.g., on-field dizziness, posttraumatic migraine) are presumed to contribute to the prolonged recoveries for some athletes (Covassin, Elbin, Harris, Parker, & Kontos, 2012; Kontos et al., 2013; Lau, Kontos, Collins, Mucha, & Lovell, 2011; Mihalik et al., 2005).

With regard to the underlying pathophysiology of concussion, symptoms and functional impairments are presumed to occur due to ionic shifts that result in metabolic changes and impaired neurotransmission following injury (Giza & Hovda, 2014). Vulnerable axonal membranes are stretched, opening voltage-dependent gates and initiating a massive efflux of potassium (K^+) into extracellular fluid. Glial cells, which are normally able to absorb excess K^+, are unable to compensate after this unregulated flux of ion concentrations (Barnett & Singman, 2015; Giza & Hovda, 2014). Glutamate, an excitatory amino acid, floods the brain, creating an excitotoxic response that suppresses neuronal activity and results in a "spreading-depression-like" state (Giza & Hovda, 2014; Kontos, Reches, et al., 2016). This unalterable depolarization is amplified by increased intracellular calcium (Ca^{2+}) accumulation, which enters through channels opened by glutamate binding to N-methyl-D-aspartate receptors. Increased intracellular Ca^{2+} levels can induce microtubule disassembly breakdown and alteration of cytoskeleton integrity, which can interrupt axonal connection and neurotransmission (Barnett & Singman, 2015; Giza & Hovda, 2014). In an attempt to restore the brain to homeostatic levels, cells must activate ionic pumps. This creates an increased demand for cellular metabolism and glycolysis, the process through which glucose is broken down to create energy to fuel the ionic pumps. Lactate, a by-product of this energetic process, accumulates in the cell, impairing mitochondrial function. Mitochondria are the organelle responsible for adenosine triphosphate (ATP) production, the neuron's primary, and preferred, source of energy. The increased energy demand coupled with the decreased energy supply (in the form of decreased regional cerebral blood flow and ATP production) causes an energy crisis in the brain that can last for days or weeks postinjury (Giza & Hovda, 2014; Barnett & Singman, 2015).

Metabolic changes after concussion may also be mediated by genetic influences (Giza & Hovda, 2014). Concussive injuries are known to alter levels of glutamate, epinephrine, and acetylcholine, which may underlie cognitive problems (e.g., learning, memory) and the painful symptoms associated with migraine (i.e., headache, nausea, photophobia, phonophobia; Kontos, Reches, et al., 2016). Recent studies have also implicated cervical muscles, nociceptive neuropeptides in the brainstem, and cerebral inflammatory processes in the experience of postconcussion symptoms (Giza & Hovda, 2014; Petraglia, Maroon, & Bailes, 2012; Zasler, 2015).

PATHOPHYSIOLOGY SIMILARITIES BETWEEN CONCUSSION AND MIGRAINE

When considering the symptoms and pathophysiology of concussion and migraine, there is significant overlap. Migraine and concussion both result in similar symptoms (see reported frequencies in concussion patients in what follows, when available): pain in the head or neck (25%–50%); nausea, vomiting, and visual changes (15%–25%); phonophobia and cognitive impairment (25%–50%); dizziness (20%–30%); mood changes (15%–50%); and fatigue (40%–45%; Giza & Hovda, 2014; Junn, Bell, Shenouda, & Hoffman, 2015). With regard to the underlying pathophysiology, both concussion and migraine involve a spreading depression within the cerebral cortex (Burstein et al., 2015; Giza & Hovda, 2014). Additionally, Packard and Ham (1997) outlined the shared biochemical alterations including depolarization, excessive excitatory amino acids, increased calcium/magnesium ratio, impaired glucose utilization, and abnormalities in various neuropeptides. There is also a suspected genetic relationship between ionic compensatory mechanisms and cerebral responses to concussion because individuals with the familial hemiplegic migraine ion channelopathy have been found to be prone to experiencing cerebral edema after mild traumatic brain injury (Giza & Hovda, 2014). These same genetic factors (i.e., ion channelopathies) may also help to explain why some athletes are more symptomatic after SRC as well as to experiencing cerebral edema after second-impact syndrome (Giza & Hovda, 2014).

POSTTRAUMATIC HEADACHE AND MIGRAINE AFTER SRC

After SRC, headaches are the most commonly reported symptom (Heyer, Young, Rose, McNally, & Fischer, 2016; Kontos et al., 2013). The high frequency of headaches postinjury has been speculated as relating to preinjury migraines, headaches, neck pain, and dizziness being independent risk factors for concussion (Giza et al., 2013; Gordon, Dooley, & Wood, 2006; Zasler, 2015); however, alternative explanations warranting further research include whiplash injury, athlete "preparedness" for injury, affective disorders, and sex differences (Zasler, 2015). The IHS (2013) defined posttraumatic headache (PTH) as a headache disorder developing within 7 days of injury. PTH is categorized as either acute or chronic (i.e., persisting beyond 3 months; Heyer et al., 2016). PTH is more frequently experienced during the acute recovery period, with full resolution of headache generally occurring several days to weeks postinjury. Generally, tension and migraine-type headaches are most commonly reported after SRC (Bramley et al., 2015). Research has shown that females are more likely than males to report PTH (Bramley et al., 2015). PTH has been found to occur more often in adolescents than younger children, as indicated by a significant relationship between headaches and concussion in this age-group (Blume, 2015). As with headaches in the general population, PTH can affect an athlete's ability to engage in school and extracurricular activities, which can consequently reduce their quality of life (Kacperski, Hung, & Blume, 2016).

Within the concussion literature, posttraumatic migraine (PTM) has been defined as a type of PTH developing after concussion to include a headache with associated features (i.e., nausea and/or photophobia and phonophobia; Kontos et al., 2013). Heyer and colleagues (2016) identified PTM as a distinct clinical entity, regardless of headache history, due to the strong correlations among headaches, nausea, photophobia, phonophobia, and dizziness for those with or without premorbid headaches. Interestingly, those with a history of premorbid headaches also showed strong correlations with neck pain (Heyer et al., 2016).

Studies have suggested that PTM following SRC may indicate a more severe injury due to experiencing more total postconcussion symptoms and demonstrating greater cognitive deficits acutely than individuals experiencing nonmigraine headaches or no headaches (Mihalik et al., 2005). Increased postconcussion symptoms for those experiencing PTM are expected because typical migraines can last for days to weeks and oftentimes interfere with cognitive abilities and emotional functioning, depending upon the treatment received. Results from this study identified worse performance acutely in patients with PTM for the visual memory, visual motor speed, and reaction time composites of the Immediate Post-Concussion Assessment and Cognitive Testing (ImPACT; Mihalik et al., 2005). Kontos and colleagues (2013) designed a study to further evaluate the effects of PTM beyond the acute period and across recovery. Results again showed worse performance for athletes with PTM on the visual memory and reaction time composites and greater symptom reports than those with nonmigraine headache or no headache at 1 to 7 and 8 to 14 days postinjury. Additionally, those with PTM demonstrated worse performance on the verbal memory composite than did the headache group at 8 to 14 days postinjury. In terms of recovery, athletes with

PTM were 7.3 and 2.6 times more likely to experience a protracted recovery than those without headache and with nonmigraine headache, respectively. Thus, PTM has been found to be associated with protracted recovery as well as cognitive impairments during both the acute period and across recovery.

COMORBIDITY OF SYMPTOMS WITH POSTTRAUMATIC HEADACHE AND MIGRAINE

PTH commonly occurs in combination with other postconcussion symptoms, including sleep disturbances, dizziness, and mood disorders (i.e., anxiety, depression; Blume, 2015; Choe & Blume, 2016). Although more research is necessary to understand symptom patterns, it is important that clinicians understand the relationship between symptom clusters. For example, comorbid balance, dizziness, anxiety, and migraine symptoms are commonly experienced after SRC (Furman, Balaban, Jacob, & Marcus, 2005). The comorbidity of these symptoms has been identified as relating to overlap of the vestibular and pain pathways with the regulation, perception, and generation of emotion and affect (Balaban, Jacob, & Furman, 2011). In complex cases involving multiple symptoms, as outlined in the preceding example, clinicians must determine whether one symptom should be treated more aggressively, or if all should be treated simultaneously. For instance, vestibular rehabilitation as completed by a physical therapist may be warranted to address vestibular dysfunction.

Nevertheless, patients with a large anxiety response to visual motion stimulation (i.e., a type of vestibular dysfunction) may be limited in their ability to progress in therapy or resume work activities. As such, recognizing the patient's anxiety response and treating the anxiety with medication, therapy, or both is critical to the patient's recovery and engagement in treatment. Likewise, patients with migraine may also experience dizziness with migraine episodes, sensitivity to visual motion stimulation, and concurrent anxiety (Furman et al., 2005). Therefore, as clinicians it is important to understand all potential causes of post-traumatic headaches and migraines following SRC as well as the appropriate manner and order in which to treat comorbid symptoms. In these situations, a multidisciplinary approach to the management of concussion is crucial (Reynolds, Collins, Mucha, & Troutman-Ensecki, 2014).

Vestibular Migraine

Vestibular migraine is a newly recognized diagnostic entity (Lempert et al., 2012). This diagnosis remains challenging because many patients with migraine headaches also experience vestibular symptoms (Furman et al.,

2005). Similarly, people with vestibular diagnoses also commonly experience migraines. The diagnosis of vestibular migraine largely remains a diagnosis of exclusion. Vestibular migraine can include symptoms of vertigo, dizziness, imbalance, and spatial disorientation (Furman & Balaban, 2015). To fit diagnostic criteria, at least 50% of the vestibular episodes must include one or more migraine features (Lempert et al., 2012). Prophylactic pharmacotherapy treatment of migraine has been effective in treatment of vestibular migraine (Baier, Winkenwerder, & Dieterich, 2009). For patients experiencing the temporal features of dizziness and visual motion sensitivity, vestibular rehabilitation has shown positive outcomes (Whitney, Wrisley, Brown, & Furman, 2000).

After SRC, patients with or without a history of migraine can develop PTM. Patients may also experience vestibular dysfunction, which can result in symptoms of dizziness, imbalance, and spatial disorientation. Current treatment of vestibular symptoms after SRC includes vestibular rehabilitation. On occasion, patients may return several months after completion of vestibular rehabilitation due to return of symptoms in the absence of reinjury. These patients may be experiencing untreated migraines headaches. In that case, clinicians should consider a differential diagnosis of vestibular migraine and subsequently refer for migraine treatment.

Other Types of Posttraumatic Headaches After SRC

Occipital Neuralgia

Occipital neuralgia can occur after SRC, resulting in chronic headaches. According to the IHS (2013), occipital neuralgia can present as unilateral or bilateral shooting or stabbing pain following the greater, lesser, or third occipital nerve distribution. The pain can be referred from the occipital head region to the fronto-orbital region. To meet diagnostic criteria for occipital neuralgia, the pain must have two of the following three characteristics: recurring attacks lasting from seconds to minutes, severe intensity, and shooting, stabbing, or sharp quality pain (IHS, 2013). The pain must be associated with reduced sensation or allodynia during innocuous stimulation of the scalp or hair. The patient must also experience one or both of the following: tenderness over the affected nerve branches or trigger points at the emergence of the greater occipital nerve or in the area of distribution of C2 (IHS, 2013). If headache is caused by occipital neuralgia, anesthetic block of the affected nerve can temporarily ease the pain (IHS, 2013). Differential diagnosis of occipital neuralgia includes referred pain from the atlantoaxial or upper zygapophyseal joints and trigger points in the suboccipital and upper neck muscles (IHS, 2013). Clinically, the pain can be differentiated by neuropathic pain quality compared with musculoskeletal pain. Musculoskeletal pain is differentiated because it is elicited when moving the affected joint (IHS, 2013).

Cervicogenic Headache

Cervicogenic headache can also plague SRC patients due to the high incidence of whiplash injury to the cervical spine. According to the IHS (2013), cervicogenic headache can involve bony, muscular, and soft tissue elements in the neck that cause headache. Diagnostic criteria for cervicogenic headache include clinical, laboratory, or imaging evidence of a disorder or lesion within the cervical spine or soft tissues which could cause headache (IHS, 2013). Evidence of at least two of these clinical findings is enough to meet diagnostic criteria: headache developed during onset of cervical disorder or appearance of the lesion, headache improved or resolved with improvement in or resolution of cervical disorder or lesion, cervical range of motion reduced and headache is significantly worse with provocation maneuver, or abolishment of headache after blockade of cervical structure or its nerve supply (IHS, 2013). To treat cervical headaches, the cervical disorder must be diagnosed and treated. Of note, orthopedic rehabilitation for cervical dysfunction can take place concurrently with other necessary treatments, including vision, cognitive, or vestibular rehabilitation.

MANAGEMENT OF POSTTRAUMATIC HEADACHE AND MIGRAINE AFTER SRC

Behavioral Management

After SRC, one of the most important but understudied treatment strategies for PTH and PTM involves implementation of healthy lifestyle habits for overall symptom reduction and management. Unfortunately, many patients assume that strict rest is key after SRC, which can lead to altered sleep patterns, skipping meals, stress, and avoidance of physical activity. These unhealthy lifestyle habits subsequently serve as a trigger for PTH and PTM, especially in individuals with a positive personal or family history. The consequences of recommending strict rest over usual care was recently investigated in a randomized controlled trial of adolescents presenting to the emergency department (Thomas, Apps, Hoffmann, McCrea, & Hammeke, 2015). No clinically significant differences were observed in terms of neurocognitive functioning or balance outcomes between groups, although the strict rest group reported more daily postconcussion symptoms and demonstrated a prolonged recovery (Thomas et al., 2015). Results were speculated to occur secondary to development of physical and emotional symptoms as triggered by missing school, falling behind academically, activity restrictions, lack of exercise, and reduced social interactions (Thomas et al., 2015). Overall, results emphasized the importance of maintaining a regulated and healthy lifestyle following SRC as opposed to strict rest.

Healthy lifestyle habits after SRC should include a regular sleep–wake schedule, regular meals, adequate fluid hydration, regular exercise, and practice of stress management techniques. Previous research has highlighted the relationships among altered sleep schedules, skipping meals, dehydration, lack of physical activity, and stress in the development of frequent headaches and other postconcussion symptoms (Choe & Blume, 2016; Kacperski et al., 2016). Implementation of healthy lifestyle habits immediately after concussion may reduce the development of headaches or PTM as well as the need for medication in select cases. With regard to specific healthy lifestyle habits, recommendations have been made based on research into each habit and as supported specifically within both the concussion and headache/migraine literature.

Regular Sleep–Wake Schedule

Dysregulation of sleep (e.g., sleep deprivation, oversleeping, disturbed or interrupted sleep) is recognized as a common headache trigger, particularly for chronic daily, awakening, and morning headache patterns (Rains, Poceta, & Penzien, 2008). In a large clinical study of 1,283 patients presenting for treatment of migraine, the following sleep complaints were reported: morning headaches (71%), difficulty initiating sleep (53%), difficulty maintaining sleep (61%), and chronically shortened sleep patterns (38%; Kelman & Rains, 2005). Greater migraine frequency and severity has also been found to be associated with shorter sleep durations (Boardman, Thomas, Millson, & Croft, 2005). Interestingly, Boardman and colleagues (2005) identified a dose–response relationship between headache severity and sleep complaints such that headache frequency was associated with slight (odds ratio [OR] = 2.4), moderate (OR = 3.6), and severe (OR = 7.5) sleep complaints in 2,662 participants. Within this study, a causal link to anxiety was also observed, which is not surprising given that psychiatric disorders, particularly affective disorders, are commonly comorbid with headache (i.e., especially migraines and chronic daily headaches) and sleep disorders (Boardman et al., 2005). Therefore, to reduce the likelihood of headaches or migraines after SRC, it is recommended that patients follow a regulated sleep schedule to include a similar sleep and wake time each day as well as a weekend sleep schedule mimicking the weeknight schedule (Kacperski et al., 2016). It is also recommended that patients avoid naps, unless napping was part of their typical schedule before injury. Naps can lead to difficulty falling asleep and poor-quality sleep that can prolong recovery and result in additional post-concussion symptoms. Other sleep-related problems (i.e., difficulty with sleep initiation or maintenance) are sometimes contributory to headaches and can be managed with melatonin (Choe & Blume, 2016).

Regular Meals

Following a routine eating schedule is important to keep the brain and body fueled during the recovery process. Additionally, irregular meals are one of most common headache triggers in individuals who experience migraine or tension-type headaches (Spierings, Ranke, & Honkoop, 2001). Therefore, we recommend not skipping meals, especially breakfast, and consuming a well-balanced diet (Kacperski et al., 2016). Of note, it is estimated that 8% to 12% of school-age children and 20% to 30% of adolescents skip breakfast (HealthyChildren.org, 2015); for this reason, it is important to discuss this issue with young athletes after SRC. Breakfast is specifically emphasized because of the known beneficial effects on cognitive functioning, energy, ability to focus, and overall academic performance (Adolphus, Lawton, & Dye, 2013). To date, there has been little research in terms of specific foods to consume or avoid following SRC. From a migraine perspective, certain foods and beverages, including red wine, aspartame sweetener, products with caffeine, aged cheeses, chocolate, and nitrates, may trigger headaches (Schulte, Jürgens, & May, 2015). Although it has been recommended that migraine sufferers reduce exposure to triggers, elimination long term has not been recommended (Martin, 2010a, 2010b).

Adequate Fluid Hydration

Dehydration is caused by an inadequate amount of total body water for proper functioning (Kenney, Long, Cradock, & Gortmaker, 2015; Popkin, D'Anci, & Rosenberg, 2010). Rates of dehydration in a recent study with participants aged 6 to 19 years old demonstrated inadequate hydration in 54.5% of the sample (Kenney et al., 2015). The rates of dehydration were significantly higher among boys, non-Hispanic Black participants, and younger children compared with girls, White participants, and older children (Kenney et al., 2015). Although severe dehydration can be associated with serious health problems (e.g., delirium), mild dehydration is also a concern and can be associated with headaches, dizziness, irritability, poor physical performance, and reduced cognitive functioning (Kenney et al., 2015). Of importance, many of the concerns resulting from mild dehydration are also reported after concussion. Water deprivation can serve as a trigger for headaches and migraines as well as a prolonged migraine experience (Popkin et al., 2010).

For headaches triggered by dehydration, relief can be experienced within 30 minutes to 3 hours after consuming water (Popkin et al., 2010). Although there is not strong literature regarding increased hydration as prevention for migraines, research has suggested that adequate fluid hydration can assist with reduced headache intensity and duration (Kacperski et al., 2016).

Regular Exercise

Aerobic exercise is known to have beneficial effects for pain and mood-related symptoms. For that reason, the American Headache Society currently recommends regular exercise to decrease the frequency and intensity of headaches and migraines (Rathier, 2015). Many research studies have focused on exercise and its beneficial effects on migraine. For example, exercise was investigated for migraine prophylaxis in a randomized controlled study using relaxation and topiramate as controls (Varkey, Cider, Carlsson, & Linde, 2011). In this study, 91 patients exercised for 40 minutes per day, three times per week, and this exercise was found to be as effective as relaxation and topiramate treatment for migraine reduction. Eight subjects in the topiramate-treatment group experienced adverse events, compared with no adverse events in the exercise group (Varkey et al., 2011). These studies highlight the importance of exercise in the management of migraine. Although patients may experience increased headache and migraine severity with exercise, avoiding exercise because of symptom provocation is not recommended (Choe & Blume, 2016; Rathier, 2015). In cases in which patients frequently experience headaches or migraines with exercise, focus should be placed on headache prevention, including possible pharmacological treatment of migraine.

Although it remains unclear how exercise should be applied in patients with headache, research has suggested that submaximal aerobic exercise (i.e., exercise in which symptom exacerbation does not occur) may be the best option in migraine prophylaxis, at least initially (Choe & Blume, 2016). Specifically, submaximal aerobic exercise has been found beneficial in terms of reducing the frequency and intensity of headache and migraine attacks while also improving quality of life (Dittrich et al., 2008). Another study by Varkey, Cider, Carlsson, and Linde (2009) demonstrated the feasibility of an indoor cycling program performed three times per week in reducing the frequency and intensity of migraine attacks. In this study, only one subject experienced a migraine from exercise during a 12-week period (Varkey et al., 2009). As highlighted in these two studies, the exercise program should be individualized to the patient and allow for recovery periods to avoid increased stress and reach optimal functioning (Daenen, Varkey, Kellmann, & Nijs, 2015). During the initial exercise stages, increased symptoms may occur because exercise can be a trigger for headaches; however, symptoms generally decrease after a few weeks when a routine is established and migraine risk is decreased (Daenen et al., 2015). The aforementioned exercise recommendations are made to habituate rather than avoid specific triggers and sensory signals disturbed by migraine processes (Martin, 2010a).

Due to similar pathophysiology, the same habituation is applied with exercise after SRC to overcome PTH and PTM. Exercise is initiated through formal exertion therapy, daily activities with the athletic trainer or as recommended by the patient's physician. It is generally recommended that the athlete initially engage in light noncontact, nonrisk physical activity every day (e.g., walk or stationary bike ride) while following an exposure-recovery model (i.e., taking short breaks as symptoms increase to a moderate severity; Reynolds et al., 2014). As the athlete tolerates physical activity, a graded exertion progression should be followed to include activities, such as dynamic movements, cardio, and sport-specific exercises (Reynolds et al., 2014). Of note, it is important to identify other comorbid symptoms, such as vestibular dysfunction, to determine which type of physical activity may be most beneficial. Screening assessments and formal vestibular rehabilitation evaluations can be helpful in this regard. For those athletes without evidence of vestibular impairment, most exercise activities can be incorporated by following a gradual progression and using recovery periods.

Regular Practice of Stress Management and Relaxation Techniques

Both physical and emotional stress can trigger and exacerbate posttraumatic headaches and migraines. Athletes with a history of psychiatric conditions or those experiencing vestibular dysfunction may be prone to experiencing increased mood-related symptoms after an injury. In many cases, stress and mood-related symptoms are elicited due to concerns regarding the long-term impacts of concussion, lack of information regarding symptoms, activity restrictions, lack of exercise, and reduced social interactions. As such, it is important for clinicians to consider the beneficial effects of education regarding concussion and expected recovery rates to prepare families for the recovery process (Choe & Blume, 2016). Additionally, clinicians should be mindful in recognizing all potential situational and environmental stressors, especially related to restrictions imposed after concussion.

Even with these efforts, stress and mood-related symptoms may persist and contribute to continued headaches and migraines. Therefore, therapeutic interventions, including relaxation training, meditation training, biofeedback, or cognitive behavior therapy, may be recommended (Brody, 2014). Other potential treatment options that may be helpful in reducing stress include academic accommodations or work restrictions, although long-term use is not typically recommended; instead, it is generally recommended that athletes return to school after a specific outlined plan (e.g., "return to learn" program) as soon as possible to mitigate stress and reduce symptom exacerbation (Gioia, 2016). If stress and mood-related symptoms remain uncontrolled with the aforementioned nonpharmacological treatments, pharmacological treatments may be considered.

Medication Management

Rebound Headaches

Because analgesics are commonly recommended after SRC, the risk for rebound headaches (i.e., medication-overuse headaches) exists, especially in susceptible individuals. A *rebound headache* has been defined as a headache present 15 or more days per month that has developed or worsened during analgesic overuse, resolves within 2 months after discontinuation of analgesics, and meets at least one of the following characteristics: bilateral, pressing/tightening quality, or mild/moderate intensity (Heyer & Idris, 2014; IHS, 2013). These headaches can also result in other symptoms, including morning headaches, neck pain, nonrestorative sleep, and vasomotor instability (Tepper & Tepper, 2010). Rebound headaches occur most commonly in individuals with a history of episodic migraine (i.e., less than 15 headache days per month), although the exact reasoning for susceptibility remains unclear (Tepper & Tepper, 2010). Rebound headaches can be caused by other medications (e.g., butalbital, opioids, triptans), but most commonly this phenomenon is observed with analgesic overuse after SRC (Heyer & Idris, 2014; Tepper & Tepper, 2010). Treatment for rebound headaches involves weaning from the overused medication and possibly beginning a prophylaxis medication regimen. Unrelated to concussion, rebound headaches have been estimated as resulting in chronic headaches for 20% to 30% of children and adolescents (Heyer & Idris, 2014).

Heyer and Idris (2014) further evaluated rebound headaches in a sample of 104 adolescent concussion patients. Of the 104 adolescents, 77 had experienced chronic posttraumatic headaches for 3 to 12 months with 54 (70.1%) meeting criteria for rebound headaches. After discontinuing analgesics, 37 patients (68.5%) had resolution of headaches or improvements to preinjury headaches, seven (13%) had no change, and 10 (18.5%) did not discontinue analgesics or did not complete follow-up evaluations. High rates (49%) of rebound headaches have also been identified in U.S. soldiers secondary to using abortive medications more days than not over a 3-month span following concussion (Theeler, Flynn, & Erickson, 2012). Thus, results from these studies suggest that analgesic detoxification should be recommended when medication overuse is suspected. In terms of general management after SRC, it is recommended that clinicians discuss potential medication overuse with young athletes and their parents early in the treatment process. It is generally recommended that over-the-counter medications be used only two to three times per week (Tepper & Tepper, 2010).

Medication Options

The goal of headache and migraine treatment follows a prevention or abortion approach during the acute and chronic phases of migraines. Specifically, treatment is aimed at preventing or reducing the frequency of episodes or aborting the pain should it occur. Generally, prescription medications are not used during the acute recovery period because of the likelihood for headaches and migraines to improve over time. In considering medications, it is important for clinicians to understand that the most common medication side effects in concussion patients involve cognitive and mood-related symptoms (Brody, 2014). Additionally, when considering use of medications, it is important for clinicians to understand the role of vestibular-oculomotor dysfunction in headaches to ensure the underlying dysfunction is also being managed before or concurrent with pharmacological treatment.

Research regarding medication management after concussion has historically been weaker than would be expected, in part because of the heterogeneity of concussion, heterogeneous populations, and lack of adequate control groups (Brody, 2014; Petraglia et al., 2012). With that said, a few studies have focused on common medications used postconcussion. In one study, 18% of adolescents receiving treatment at a regional concussion program were prescribed amitriptyline due to PTH with reduced headaches reported in 82% of those patients (Bramley et al., 2015). Kuczynski, Crawford, Bodell, Dewey, and Barlow (2013) also investigated pharmacological treatment in children presenting to a pediatric clinic with headaches that had lasted longer than 3 months. In this sample, pharmacological interventions included amitriptyline, melatonin, topiramate, nortriptyline, indomethacin, and flunarizine from which 64% reported headache improvement and 45% reported complete resolution. Amitriptyline (68% improvement) and melatonin (75%) were found to be most effective for this pediatric sample. Both of these studies show that amitriptyline is generally well-tolerated and beneficial for patients experiencing PTH or PTM. Finally, a retrospective study of adult military populations revealed a 48% improvement rate in terms of headache days per month with topiramate. Other treatments including antidepressants (29%), propranolol (33%), and valproic acid (20%) were not as effective in this population (Erickson, 2011). Interestingly, those with blast-related injuries were less likely to improve than those with nonblast injuries. This research supports the idea that medications for PTH and PTM must be chosen individually for the patient in the context of headache or migraine, personal, and injury-specific characteristics.

When headaches or migraines persist or prevent engagement in the recommended treatments, prophylactic medications, including analgesics (e.g., acetaminophen, aspirin), nonsteroidal anti-inflammatory drugs (e.g., ibuprofen, naproxen), antidepressants (e.g., amitriptyline, nortriptyline), anticonvulsants (e.g., topiramate, valproic acid, gabapentin), β-adrenergic antagonists (e.g., propranolol), vestibular suppressants (e.g., meclizine), benzodiazepines (e.g., lorazepam, clonazepam, diazepam), and neurostimulants (e.g., amantadine, methylphenidate, dextroamphetamine, atomoxetine), may be used (Petraglia et al., 2012). Common abortive medications include triptans (e.g., sumatriptan, rizatriptan). Other recommendations from a prevention standpoint have included naturopathic options such as supplementation with magnesium, vitamin B, riboflavin, coenzyme Q10, and fish oil (Petraglia et al., 2012).

CASE STUDY: BEHAVIORAL MANAGEMENT OF POSTTRAUMATIC HEADACHES AND MIGRAINES

This case study discusses care provided to a 12-year-old girl who presented to a specialized concussion clinic for evaluation and management of a SRC. Each visit at the clinic included completion of a clinical interview, administration of ImPACT, and a vestibular-oculomotor screening (VOMS) assessment. ImPACT was used as a brief computerized neurocognitive battery to help in diagnosing and evaluating recovery from concussion. ImPACT involves completion of the Post-Concussion Symptom Scale (PCSS) including self-report of 22 symptoms associated with concussion and six subtests measuring four cognitive domains (i.e., verbal memory, visual memory, visual motor speed, and reaction time) typically affected by concussion. The VOMS assessment was used as a brief screening tool for the vestibular and oculomotor systems, which are commonly affected after concussion (Mucha et al., 2014). During the VOMS, patients rate baseline symptoms of headache, dizziness, nausea, and fogginess. Patients then report subjective change in symptoms after a series of eye and head movements (e.g., pursuits, saccades, vestibular-ocular reflex, visual motion sensitivity, and near point of convergence).

Initial Evaluation

Background Information

The 12-year-old girl selected for this case study first presented to clinic for evaluation of a SRC 3 days postinjury. The patient reported playing basketball when another player unexpectedly passed the ball, which struck the right side of that patient's head. There were no acute markers of injury (i.e., loss of consciousness, posttraumatic amnesia, disorientation, or confusion). Acute symptoms included a moderate headache, and she immediately discontinued play. Later that day, she experienced onset of nausea and fatigue while at a restaurant. Before evaluation, the nausea subsided; however, the patient continued to experience headaches (exacerbated by light or noise), photophobia, phonophobia, and slowed thinking. The patient denied mood changes; however, her mother reported lethargy. Consistent with her mother's report, the patient endorsed increased sleep, including frequent naps that were resulting in skipped meals. Medical and personal history were remarkable for motion sickness, headaches (with one previous migraine), and oculomotor dysfunction. Neither the patient nor her parents recalled the specific oculomotor diagnosis; however, vision therapy was required at a young age. Family history of migraine was also reported. Academically, the patient reported being a seventh-grader at a local suburban public school. She also reported a history of reading disability and use of an individualized education plan (IEP) in school. Extracurricular activities were reported as swimming and lacrosse.

Test Results

On the date of the initial evaluation, ImPACT yielded impaired verbal memory (below 1st percentile), impaired visual memory (below 1st percentile), high average visual motor speed (81st percentile) and average reaction time (33rd percentile). Total symptom score on the PCSS was a 24. Before the VOMS, she reported a moderate headache (4/10 severity). There was no symptom provocation during the oculomotor components (i.e., pursuits, saccades), but she reported increased headache (5/10 severity) during the vestibular components (i.e., vestibular-oculomotor reflex [VOR], visual motion sensitivity [VMS]) of the VOMS. Near point of convergence (NPC) and accommodation were within normal limits.

Impression and Plan

Given the aforementioned findings including an identifiable mechanism, ongoing symptoms, and abnormal neurocognitive data, the patient was diagnosed with an SRC. Treatment recommendations included cognitive and physical rest within the context of a strict behavioral management plan (i.e., adhering to a regulated schedule in terms of diet, hydration, sleep, and obtaining light physical activity). We also encouraged her to remain social and engage in pleasurable activities to minimize stress. We provided her with academic accommodations and restrictions for physical activity to minimize the risk of reinjury or exacerbation of migraine symptoms. Specifically, we encouraged her to continue with activities when symptoms were mild (i.e., 2/10–4/10 severity); however, if symptoms increased (i.e., 5/10–6/10 severity), she was instructed to build in breaks to allow for natural dissipation. She was instructed to follow up in 7 to 10 days for treatment updates.

Follow-Up Phone Call

Approximately 5 days after the initial evaluation, the patient's mother called the clinic as she had been suffering from severe headaches (8/10 severity) and irregular sleep patterns (i.e., sleeping in, napping), which was consequently resulting in fluctuating school attendance (i.e., going in late, leaving early). Specifically, her technical education class was identified as triggering an exacerbation of symptoms. As such, the academic accommodations were updated to excuse her from technical education class. Ultimately, this change was helpful in mitigating stress and preventing exacerbation of symptoms. In addition, we emphasized the importance of maintaining a regulated schedule as the first line of defense against migraine.

Second Evaluation

Updated Information

The patient and her parents returned to clinic 10 days after the first visit, during which she reported symptom improvement after adhering to the regulated schedule. Since the phone call, she had maintained regular school attendance and participated in play practice to remain social and engaged. In terms of symptoms, she continued to report primarily mild headaches but with occasional severe headaches triggered by loud noises. She also endorsed dizziness (with intense concentration) and fatigue.

Test Results

ImPACT revealed a similar pattern: impaired verbal memory (below 1st percentile), impaired visual memory (below 1st percentile), average visual motor speed (83rd percentile), and average reaction time (40th percentile). Total symptom score on the PCSS was stable at a 24. During the VOMS, she endorsed mild headache provocation that increased from a 3/10 to a 4/10 severity with the vestibular components (i.e., VOR and VMS); the rest of the exam was nonprovocative. NPC was again within normal limits across three trials.

Impression and Plan

Given findings during this evaluation, it was evident that symptoms were improving and remained consistent with a postconcussion migraine profile. Due to lack of vestibular, ocular, or anxiety or mood findings, we again emphasized the behavioral management strategies although it was recommended that she increase engagement in physical activity (e.g., swimming, noncontact physical education class). We asked her to return in approximately 2 weeks for further recommendations.

Third Evaluation

Updated Information

The patient continued to report improvements at her follow-up visit. Unfortunately, she fell ill the previous week and missed some school; however, she felt confident in making up missed exams when she returned to school. Physically, she had tolerated swimming and noncontact lacrosse practice, with occasional mild headache provocation. She also endorsed photophobia when looking at the Promethean board (an interactive whiteboard used in classrooms).

Test Results

ImPACT was significantly improved, as follows: low average verbal memory (17th percentile), borderline visual memory (3rd percentile), low average visual motor speed (17th percentile), and borderline reaction time (6th percentile). Total symptom score on the PCSS was improved to 11. She denied all symptoms before the VOMS, and the exam yielded no symptom provocation. Convergence was again within normal limits across three trials.

Impression and Plan

Given the findings during this evaluation, the athlete continued to show improvements in symptoms and neurocognitive data. Recommendations included removal of academic accommodations, continued noncontact and nonrisk physical activity, and continued regulation of her daily schedule. It was recommended that she follow-up in 2 weeks, at which time she would also complete an exertion exit test. An exertion exit test is a standardized workout overseen by a physical therapist to ensure the athlete remains asymptomatic with cardio, dynamic, and sport-specific exercise.

Final Evaluation

Updated Information

At the next clinical appointment, the patient reported symptoms as being resolved. She had been asymptomatic for approximately 10 days.

Physically, she had participated in swim-team tryouts and lacrosse practice without any symptom provocation. Additionally, she successfully passed an exertion exit test with a physical therapist. Academically, she had been attending school full time and was fully caught up on her missed work. She had not been using any academic accommodations. She remained social during spring break and had plans to attend a birthday party the following night.

Test Results

Compared with the previous visit, visual memory (72nd percentile) and visual motor speed (50th percentile) were improved to the average range. Reaction time (1st percentile) and verbal memory (7th percentile) remained lower than expected; however, in the context of her diagnosed reading disability and cautious test-taking approach (i.e., Impulse Control Composite = 1) scores were overall improved. VOMS was entirely nonprovocative.

Impression and Plan

During this evaluation, the patient presented as asymptomatic at rest as well as with cognitive and physical activities. ImPACT scores, as mentioned, were attributed to her preexisting reading disorder. The VOMS examination was nonprovocative without evidence of vestibular-oculomotor dysfunction. As such, the patient met requirements for clearance and was returned to all academic and contact sports without accommodations.

Summary

Often, patients present to a specialty clinic with a constellation of symptoms that require specialty intervention, such as vestibular rehabilitation or cervicogenic treatment. We chose this case because it reflected rather pure PTM. In addition, it demonstrated the efficacy of behavioral regulation as a treatment method. This was highlighted between the first and second clinic visits as the patient deteriorated with dysregulation and was then able to gain some relief from symptoms with implementation of a strict schedule. Adhering to this schedule over time along with a graded progression in terms of physical activity allowed her to recover completely from the postconcussion symptoms without any pharmacologic intervention. However, with this patient's history of vision problems, reading disability, and an IEP in school, her test scores were somewhat inconsistent. In cases with preexisting learning disorder, trained neuropsychologists should be involved as part of the multidisciplinary team to interpret neuropsychological data in the context of the patient's current situation and premorbid factors.

CLINICAL TAKE-HOME POINTS

1. *Concussion and migraine share similar pathophysiology, possibly responsible for the high rates of posttraumatic headaches and migraines following SRC.*
2. *Headaches can be caused by a multitude of factors, and therefore, understanding the potential underlying mechanisms is important for proper management and treatment.*
3. *Implementation of healthy lifestyle habits immediately after concussion may reduce the development of PTH or PTM, as well as the need for medication in select cases.*

KEY QUESTIONS TO BE ADDRESSED IN THE NEXT 5 YEARS

Within the next 5 years, it will be important to answer the following questions.

1. *What is the relationship between underlying genetic vulnerabilities and development of PTH or PTM following SRC?* Investigation of this question would help determine which genetic vulnerabilities put an individual at risk for experiencing PTH or PTM after concussion. Specifically, PTH and PTM after SRC are commonly reported in those individuals with a personal history of headaches or migraines, family history of headaches or migraines, anxiety, or high stress levels. At this time, it remains unknown which of these mechanisms is the most predominant or strongest in relating to development of PTH or PTM (Balaban, Jacob, & Furman, 2011; Kacperski et al., 2016). Although some research has focused on the relationship between the apolipoprotein E gene in development of migraine and tension-type headaches, results have been conflicting (Giza et al., 2013; Miao, Wang, Zheng, & Zhuang, 2015). Additionally, Giza and Hovda (2014) have highlighted the relationship between genetic factors related to ion channel dysfunction (e.g., familial hemiplegic migraine) and increased symptomatology in athletes after SRC. As such, focus on these and other genetic vulnerabilities could be helpful in better informing identification, treatment, and management of PTH and PTM following SRC (see Merritt & Arnett, Chapter 4 in this volume, on genetic factors involved in SRC, which discusses genetic vulnerability to headache in more detail).
2. *What is the relationship between PTH and PTM with other common postconcussion symptoms (e.g., anxiety) and findings (e.g., vestibular*

dysfunction, ocular abnormalities)? The answer to this question will be important in terms of determining whether a unifying biological substrate can explain the comorbid symptom patterns observed after SRC. Specifically, posttraumatic vision or oculomotor problems have been reported in up to 60% of pediatric patients following SRC, with comorbid symptoms including headache, fatigue, tracking difficulties, and photophobia (Pearce et al., 2015). The high prevalence of vision symptoms (or dysfunction) after concussion is reflective of the vast neuroanatomy of the visual system that includes brainstem, cortical, and subcortical structures (Master et al., 2016). Additionally, approximately 40% to 50% of athletes report balance problems and dizziness after SRC, likely linked to underlying vestibular dysfunction (Kontos, Sufrinko, Elbin, Puskar, & Collins, 2016). Balaban and colleagues (2011) have published regarding the underlying pathways of the vestibular, migraine, and anxiety relationship; however, further work is necessary to inform the other comorbid symptom relationships involving PTH and PTM after SRC.

3. *What are the behavioral treatments and intervention time points necessary to avoid chronic postconcussion symptoms, including PTH and PTM?* On the basis of the research presented in this chapter, particularly within the regular exercise section, it is evident that a habituation-based approach to overcoming triggers is important in the management and treatment of headaches and migraines (Martin, 2010a). Research surrounding this question would help clinicians in better understanding when to begin the exposure process and the role of exertion in overcoming PTH and PTM after SRC. Varkey and colleagues have conducted such studies within the migraine literature, although the research remains sparse with regard to those individuals experiencing postconcussion symptoms. In addressing this question, it will also be important for researchers to understand comorbid symptom relationships and concussion profiles (Reynolds et al., 2014), as clinicians would benefit from better understanding whether one symptom should be treated more aggressively or if all should be treated simultaneously.

REFERENCES

Adolphus, K., Lawton, C. L., & Dye, L. (2013). The effects of breakfast on behavior and academic performance in children and adolescents. *Frontiers in Human Neuroscience, 7,* 425. http://dx.doi.org/10.3389/fnhum.2013.00425

Baier, B., Winkenwerder, E., & Dieterich, M. (2009). "Vestibular migraine": Effects of prophylactic therapy with various drugs. A retrospective study. *Journal of Neurology, 256*, 436–442. http://dx.doi.org/10.1007/s00415-009-0111-3

Balaban, C. D., Jacob, R. G., & Furman, J. M. (2011). Neurologic bases for comorbidity of balance disorders, anxiety disorders and migraine: Neurotherapeutic implications. *Expert Review of Neurotherapeutics, 11*, 379–394. http://dx.doi.org/10.1586/ern.11.19

Barnett, B. P., & Singman, E. L. (2015). Vision concerns after mild traumatic brain injury. *Current Treatment Options in Neurology, 17*, 329. http://dx.doi.org/10.1007/s11940-014-0329-y

Blau, J. N. (1980). Migraine prodromes separated from the aura: Complete migraine. *British Medical Journal, 281*, 658–660. http://dx.doi.org/10.1136/bmj.281.6241.658

Blume, H. K. (2015). Headaches after concussion in pediatrics: A review. *Current Pain and Headache Reports, 19*, 42. http://dx.doi.org/10.1007/s11916-015-0516-x

Boardman, H. F., Thomas, E., Millson, D. S., & Croft, P. R. (2005). Psychological, sleep, lifestyle, and comorbid associations with headache. *Headache, 45*, 657–669. http://dx.doi.org/10.1111/j.1526-4610.2005.05133.x

Bramley, H., Heverley, S., Lewis, M. M., Kong, L., Rivera, R., & Silvis, M. (2015). Demographics and treatment of adolescent posttraumatic headache in a regional concussion clinic. *Pediatric Neurology, 52*, 493–498. http://dx.doi.org/10.1016/j.pediatrneurol.2015.01.008

Brody, D. L. (2014). *Concussion care manual: A practical guide.* Oxford, England: Oxford University Press. http://dx.doi.org/10.1093/med/9780199383863.001.0001

Burstein, R., Noseda, R., & Borsook, D. (2015). Migraine: Multiple processes, complex pathophysiology. *The Journal of Neuroscience, 35*, 6619–6629. http://dx.doi.org/10.1523/JNEUROSCI.0373-15.2015

Choe, M. C., & Blume, H. K. (2016). Pediatric posttraumatic headache: A review. *Journal of Child Neurology, 31*, 76–85. http://dx.doi.org/10.1177/0883073814568152

Covassin, T., Elbin, R. J., Harris, W., Parker, T., & Kontos, A. (2012). The role of age and sex in symptoms, neurocognitive performance, and postural stability in athletes after concussion. *The American Journal of Sports Medicine, 40*, 1303–1312. http://dx.doi.org/10.1177/0363546512444554

Cuvellier, J. C., Mars, A., & Vallée, L. (2009). The prevalence of premonitory symptoms in paediatric migraine: A questionnaire study in 103 children and adolescents. *Cephalalgia, 29*, 1197–1201. http://dx.doi.org/10.1111/j.1468-2982.2009.01854.x

Daenen, L., Varkey, E., Kellmann, M., & Nijs, J. (2015). Exercise, not to exercise, or how to exercise in patients with chronic pain? Applying science to practice. *The Clinical Journal of Pain, 31*, 108–114. http://dx.doi.org/10.1097/AJP.0000000000000099

Dittrich, S. M., Günther, V., Franz, G., Burtscher, M., Holzner, B., & Kopp, M. (2008). Aerobic exercise with relaxation: Influence on pain and psychological well-being in female migraine patients. *Clinical Journal of Sport Medicine, 18,* 363–365. http://dx.doi.org/10.1097/JSM.0b013e31817efac9

Echemendia, R. J. (2012). Cerebral concussion in sport: An overview. *Journal of Clinical Sport Psychology, 6,* 207–230. http://dx.doi.org/10.1123/jcsp.6.3.207

Erickson, J. C. (2011). Treatment outcomes of chronic post-traumatic headaches after mild head trauma in U.S. soldiers: An observational study. *Headache, 51,* 932–944. http://dx.doi.org/10.1111/j.1526-4610.2011.01909.x

Furman, J. M., & Balaban, C. D. (2015). Vestibular migraine. *Annals of the New York Academy of Sciences, 1343,* 90–96. http://dx.doi.org/10.1111/nyas.12645

Furman, J. M., Balaban, C. D., Jacob, R. G., & Marcus, D. A. (2005). Migraine–anxiety associated dizziness (MARD): A new disorder? *Journal of Neurology, Neurosurgery, & Psychiatry, 76,* 1–8. http://dx.doi.org/10.1136/jnnp.2004.048926

Gioia, G. A. (2016). Medical-school partnership in guiding return to school following mild traumatic brain injury in youth. *Journal of Child Neurology, 31,* 93–108. http://dx.doi.org/10.1177/0883073814555604

Giza, C. C., & Hovda, D. A. (2014). The new neurometabolic cascade of concussion. *Neurosurgery, 75*(Suppl. 4), S24–S33. http://dx.doi.org/10.1227/NEU.0000000000000505

Giza, C. C., Kutcher, J. S., Ashwal, S., Barth, J., Getchius, T. S., Gioia, G. A., . . . Zafonte, R. (2013). Summary of evidence-based guideline update: Evaluation and management of concussion in sports: Report of the Guideline Development Subcommittee of the American Academy of Neurology. *Neurology, 80,* 2250–2257. http://dx.doi.org/10.1212/WNL.0b013e31828d57dd

Gordon, K. E., Dooley, J. M., & Wood, E. P. (2006). Is migraine a risk factor for the development of concussion? *British Journal of Sports Medicine, 40,* 184–185. http://dx.doi.org/10.1136/bjsm.2005.022251

HealthyChildren.org. (2015). The case for eating breakfast. *Healthy Children Magazine.* Retrieved from https://www.healthychildren.org/English/healthy-living/nutrition/Pages/The-Case-for-Eating-Breakfast.aspx

Henry, L. C., Elbin, R. J., Collins, M. W., Marchetti, G., & Kontos, A. P. (2016). Examining recovery trajectories after sport-related concussion with a multimodal clinical assessment approach. *Neurosurgery, 78,* 232–241. http://dx.doi.org/10.1227/NEU.0000000000001041

Heyer, G. L., & Idris, S. A. (2014). Does analgesic overuse contribute to chronic post-traumatic headaches in adolescent concussion patients? *Pediatric Neurology, 50,* 464–468. http://dx.doi.org/10.1016/j.pediatrneurol.2014.01.040

Heyer, G. L., Young, J. A., Rose, S. C., McNally, K. A., & Fischer, A. N. (2016). Post-traumatic headaches correlate with migraine symptoms in youth with concussion. *Cephalalgia, 36,* 309–316.

International Headache Society. (2013). The International Classification of Headache Disorders, 3rd edition (beta version). *Cephalalgia, 33,* 629–808. http://dx.doi.org/10.1177/0333102413485658

Junn, C., Bell, K. R., Shenouda, C., & Hoffman, J. M. (2015). Symptoms of concussion and comorbid disorders. *Current Pain and Headache Reports, 19*, 46. http://dx.doi.org/10.1007/s11916-015-0519-7

Kacperski, J., Hung, R., & Blume, H. K. (2016). Pediatric posttraumatic headache. *Seminars in Pediatric Neurology, 23*, 27–34. http://dx.doi.org/10.1016/j.spen.2015.08.005

Kelman, L., & Rains, J. C. (2005). Headache and sleep: Examination of sleep patterns and complaints in a large clinical sample of migraineurs. *Headache, 45*, 904–910. http://dx.doi.org/10.1111/j.1526-4610.2005.05159.x

Kenney, E. L., Long, M. W., Cradock, A. L., & Gortmaker, S. L. (2015). Prevalence of inadequate hydration among U.S. children and disparities by gender and race/ethnicity: National health and nutrition examination survey, 2009–2012. *American Journal of Public Health, 105*, e113–e118. http://dx.doi.org/10.2105/AJPH.2015.302572

Kontos, A. P., Elbin, R. J., Lau, B., Simensky, S., Freund, B., French, J., & Collins, M. W. (2013). Posttraumatic migraine as a predictor of recovery and cognitive impairment after sport-related concussion. *The American Journal of Sports Medicine, 41*, 1497–1504. http://dx.doi.org/10.1177/0363546513488751

Kontos, A. P., Reches, A., Elbin, R. J., Dickman, D., Laufer, I., Geva, A. B., . . . Collins, M. W. (2016). Preliminary evidence of reduced brain network activation in patients with post traumatic migraine following concussion. *Brain Imaging and Behavior, 10*, 594–603.

Kontos, A. P., Sufrinko, A., Elbin, R. J., Puskar, A., & Collins, M. W. (2016). Reliability and associated factors for performance on the vestibular/ocular motor screening (VOMS) tool in healthy collegiate athletes. *The American Journal of Sports Medicine, 44*, 1400–1406. http://dx.doi.org/10.1177/0363546516632754

Kuczynski, A., Crawford, S., Bodell, L., Dewey, D., & Barlow, K. M. (2013). Characteristics of post-traumatic headaches in children following mild traumatic brain injury and their response to treatment: A prospective cohort. *Developmental Medicine & Child Neurology, 55*, 636–641. http://dx.doi.org/10.1111/dmcn.12152

Lashley, K. S. (1941). Patterns of cerebral integration indicated by the scotomas of migraine. *Archives of Neurology & Psychiatry, 46*, 331–339. http://dx.doi.org/10.1001/archneurpsyc.1941.02280200137007

Lau, B. C., Kontos, A. P., Collins, M. W., Mucha, A., & Lovell, M. R. (2011). Which on-field signs/symptoms predict protracted recovery from sport-related concussion among high school football players? *The American Journal of Sports Medicine, 39*, 2311–2318. http://dx.doi.org/10.1177/0363546511410655

Lempert, T., Olesen, J., Furman, J., Waterston, J., Seemungal, B., Carey, J., . . . Newman-Toker, D. (2012). Vestibular migraine: Diagnostic criteria. *Journal of Vestibular Research, 22*, 167–172.

Linde, M., Mellberg, A., & Dahlöf, C. (2006). The natural course of migraine attacks. A prospective analysis of untreated attacks compared with attacks treated with a triptan. *Cephalalgia, 26,* 712–721. http://dx.doi.org/10.1111/ j.1468-2982.2006.01097.x

Martin, P. R. (2010a). Behavioral management of migraine headache triggers: Learning to cope with triggers. *Current Pain and Headache Reports, 14,* 221–227. http://dx.doi.org/10.1007/s11916-010-0112-z

Martin, P. R. (2010b). Managing headache triggers: Think "coping" not "avoidance." *Cephalalgia, 30,* 634–637. http://dx.doi.org/10.1111/j.1468-2982.2009.01989.x

Master, C. L., Scheiman, M., Gallaway, M., Goodman, A., Robinson, R. L., Master, S. R., & Grady, M. F. (2016). Vision diagnoses are common after concussion in adolescents. *Clinical Pediatrics, 55,* 260–267. http://dx.doi.org/ 10.1177/0009922815594367

McCrory, P., Meeuwisse, W. H., Aubry, M., Cantu, B., Dvorák, J., Echemendia, R. J., . . . Turner, M. (2013). Consensus statement on concussion in sport: The 4th International Conference on Concussion in Sport held in Zurich, November 2012. *The British Journal of Sports Medicine, 47,* 250–258. http:// dx.doi.org/10.1136/bjsports-2013-092313

McCrory, P., Meeuwisse, W., Dvorák, J., Aubry, M., Bailes, J., Broglio, S., . . . Vos, P. E. (2017). Consensus statement on concussion in sport—The 5th international conference on concussion in sport held in Berlin, October 2016. *British Journal of Sports Medicine, 51,* 838–847.

Miao, J., Wang, F., Zheng, W., & Zhuang, X. (2015). Association of the apolipoprotein E polymorphism with migraine: A meta-analysis. *BMC Neurology, 15,* 138. http://dx.doi.org/10.1186/s12883-015-0385-2

Mihalik, J. P., Stump, J. E., Collins, M. W., Lovell, M. R., Field, M., & Maroon, J. C. (2005). Posttraumatic migraine characteristics in athletes following sports-related concussion. *Journal of Neurosurgery, 102,* 850–855. http://dx.doi.org/ 10.3171/jns.2005.102.5.0850

Mild Traumatic Brain Injury Committee of the Head Injury Interdisciplinary Special Interest Group of the American Congress of Rehabilitation Medicine. (1993). Definition of mild traumatic brain injury. *Journal of Head Trauma Rehabilitation, 8,* 86–87.

Mucha, A., Collins, M. W., Elbin, R., Furman, J. M., Troutman-Enseki, C., DeWolf, R. M., . . . Kontos, A. P. (2014). A brief Vestibular/Ocular Motor Screening (VOMS) assessment to evaluate concussions preliminary findings. *American Journal of Sports Medicine, 42,* 2479–2486.

Packard, R. C., & Ham, L. P. (1997). Pathogenesis of posttraumatic headache and migraine: A common headache pathway? *Headache, 37,* 142–152. http:// dx.doi.org/10.1046/j.1526-4610.1997.3703142.x

Patel, M. V., Patel, H. B., Thakkar, S., Shah, V., Suratia, B., Thummar, S., . . . Vadodaria, B. (2016). Study of prevalence of headache and its various facets among 200 medical students of SBKS MI RC Sumandeep Vidyapeeth. *International Journal of Biomedical and Advance Research, 7,* 72–75. http://dx.doi.org/ 10.7439/ijbar.v7i2.2923

Pearce, K. L., Sufrinko, A., Lau, B. C., Henry, L., Collins, M. W., & Kontos, A. P. (2015). Near point of convergence after a sport-related concussion: Measurement reliability and relationship to neurocognitive impairment and symptoms. *The American Journal of Sports Medicine, 43,* 3055–3061. http://dx.doi.org/10.1177/0363546515606430

Petraglia, A. L., Maroon, J. C., & Bailes, J. E. (2012). From the field of play to the field of combat: A review of the pharmacological management of concussion. *Neurosurgery, 70,* 1520–1533. http://dx.doi.org/10.1227/NEU.0b013e31824cebe8

Popkin, B. M., D'Anci, K. E., & Rosenberg, I. H. (2010). Water, hydration, and health. *Nutrition Reviews, 68,* 439–458. http://dx.doi.org/10.1111/j.1753-4887.2010.00304.x

Rains, J. C., Poceta, J. S., & Penzien, D. B. (2008). Sleep and headaches. *Current Neurology and Neuroscience Reports, 8,* 167–175. http://dx.doi.org/10.1007/s11910-008-0027-9

Rathier, L. (2015, November 1). *Effects of exercise on headaches and migraines.* Retrieved from http://www.achenet.org/resources/effects_of_exercise_on_headaches_and_migraines/

Reynolds, E., Collins, M. W., Mucha, A., & Troutman-Ensecki, C. (2014). Establishing a clinical service for the management of sports-related concussions. *Neurosurgery, 75*(Suppl. 4), S71–S81. http://dx.doi.org/10.1227/NEU.0000000000000471

Schulte, L. H., Jürgens, T. P., & May, A. (2015). Photo-, osmo- and phonophobia in the premonitory phase of migraine: Mistaking symptoms for triggers? *The Journal of Headache and Pain, 16,* 14. http://dx.doi.org/10.1186/s10194-015-0495-7

Silberstein, S. D. (2004). Migraine pathophysiology and its clinical implications. *Cephalalgia, 24*(Suppl. 2), 2–7. http://dx.doi.org/10.1111/j.1468-2982.2004.00892.x

Spierings, E. L., Ranke, A. H., & Honkoop, P. C. (2001). Precipitating and aggravating factors of migraine versus tension-type headache. *Headache, 41,* 554–558. http://dx.doi.org/10.1046/j.1526-4610.2001.041006554.x

Tepper, S. J., & Tepper, D. E. (2010). Breaking the cycle of medication overuse headache. *Cleveland Clinic Journal of Medicine, 77,* 236–242. http://dx.doi.org/10.3949/ccjm.77a.09147

Theeler, B. J., Flynn, F. G., & Erickson, J. C. (2012). Chronic daily headache in U.S. soldiers after concussion. *Headache, 52,* 732–738. http://dx.doi.org/10.1111/j.1526-4610.2012.02112.x

Thomas, D. G., Apps, J. N., Hoffmann, R. G., McCrea, M., & Hammeke, T. (2015). Benefits of strict rest after acute concussion: A randomized controlled trial. *Pediatrics, 135,* 213–223. http://dx.doi.org/10.1542/peds.2014-0966

Varkey, E., Cider, A., Carlsson, J., & Linde, M. (2009). A study to evaluate the feasibility of an aerobic exercise program in patients with migraine. *Headache, 49,* 563–570. http://dx.doi.org/10.1111/j.1526-4610.2008.01231.x

Varkey, E., Cider, A., Carlsson, J., & Linde, M. (2011). Exercise as migraine prophylaxis: A randomized study using relaxation and topiramate as controls. *Cephalalgia, 31*, 1428–1438. http://dx.doi.org/10.1177/0333102411419681

Whitney, S. L., Wrisley, D. M., Brown, K. E., & Furman, J. M. (2000). Physical therapy for migraine-related vestibulopathy and vestibular dysfunction with history of migraine. *The Laryngoscope, 110*, 1528–1534. http://dx.doi.org/10.1097/00005537-200009000-00022

Wöber-Bingöl, C. (2013). Epidemiology of migraine and headache in children and adolescents. *Current Pain and Headache Reports, 17*, 341. http://dx.doi.org/10.1007/s11916-013-0341-z

Zasler, N. D. (2015). Sports concussion headache. *Brain Injury, 29*, 207–220. http://dx.doi.org/10.3109/02699052.2014.965213

3

ASSESSMENT OF DEPRESSION AND ANXIETY IN SPORTS CONCUSSION EVALUATIONS

PETER A. ARNETT, ERIN GUTY, AND MEGAN BRADSON

In this chapter, we discuss the assessment of anxiety and depression in sports concussion evaluations. Although there is a developing literature on the long-term effects of concussion on mood and affective functioning more generally (Kerr, Marshall, Harding, & Guskiewicz, 2012; McCrory, Meeuwisse, Kutcher, Jordan, & Gardner, 2013; Strain et al., 2013), as well as studies showing that history of concussion is a risk factor for later depression in adolescents (Chrisman & Richardson, 2014), the focus of our chapter is mostly on the relatively acute period postconcussion. First, we review whether anxiety and depression are elevated in the sports concussion context. Second, we summarize some strategies for measuring depression and anxiety postconcussion. Third, we discuss how anxiety and depression may influence cognitive functioning and, as such, complicate return-to-play decisions. Fourth, we include a case study that illustrates some of the themes discussed in the chapter. Fifth, we outline four take-home points for clinicians relating to the assessment of anxiety and depression. Finally, we identify

http://dx.doi.org/10.1037/0000114-004
Neuropsychology of Sports-Related Concussion, P. A. Arnett (Editor)

six key questions in this area of study that we feel are most pressing to be addressed in the next 5 years. Because there are relatively few studies examining depression or anxiety specifically in sports-related concussion (SRC) populations (although many studies have been conducted on mild traumatic brain injury [mTBI] populations with different injury mechanisms), some reference is made here to the broader mTBI literature.

DEPRESSION AND ANXIETY POSTCONCUSSION

Depression

Depression is relatively common after mTBI. An older meta-analysis by Busch and Alpern (1998) based on a review of 12 studies comprising a total of 218 participants showed prevalence estimates ranging from 22% to 42%, with a mean of 32%. Of note, however, only 2% of these participants ($n = 4$) had specifically suffered from sports-related injuries. Using rigorous diagnostic criteria (*Diagnostic and Statistical Manual of Mental Disorders*, 4th ed.; American Psychiatric Association, 1994), Rapoport and colleagues (2006) found that 15% of their sample met criteria for major depression. However, it is important to highlight that all of these participants were age 50 or older (mean = 67) and were seen and assessed for depression an average of 46.9 days ($SD = 34$) postinjury, thus not a typical age range for sports concussion studies. Also, it is unclear how many participants suffered from injury via their participation in sports. As such, the applicability of these data to a typical sports concussion context is unclear.

In a population-based study, Jorge and Robinson (2002) estimated that about 6% of the mTBIs that occur annually result in clinical depression. However, given the likelihood of underreporting and the results of other studies, it is likely that this lower figure is an underestimate of the true point prevalence of depression postconcussion.

In a study with more direct applicability to concussion, we recently examined depression at baseline and postconcussion in a sample of collegiate athletes (Vargas, Rabinowitz, Meyer, & Arnett, 2015). We assessed 84 athletes at baseline and then again postconcussion. Most of the participants (71%) were tested within 5 days postconcussion, and only three athletes reported having had some psychiatric treatment before their concussion. The depression outcome measure was the Beck Depression Inventory—Fast Screen (BDI–FS; Beck, Steer, & Brown, 2000). We compared this athlete group with a control group of 42 undergraduates who were also tested at 2 time points, an average of 6.8 weeks apart. These latter participants all reported being involved in "formal, recreational, or pick-up sports," so this achieved our goal of including an athletic control group.

Of note, the BDI–FS was developed primarily for use in medical populations, with seven items that measure sadness, hopelessness, feeling like a failure, anhedonia (loss of pleasure), self-esteem, self-blame, and suicidality. Excluded among these depression symptoms are neurovegetative symptoms of depression including difficulty concentrating, trouble sleeping, and fatigue, among others. Excluding these latter symptoms is a useful feature for measuring depression in concussed samples because such neurovegetative symptoms in this context may be indicative of postconcussion symptoms rather than depression per se. On the basis of recommendations from the BDI–FS manual, a cutoff of 4 and above was used because this has been shown to be highly associated with diagnostic criteria for major depression in other samples.

At baseline, we found that 11% of athletes scored above the cutoff on the BDI–FS. Postconcussion, however, 23% met this cutoff, a significant increase from the number who reported depression at baseline. Comparatively, 7% of the control group was depressed when initially tested and then 10% when tested about 6 to 7 weeks later, a nonsignificant change in the number reporting depression. Of note, the duration of the test–retest interval was not significantly correlated with the BDI–FS at either time point in the athletes or the controls.

In terms of examining change in individuals over time, we also assessed reliable change in BDI–FS scores. Significantly more athletes (20%) compared with control subjects (5%) displayed a reliable increase in BDI–FS scores between the 2 time points. Seventeen athletes (20%) showed a reliable increase in BDI–FS score, eight had a reliable decrease, and 59 athletes had no reliable change. In the control group, two participants (5%) showed a reliable increase in BDI–FS score, three had a reliable decrease, and 37 showed no reliable change.

In summary, our study showed that 23% of concussed athletes displayed clinically significant depression symptoms, compared with only 11% at baseline. Thus, roughly twice as many athletes reported such depression postconcussion compared with their reports at baseline. Furthermore, 20% of concussed athletes showed a reliable increase in depression from their baseline scores, 4 times the rate of control subjects (5%). Therefore, it is reasonable to conclude from our study that the prevalence of depression postconcussion is substantially elevated over what it is at baseline.

As to the mechanism of higher depression rates postconcussion, this is unclear. However, in our study, we did find several significant predictors of post-concussion depression. In particular, we found that those individuals at greatest risk for postconcussion depression had higher baseline BDI–FS scores and a higher score at baseline on a postconcussion symptom measure, as well as lower estimated FSIQ. Surprisingly, compared with athletes not showing a reliable increase in depression postconcussion, athletes who displayed a reliable increase did not have significantly higher depression scores at baseline.

In another prospective study on 75 high school ($n = 54$) and collegiate ($n = 21$) athletes, Kontos, Covassin, Elbin, and Parker (2012) administered the ImPACT, as well as the Beck Depression Inventory—II (BDI–II; Beck, Steer, & Brown, 1996) at baseline and postconcussion at 2-day, 5- to 7-day, and 10- to 14-day intervals. One nice feature of this study was that the investigators identified 10 postconcussion symptoms not typically thought to overlap with depression symptoms (e.g., mental fogginess, visual problems, dizziness) and created a scale that they then used as a covariate in their analyses to control for general symptom reporting. Another novel feature of this study is that the authors divided the BDI–II into "affective" (e.g., worthlessness, pessimism) and "somatic" (e.g., loss of energy, fatigue) scales. Of note, a majority of the athletes ($n = 40$, 53%) had a score of "0" on the BDI–II at baseline, with the rest falling in the 1 to 13 range (deemed "minimal depression" by the investigators). Thus, none of the athletes met criteria for even mild clinical depression at baseline (scores must be >13 to be in the mild depression range on the BDI–II). These investigators found that the athletes had significantly higher mean BDI–II scores compared with baseline at all time points postconcussion. Interestingly, the collegiate athletes continued to show an increase in depression at 14 days postconcussion, whereas the high school athletes started to decline at this point. Another interesting finding from this study is that visual memory and reaction time were significantly correlated with depression at 2 and 7 days postconcussion.

One limitation of Kontos, Covassin, and colleagues' (2012) study is that few athletes reported clinically significant depression at any time point. The highest level of even mild clinical depression was found at 2 days postconcussion, when only 7% (five of 75) of the athletes reported BDI–II scores above the minimal depression range. The authors speculate that these generally low clinical scores could be due to underreporting tendencies in the athletes. There will be more discussion of this issue later in the chapter when we discuss Ramanathan, Rabinowitz, Barwick, and Arnett's (2012) study using a performance-based measure to assess depression in athletes.

Mainwaring and colleagues (Mainwaring, Hutchison, Bisschop, Comper, & Richards, 2010) used a clever methodological element in their study of emotional functioning in athletes postconcussion. Specifically, in addition to examining concussed athletes, they assessed emotional functioning in a group of athletes with anterior cruciate ligament (ACL) injuries and compared both with a noninjured control group. These investigators assessed emotional functioning with the Profile of Mood States (POMS; McNair,

Lorr, & Droppleman, 1971), a measure that has an overall index of mood disturbance that subtracts positive from negative emotional functioning, as well as a scale specific to depression. There were no group differences on the POMS scales at baseline. However, compared with the control group, both injured groups displayed significantly higher scores on the depression scale, as well as a significant increase in depression from baseline to the first time point postinjury. The depression scores of the concussed group also returned to baseline levels by the second time point postinjury (7 days). Also, whereas the concussed group displayed about a threefold increase, the ACL group showed around a sevenfold increase in depression scores. The concussed group additionally displayed significantly higher overall mood disturbance at the first time point compared with the control group, as well as a dramatic increase in mood disturbance from baseline to the first time point postconcussion. Finally, similar to their score on the depression scale over time, the scores of the concussed group on overall mood disturbance had returned to baseline levels by 7 days postinjury.

Mainwaring and colleagues' (2010) study provides thought-provoking data. Given that both the concussed and ACL groups displayed increased depression and mood disturbance postinjury, these data would seem to suggest that the main causal factor involved in both groups is simply being injured, regardless of the nature of that injury. However, it is certainly possible that different mechanisms underlie the emotional disturbances of these groups. For example, there are functional magnetic resonance imaging studies of concussed athletes showing reduced dorsolateral prefrontal cortex activity and increased anterior cingulate and medial orbitofrontal region activity (Chen, Johnston, Petrides, & Ptito, 2008), comparable to what has often been found in individuals with major depression. Removal from play could be the factor underlying both groups' increase; however, Mainwaring and colleagues dismissed this interpretation from their data by showing that both injured groups returned to normal mood functioning before they returned to play. Still, this pattern could simply reflect the fact that both groups were quickly able to cope with their removal from play, with the initial removal still underlying their emotional dysfunction in the acute period postinjury. In the final analysis, Mainwaring et al.'s study provides a good methodological template for other studies to follow by including another type of injured athlete group for comparison to make it possible to tease out the specific emotional effects of concussion versus more general effects of simply being injured more generally. Again, using Mainwaring et al.'s study as a model, it would also be useful for future work to include more commonly used and practical clinically oriented measures of emotional functioning. Although the POMS is a reliable and valid measure of emotional functioning and assesses a broader range of emotional functioning than measures like the BDI or the Center for

Epidemiological Studies—Depression scale (CES–D; Radloff, 1977), it may have limited practicality in most sports concussion settings given its length. The long form contains 65 items and the short form contains 37 items.

In another related study conducted by Mainwaring's group on collegiate athletes, Hutchison and colleagues (Hutchison, Mainwaring, Comper, Richards, & Bisschop, 2009) also assessed the same three groups as Mainwaring et al. (2010) on the POMS. This study included 20 athletes with concussions, 14 with musculoskeletal injuries, and 19 healthy athletic control subjects. The groups did not differ on any of the POMS subscales at baseline. However, the concussed group displayed significantly increased fatigue and decreased vigor and energy at the first postbaseline time point (about 3 days) compared with both the musculoskeletal injury group and the athletic healthy control group. The musculoskeletal group showed increased anger postinjury compared with the other groups. Although both of the injury groups displayed a large increase in depression at the first postinjury time point (about an average of 3 POMS raw score points—see their Figure 6), they did not differ from one another.

Roiger, Weidauer, and Kern (2015) conducted a study mirroring the methodology of investigations by the Mainwaring et al. (2010) and Hutchison et al. (2009) studies in a Division I National Collegiate Athletic Association sample using a longitudinal design. Their study included seven participants in each of the groups, with one group having SRC, another group with injuries other than concussion, and a third group of sport-matched healthy control subjects. They used the CES-D to measure depression and assessed the injured athletes at baseline, 7 days, 1 month, and 3 months postinjury. The noninjured control group was only tested at baseline. Participants with any baseline mental health problems (depression, anxiety) were excluded, so the authors' sample was not representative of athletes more generally.

These investigators found that the three groups did not differ at baseline; however, both of the injured groups displayed significant increases from baseline to the 1-week postinjury time point but did not differ from one another in the degree of increase on the CES-D. The nonconcussed injured group also showed a significant increase from baseline at the 1-month postinjury time point, indicating that it took them longer to get back to baseline than the concussed injury group. Both groups were back to their baseline depression scores at 3 months postinjury. Neither of the injured groups differed from one another at either time point. In terms of clinically related depression, the authors noted that two of the 14 injured athletes scored above the clinical threshold on the CES–D (score ≥16) at 1-week postinjury (14.2% of the sample), but they never reported the group(s) of these athletes (Roiger et al., 2015).

In a study focusing on neuroimaging parameters and emotional functioning in collegiate athletes, Meier et al. (2015) compared 17 concussed football players and 27 noninjured football team controls on the Hamilton

Depression (HAM–D; Hamilton, 1967) and the Hamilton Anxiety (HAM–A; Maier, Buller, Philipp, & Heuser, 1988) rating scales. The concussed players were tested at 1 day, 1 week, and 1 month postconcussion, but not at baseline. The noninjured athletes were tested once. These investigators found that the concussed athletes had significantly higher scores on both the HAM–D and the HAM–A at 1-day post-concussion. The concussed athletes were also higher than healthy athletes at 1 week and 1 month postconcussion; they were also higher at 1 week on the HAM–A. These researchers also found that the scores on both the HAM–D and HAM–A were significantly improved at 1 month compared with both 1 day and 1 week postconcussion.

Although the authors do not speak directly to the clinical significance of their findings, some interesting patterns can be derived from their Figure 1. Using the standard cutoff on the HAM–D of 17 or greater indicating at least moderate clinical depression, about 18% of the sample (three of 17) would qualify as depressed at 1 day post-concussion but only about 7% (one of 15) by 1 week and then none qualifying by 1 month postconcussion. In terms of the HAM–A, using the same 17 or greater value to indicate at least moderate clinical anxiety, 35% of the sample (six of 17) qualify as anxious at 1 day post-concussion, with this decreasing to 7% (one of 15) at 1 week and then none qualifying by 1 month. Also of interest, the authors found that higher HAM–A and HAM–D scores at 1 day postconcussion were associated with lower dorsal midinsular cortex cerebral blood flow at 1 month postconcussion (see the authors' Figure 3B). Thus, concussed athletes' anxiety and depression reports in the acute phase after concussion predicted diminished cerebral blood flow one month later, suggesting a possible biological mechanism underlying their initial emotional disturbance.

Ellis and colleagues' (2015) study appears to be the only published study examining emotional outcomes in pediatric sports concussion patients. These investigators examined emotional symptoms using a retrospective chart review in 173 children and adolescents (all participants were age 19 and younger— mean age for sample = 14.22). The authors divided their sample into those with SRC ($n = 134$) and those with postconcussion syndrome (PCS; $n = 39$). Those with SRC were assessed at a median of 7 days postconcussion, whereas those with PCS were assessed at a median of 80 days postinjury. Thus, these two samples within their study were very different.

In terms of the assessment of postinjury psychiatric status, the authors identified increased psychiatric problems postinjury in three ways: (a) the onset of a new psychiatric disorder (NPD) postinjury (NPDs were broadly divided into anxiety and mood disorders); (b) worsening symptoms of a preinjury psychiatric disorder; or (c) the onset of acute, isolated suicidal ideation.

In terms of preinjury status, only 6.7% of the sample had a mood or anxiety disorder at baseline. As far as outcomes in emotional functioning post-concussion, these investigators found that 43.3% of the participants with acute SRC had scores of 1 or higher on the emotional symptoms scale from the Post-Concussion Symptoms Scale (PCSS; Kontos, Elbin, et al., 2012), compared with 71.8% of those with PCS (of note, the items they used for this scale are the same as those that came out of the factor analysis by Meyer & Arnett, 2015, as described later in this chapter). However, the authors did not provide any base rate data for this PCSS scale preinjury, so it is not clear how unusual a score of ≥ 1 would be postconcussion. As far as the onset of actual diagnosable postconcussion psychiatric disorders, the authors unfortunately did not parse out the SRC from PCS patients at this point as they explored their psychiatric diagnosis data. However, they did report that 11.5% of the total sample met study criteria for a postinjury psychiatric disorder, with most being NPD ($n = 14$), a few with subjective worsening symptoms of a preexisting psychiatric disorder ($n = 4$), and a couple with isolated suicidal ideation. Thus, not surprisingly, the incidence of a diagnosable disorder postinjury is much lower than simply a report of some emotional disturbance.

Ellis and colleagues' (2015) study provides a window into emotional functioning in pediatric concussion patients. However, given their focus on two extremes of the emotional functioning continuum in the study ranging from any report of emotional symptoms to a diagnosable psychiatric condition, comparison with other studies is difficult. It is not possible to draw any clear conclusions from their data regarding whether emotional functioning problems in pediatric concussion patients are more or less prevalent than in older samples. These authors' focus on diagnosable psychiatric conditions is rigorous; however, the practicality of having a psychiatrist available to conduct a diagnostic interview and make a formal psychiatric diagnosis is an unlikely scenario for most sports concussion programs. Also, the authors' method of combining acute SRC patients with PCS patients in most analyses makes it difficult to draw clear-cut conclusions from their study. In the final analysis, Ellis et al.'s study provides an initial foray into exploring emotional functioning in pediatric concussion patients, but further work is clearly needed.

Anxiety

Anxiety has been much less intensively studied in concussed athletes compared with depression. Still, the few existing studies show that anxiety is elevated postconcussion. Covassin and her colleagues (2014) examined anxiety in collegiate athletes using the State–Trait Anxiety Inventory (STAI; Spielberger, Gorsuch, Lushene, Vagg, & Jacobs, 1983) in 63 concussed individuals and 63 athletes with orthopedic injuries. All athletes were tested within 1 week postinjury. Trait anxiety was measured at baseline and state anxiety was measured postinjury but not until the athlete was ready to return to play, which was about 8 to 9 days in both groups, on average. They found that the two injury groups had similar levels of state and trait anxiety. Compared with values from the norms in the STAI manual for college students (Spielberger, 1983), the State scores of both groups of athletes postinjury were actually about half an SD lower. In contrast, the groups' scores at baseline for Trait anxiety were more than half an SD higher than the normative group. Comparable to Mainwaring and colleagues' (2010) study described earlier relating to depression in these two types of injured patients, these injured groups did not differ on anxiety postinjury. Surprisingly, both groups reported much higher trait compared with state anxiety, even though state anxiety was assessed postinjury and trait anxiety was assessed at baseline. The authors speculated that this may be due to the increased support the athletes perceive they have after injury.

Covassin et al.'s (2014) study also examined social support after injury using the Social Support Questionnaire (Sarason, Levine, Basham, & Sarason, 1983), a measure of perceived social support. They found that the groups identified similar sources of support but that the orthopedic control subjects expressed more satisfaction in their support compared with the concussed group. Interestingly, satisfaction in social support from family at baseline significantly predicted state anxiety at the time of return to play only in the concussed group. Thus, concussed athletes with greater satisfaction in family support at baseline were less likely to report state anxiety postconcussion.

Being one of the only published studies examining anxiety in concussed athletes, Covassin et al.'s (2014) study is important. A strength of the study, as with some of the studies from Mainwaring's group discussed earlier, is that it included an orthopedic control group. The study also included fairly large numbers of injured athletes. One limitation of the study, acknowledged by the authors, is that the participants were all tested within a short window after their injury at the time they returned to play. Thus, such a methodology involved the exclusion of those athletes who may have more complicated recoveries. A future study that included all athletes postinjury during an acute period before their return to play would further explicate the nature of anxiety postinjury. Also, given that anxiety and depression are often comorbid after injury (Yang, Peek-Asa, Covassin, & Torner, 2015; discussed subsequently), the measurement of depression may have further elucidated the nature of anxiety experienced by athletes postconcussion. Finally, studies that include clinical cutoffs for measures of either anxiety or depression are useful in showing just how many athletes are at risk for these conditions postconcussion.

Yang and colleagues (2015) measured anxiety and depression at baseline and 7 days postconcussion in 71 athletes. They assessed depression using the CES-D and anxiety with the STAI, measuring trait anxiety at baseline and state anxiety postconcussion. They found that nearly 20% of the athletes reported some depression postconcussion and about 33% reported anxiety (the cutoff for depression and anxiety was not specified). Similar to Vargas and colleagues (2015), these investigators found that depression at baseline was a risk factor for depression postconcussion. Specifically, athletes who had depression symptoms at baseline were 4.59 times more likely to experience depression symptoms postconcussion. Depression at baseline was also a risk factor for anxiety postconcussion, with athletes reporting depression at baseline being 3.40 times more likely to report state anxiety postconcussion. All comparisons were with athletes who did not report any depression at baseline. Interestingly, baseline trait anxiety did not predict either depression or anxiety postconcussion.

Yang et al.'s (2015) study is important in showing that depression at baseline is a risk factor not only for depression but also for anxiety postconcussion. Also, given the high variability in the prevalence of depression reported postconcussion among the few studies that have assessed it, the study provides some nice symmetry with another recent study in the literature showing similar prevalence of depression postconcussion (Vargas et al., 2015; 23%). However, a limitation of this study is that it was never explicitly reported what cutoff the authors used for anxiety or depression at either time point. It would be useful to know whether typical clinical cutoffs or some other strategy was used.

COMMON STRATEGIES FOR MEASURING DEPRESSION POSTCONCUSSION

In the most recent consensus statement on concussion in sport (McCrory et al., 2017), depression as a postconcussion symptom is recognized. Also, the importance of assessing and treating depression is mentioned, and some appreciation for its possible moderating effect on concussion outcomes is discussed. However, no specific measurement tools are discussed, and no particular guidelines for assessing depression postconcussion are mentioned. In the prior consensus statement (McCrory et al., 2013), the authors noted, "Although such mental health issues may be multifactorial in nature, it is recommended that the treating physician consider these issues in the management of concussed patients." However, no such passage appears in the updated statement. Surprisingly, even though both of these articles also highlight the potential importance of neuropsychologists in the sports concussion context more generally, no mention is made of the role that clinical neuropsychologists might play in diagnosing and managing depression in these individuals. This is despite the fact that clinical neuropsychologists, by virtue of their usual training in clinical psychology and treatment approaches for a variety of psychiatric conditions, would seem to be ideally suited for this role.

Moving forward, this is an area within the sports concussion context where clinical neuropsychologists could play a greater role and would generally have much more experience in addressing such issues than "the treating physician," whose focus and training are more likely to center around diagnosing and treating the neurological and physical sequelae of concussion than addressing psychiatric issues.

As noted, the recent consensus statements on sports concussion (McCrory, Meeuwisse, Dvorák, et al., 2017; McCrory, Meeuwisse, Kutcher, et al., 2013) offer no suggestion of a formal measure to assess depression postconcussion. A number of studies have used some variant of the Beck Depression Inventory (e.g., BDI–II, BDI–FS), and they appear to have some validity in this context. Vargas et al. (2015) used the BDI–FS, and there is much to recommend its use. First, it is brief, including only seven items that can be completed in a couple of minutes. Second, it has been widely used, and a number of published studies have demonstrated that it has good psychometric properties, including good reliability and validity (Beck et al., 2000). Third, it has a well-established cutoff (≥ 4) that has been validated in a number of contexts. With that said, to our knowledge, there has been no full validation study of the BDI–FS published in the sports concussion literature that provides specificity and sensitivity values. Still, the cutoff of 4 or greater has been replicated in other neurological populations (Benedict, Fishman, McClellan, Bakshi, & Weinstock-Guttman, 2003; Strober & Arnett, 2015).

Another possible approach to assessing affective functioning postconcussion is to use the affective items included in most postconcussion symptom scales. For example, several studies have now shown that there is a distinct affective cluster of symptoms in the most commonly used PCSS (Kontos, Elbin, et al., 2012; Merritt & Arnett, 2014; Pardini et al., 2004). Furthermore, Kontos, Deitrick, and Reynolds (2016) suggested the possibility of using such scales as a way of screening affective functioning postconcussion. However, more research is needed to explore exactly how such a scale would be used clinically, in terms of establishing some type of cutoff score that would indicate elevated risk for depression postconcussion. To our knowledge, the only study providing this information is one recently published study from our lab (Merritt, Bradson, Meyer, & Arnett, 2018). In this test–retest reliability study of the PCSS in athletic college students, we provide reliable change indices for the affective symptom cluster from the PCSS for 80%, 90%, and 95% confidence intervals (CIs). Specific items included in the affective symptom cluster from a prior factor analysis (see Merritt & Arnett, 2014) were irritability, sadness, nervousness, and feeling more emotional than usual. Using the midpoint of these values (the 90% CI), for example, an increase in the affective symptoms of 4 or more raw score points from baseline to postconcussion (see Table 5 in the article) would represent a reliable increase in affective symptoms. An athlete showing this pattern of change on the PCSS would thus be identified as someone who might be at risk for affective problems postconcussion and thus be targeted for appropriate follow-up and intervention, as clinically indicated. With this said, however, these values are only based on this one study with a relatively small sample size ($n = 38$), so further work is clearly necessary to determine whether these data are replicable in at least one other (preferably larger) sample from another lab before clinical application occurs.

As far as how to proceed with using such an affective scale from the PCSS when no baseline is available whereby change from baseline cannot be determined, a base rate approach could be pursued. Similar to what has been proposed for using base rates to assess cognitive functioning when no baseline is available (e.g., Arnett, Meyer, Merritt, & Guty, 2016), the base rates of particular values on the affective scale in nonconcussed athletes could be determined and then an appropriate cutoff identified. For example, if a score of 4 or higher on the affective scale was above the 90th percentile, then this could be used as the cutoff. In this instance, it would indicate that scores this high occurred in less than 10% of the baseline nonconcussed sample and thus might be a reasonable screening cutoff for risk of affective problems.

The CES–D is a widely used clinical measure of depression and has been used in at least two studies on sports-related concussion (see Roiger et al., 2015, and Yang et al., 2015, discussed earlier); however, it contains 20 items and so is a less practical option than the BDI–FS. The POMS has been used in several sports concussion studies and has good reliability and validity; it also assesses a broader range of emotional functioning than measures such as the BDI or the CES–D. However, as noted earlier, it is likely to have limited utility in most sports concussion settings given its length, with 65 items on the long form and 37 on the short form. As mentioned in the discussion of Ellis et al.'s (2015) study on pediatric concussion, use of routine psychiatric interviewing is also likely to be very impractical in these settings.

In the final analysis in terms of measurement selection, the BDI-FS seems most practical in this context. It is brief, has well-established reliability and validity, has been used in the sports concussion context, and can be used for individuals as young as age 13. The affective symptoms scale of the PCSS has great promise but is "not yet ready for prime time." Given that the PCSS is already routinely used in most sports-concussion contexts, it would be useful if the scale could simply be extracted out of the total PCSS and be routinely used to identify those at risk for affective problems postconcussion. However, to our knowledge, there is only one published study that provides cutoffs for this scale in the sports concussion context (Merritt et al., 2018). Furthermore, those cutoffs only relate to reliable change from baseline. Thus, it would be necessary to have baseline data for the PCSS to use these cutoffs.

Additionally, the participants from Merritt et al.'s (2018) study were all collegiate athletes, so the data would not necessarily apply to younger (or older) samples. More research in this area is clearly warranted that includes the replication of Merritt et al., the use of a broader age range of athletes, and the establishment of cutoffs that reflect base rates so that the affective scale from the PCSS could be used in cases of athletes for whom baseline data were not available.

One factor complicating the measurement of depression in sports concussion is that athletes may have a tendency to underreport symptoms in general, including depression, as they are typically keenly aware that reporting symptomatology will likely result in them being withheld from return-to-play. To circumvent this possibility, we conducted a study that employed a performance-based measure of affect (Ramanathan et al., 2012). In this study, we examined 256 collegiate athletes at baseline using the BDI–FS. Our performance-based measure, Affective Word List (AWL), involved recall of 16 affectively valenced words, with half being positive (e.g., *glad, laugh, joy, hope*), and half being negative (e.g., *doom, vile, pain, gloom*; see Meyer & Arnett, 2015). The list was read to each of the athletes for three trials and their recall recorded each time; we also included a delay trial after 20 to 25 minutes. The key scoring dependent variable was the Initial Bias Index that involved subtracting negative words from positive words recalled on initial recall trials. We then created a Positive Affect group (those who scored 1 *SD* or more above mean on the Initial Bias Index, n = 46) and a Negative Affect group (those who scored 1 *SD* or more below mean on Initial Bias Index, n = 41). To capture even those individuals reporting mild depression, we used 2 or higher as our cutoff on the BDI–FS. We found that 80% of those in the Negative Affect Group showed some depression, compared with only 20% of the Positive Affect Group, thus providing some validity for our AWL.

An important feature of Ramanathan et al.'s (2012) study is that athletes were assessed at baseline. We did this to avoid the aforementioned tendency of some athletes to underreport symptomatology that is most likely to happen postconcussion. At baseline, there are no implications for return to play, so we reasoned that most athletes would be more candid in their self-report than they would likely be postconcussion. Still, given that we have found a reasonably high number of athletes who report clinically significant depression via their self-report postconcussion in our collegiate sample (e.g., Vargas et al., 2015, where clinically significant depression was found in 23% of athletes), an important follow-up to this initial validation study will be to explore the AWL in depressed and nondepressed athletes postconcussion.

Ramanathan et al.'s (2012) study demonstrated that athletes who show negative cognitive biases at baseline are also likely to report at least mild depression. As such, using performance-based measures to identify athletes at risk for depression postconcussion may be useful. Using such approaches may identify athletes who may underreport depression postconcussion and warrant further clinical follow-up. At this early stage of study, however, it would not be appropriate to suggest the AWL for clinical use until further validation studies are conducted that show there is added value for the use of this measure, above and beyond simply asking athletes about their level of depression using a measure such as the BDI–FS.

ASSOCIATION OF DEPRESSION AND ANXIETY WITH COGNITIVE FUNCTIONING

Given the well-established association between depression and anxiety with cognitive functioning in the broader literature outside of sports-related concussion (Basso, Miller, Estevis, & Combs, 2013; Eysenck, 2013), combined with the fact that depression and anxiety appear to be fairly common post-concussion, it is surprising that there have been relatively few studies examining this issue in the sports concussion literature. As noted earlier, Kontos, Covassin, et al. (2012) found that worse visual memory and reaction time at 2 and 7 days postconcussion were associated with higher depression scores in a sample of high school and collegiate athletes. We examined this issue in a recent study examining 132 collegiate athletes at baseline and post-concussion (Meyer & Arnett, 2017). The participants were divided into depressed ($n = 29$) versus nondepressed groups ($n = 103$) postconcussion and compared on a battery of neurocognitive tests. Depression was measured with the BDI–FS, and standard cutoffs were used (≥ 4 to identify depressed athletes). Thus, 22% of this sample was depressed. The depressed athletes performed significantly worse on both the Hopkins Verbal Learning Test—Revised Total Recall (Brandt, 1991) and the ImPACT Visual Memory Composite score (Lovell, 2007). Reliable change on the cognitive test indices was also examined between groups, and we found that compared with nondepressed athletes (8%), significantly higher proportions of depressed athletes (25%) showed reliable declines on the ImPACT Verbal Memory Composite Score and the Symbol Digit Modalities Test (SDMT).

The potential impact of poor motivation on testing at baseline on neurocognitive scores has seen a fair amount of attention in the research literature (Bailey, Echemendia, & Arnett, 2006; Schatz & Glatts, 2013); however, there has been little attention to the potential influence of depression and anxiety. In a study of collegiate athletes at baseline (Bailey, Samples, Broshek, Freeman, & Barth, 2010), depression was found to be associated with some cognitive difficulties. These investigators examined cognitive functioning and depression in 47 collegiate football players at baseline. These investigators measured emotional and personality functioning using the Personality Assessment Inventory (PAI), a broad-based measure consisting of 344 items and 22 distinct subscales, 11 of which are clinical in nature. They measured cognitive functioning with the computerized Cognitive Resolution Index (CRI; Erlanger et al., 2003). The CRI includes six subtests measuring attention, reaction time, and speed of information processing. From these six tests, three composite indices are derived including simple reaction time (SRT), complex reaction time (CRT), and processing speed (PS).

Bailey et al. (2010) found significant correlations for the Anxiety scale of the PAI with the CRI–SRT and CRI–CRT composites, with effect sizes in the medium range. No significant correlations were found between the Depression scale from the PAI and any of the CRI composite indices. However, when the authors divided their sample up into those with high scores on the Suicidal Ideation Scale of the PAI, they found that it was significantly correlated with both the CRI–SRT and CRI–CRT composites.

Bailey and colleagues' (2010) results are important because they show that, even at baseline, collegiate athletes' neurocognitive difficulties are associated with increased distress. This suggests that athletes who are significantly distressed at baseline may underperform cognitively. As such, if they do not show similar levels of distress postconcussion, their scores at this post-injury time point may not provide an accurate comparison with their baseline scores. In this case, postconcussion scores could be equivalent to baseline scores because the athlete is no longer distressed, and obscure declines actually associated with their concussion. In these instances, it may be worthwhile to compare such athletes' postconcussion scores to available norms, as a way of double-checking whether they are, in fact, impaired. This study underscores the importance of assessing athletes' psychological distress not only postconcussion but also at baseline. Another reason for assessing psychiatric factors at baseline is that they are predictors of PCS (Meares et al., 2011; Ponsford et al., 2012), something that occurs in a small but significant proportion (10%–20%) of those with mTBI (Iverson & Lange, 2011).

CASE STUDY

This athlete (Mr. D) is a 19-year-old right-handed man who competes on a collegiate lacrosse team.[1] He suffered a concussion about 5 days before our evaluation during a game when he was struck in the forehead after falling to the playing surface. He remembered the hit and denied losing consciousness

---

[1]Some of the original details of this case have been changed to protect the confidentiality of the individual tested.

or any anterograde amnesia, but he experienced some retrograde amnesia, indicating that he did not remember what happened right before his head hit the playing surface. Mr. D reported experiencing moderate to severe post-concussion symptoms immediately after the impact, including disorientation (2 of 6 where 0 is *none* and 6 is *severe*), dizziness (4), balance problems (5), visual disturbance (6), feeling in a fog (3), pressure in the head (5), problems with attention (4), and headache (4). By about 12 hours postinjury, he continued to experience balance problems (3), pressure in the head (4), problems with attention (3), and headache (2). At the time of our initial testing, he reported being asymptomatic and feeling completely back to his preinjury self. He had not been exercising or physically exerting himself since his injury and indicated that he had a history of one concussion that occurred about a year earlier.

On our initial neuropsychological testing, Mr. D's performance was compared with baseline testing conducted about 16 months previously. He scored significantly below baseline on one index of visual memory (Brief Visuospatial Memory Test—Revised Delayed Recall) and three indices of sustained attention and processing speed (SDMT, Cancellation Total Correct, ImPACT Reaction Time Composite). Mr. D endorsed clinically significant depression symptoms (BDI–FS = 6), which represents a significant increase from his report of no depression (BDI–FS = 0) at baseline.

Using the evidence basis for our battery where significant declines from baseline on three or more test indices is highly unusual in nonconcussed athletes (Rabinowitz & Arnett, 2013), we concluded that Mr. D was not back to his preinjury baseline, given that he scored significantly below his baseline scores on four test indices. We hypothesized that his current depression was exacerbating his cognitive difficulties but acknowledged that it was not possible to determine the extent to which the primary effects of Mr. D's concussion or the secondary effects of his depression could account for his cognitive difficulties. We also recommended referring him back for follow-up testing when he reported that his mood functioning was back to normal. Given his report of clinically significant depression, we also suggested that he be referred for some short-term counseling either with the team psychologist or the university counseling center.

We saw Mr. D again 1 week later, and at this time he again reported being asymptomatic and denied experiencing any recurrence of symptoms in the previous week. This time on the neurocognitive testing, Mr. D showed substantial improvement, scoring significantly below baseline on one test (SDMT). Additionally, his score on the depression measure declined significantly from the previous week (BDI–FS = 2 now). Given that decline on only one test index is not unusual given established base rates of decline for our neurocognitive test battery, we concluded that Mr. D was back to his preinjury neurocognitive baseline. We also hypothesized that his improved mood since our previous meeting may have accounted for his improved cognitive functioning. However, it is certainly also possible that his mood improved because his cognitive functioning improved or because of some third variable (e.g., change in brain functioning that positively affected both cognitive functioning and mood). This case thus illustrates the fact that mood changes and cognitive changes often co-occur postconcussion but also that causal issues at work are difficult to specify.

CLINICAL TAKE-HOME POINTS

It is critical for clinicians to be aware of risk for affective problems and anxiety postconcussion. What follows are a few clinical take-home points in relation to this.

1. *Clinicians should routinely screen for depression postconcussion.* Although the state of our empirical knowledge about how best to screen for depression in concussion is not well developed, we recommend the use of the BDI–FS. It only includes seven items and can thus be completed quickly. Any athlete scoring 4 or higher on this measure should be referred for further evaluation and possible pharmacological or psychotherapeutic treatment.

2. *There is an extensive literature demonstrating that depression is associated with cognitive impairments.* Although the specific literature in relation to concussion on this topic is relatively limited, the few studies that have addressed these issues have been consistent with the broader depression literature. As such, clinicians should be aware that when depression is comorbid with cognitive impairments postconcussion, it may mediate some of the cognitive problems that are seen. As such, successful resolution of the depression may result in improved cognitive functioning. Knowledge of this relationship helps to underscore the importance of correctly assessing and treating postconcussion depression because failure to treat it may result in the delayed resolution of cognitive problems.

3. *If it is not feasible to use the BDI–FS to screen for depression, then considering the four items comprising the affective scale from the PCSS could be considered.* These items include irritability, sadness, nervousness, and feeling more emotional than usual. Any athlete increasing on this scale by 4 or more points from baseline would be considered reliably increasing on this scale, such

that further evaluation of possible affective problems after concussion and possible treatment may be warranted.

4. *On the basis of the few studies that have examined anxiety in sports concussion contexts, it appears to be about as common, or more, compared with depression.* As far as screening for anxiety, however, the state of the literature at this point is so rudimentary that no clear screening recommendations can be made. Still, clinicians screening for depression could also follow up and ask questions about possible comorbid anxiety. Compared with others working in the sports concussion context, clinical neuropsychologists would seem to be uniquely qualified to evaluate both depression and anxiety postconcussion and recommend treatment as appropriate.

KEY QUESTIONS TO BE ADDRESSED IN THE NEXT 5 YEARS

Over the next 5 years more research needs to be conducted on depression and anxiety in sports-related concussion. Specifically, researchers should consider six key questions.

1. *First, what is the accurate prevalence of depression following a sports-related concussion?* Although most studies have shown that concussed athletes show more depression overall than healthy control subjects postconcussion, studies using actual clinical cutoffs on standardized depression measures are relatively few and far between. One study using such a strategy on collegiate athletes (e.g., Vargas et al., 2015) has found clinical depression to be approximately 23% postconcussion. Another study on collegiate and high school athletes (Kontos, Covassin, et al., 2012), however, found the postconcussion rate of depression to be only 7%. Given that several other studies have consistently found higher depression in concussed athletes versus controls, it seems likely that depression is elevated postconcussion. Still, more research is needed to clarify the accurate value for depression prevalence in athletes during the relatively acute period postconcussion.

2. *Do concussion injuries specifically result in increased depression risk postconcussion, or is this increased depression simply a function of being injured more generally?* At least two studies comparing concussed athletes to orthopedic control subjects have been conducted and have shown that there is no elevated risk of

depression and emotional difficulties in concussed athletes relative to other types of injured athletes. However, more work in this domain is clearly warranted, especially with regard to different mechanisms that may be at work after sports concussion versus other types of sport-related injuries. If there are different mechanisms at work, either biologically or psychosocially, then different interventions to treat such depression will be warranted.

3. *What is the best way to measure anxiety postconcussion?* There are at least some data from the sports concussion literature to guide the selection of screening measures for depression. No such scenario exists for anxiety. Although both Covassin et al. (2014) and Yang et al. (2015) used the STAI, no particular cutoffs were recommended in either study. The STAI is also a fairly long measure for acute clinical use, with 20 items on each of the Trait and State scales. Exploration into shorter measures of anxiety with adequate psychometric properties is warranted.

4. *What is the accurate prevalence of clinical anxiety postconcussion, and do different mechanisms underlie postconcussion anxiety in concussed versus other injured athletes?* Although the literature on depression postconcussion is relatively sparse, anxiety has been even less frequently examined. One of the few studies on anxiety prevalence (Yang et al., 2015) showed that 33% of collegiate athletes reported anxiety postconcussion, and this represented a substantial increase from their baseline levels. However, although a reliable and valid measure of anxiety (STAI) was used, it was not clear what cutoff was used to denote anxiety. More research is clearly needed in this area to determine how accurate Yang et al.'s 33% value is and to clarify optimal measures and cutoffs for identifying clinically significant anxiety postconcussion.

   In addition to this, the limited studies on anxiety suggest that concussion injuries are no more likely to lead to increased anxiety than orthopedic types of injuries. If additional work confirms these initial findings, then more work exploring different mechanisms that may be at work will be warranted, similar to the logic outlined for depression in Question 2.

5. *What is the comorbidity of depression and anxiety postconcussion and is there an additional risk in outcome associated with it?* Few studies have examined the comorbidity of these conditions postconcussion. Covassin et al. (2014) and Yang et al. (2015) represent perhaps the only published studies that have

examined both depression and anxiety in concussion and found these conditions to be comorbid. Further research examining this comorbidity in more detail to determine how common it is and whether it confers greater risk in terms of either prolonged symptom resolution or greater cognitive deficits is warranted.

6. *How might performance-based measures of affect be employed in the sports concussion context?* One study from our lab (Ramanathan et al., 2012) showed that a performance-based test of affect can identify individuals at risk for at least mild depression at baseline. Given that some athletes may tend to underreport depression and other symptoms postconcussion because they know that reporting symptoms may delay their RTP, it could be useful to use performance-based measures of affect postconcussion. As such, affective problems postconcussion would not rely exclusively on athletes' self-report. More work in this area is needed to see whether there could be added value to performance-based measures of affect in concussed athletes, especially when an individual scores above the cutoff for negative recall but does not self-report any depression symptoms.

REFERENCES

American Psychiatric Association. (1994). *Diagnostic and statistical manual of mental disorders* (4th ed.). Washington, DC: Author.

Arnett, P., Meyer, J., Merritt, V., & Guty, E. (2016). Neuropsychological testing in mild traumatic brain injury: What to do when baseline testing is not available. *Sports Medicine and Arthroscopy Review, 24,* 116–122. http://dx.doi.org/10.1097/JSA.0000000000000123

Bailey, C. M., Echemendia, R. J., & Arnett, P. A. (2006). The impact of motivation on neuropsychological performance in sports-related mild traumatic brain injury. *Journal of the International Neuropsychological Society, 12,* 475–484. http://dx.doi.org/10.1017/S1355617706060619

Bailey, C. M., Samples, H. L., Broshek, D. K., Freeman, J. R., & Barth, J. T. (2010). The relationship between psychological distress and baseline sports-related concussion testing. *Clinical Journal of Sport Medicine, 20,* 272–277. http://dx.doi.org/10.1097/JSM.0b013e3181e8f8d8

Basso, M. R., Miller, A., Estevis, E., & Combs, D. (2013). Neuropsychological deficits in major depressive disorder: Correlates and conundrums. In P. A. Arnett (Ed.), *Secondary influences on neuropsychological test performance* (pp. 39–66). New York, NY: Oxford University Press.

Beck, A. T., Steer, R. A., & Brown, G. K. (1996). *Beck Depression Inventory—2 manual.* San Antonio, TX: The Psychological Corporation.

Beck, A. T., Steer, R. A., & Brown, G. K. (2000). *BDI–II Fast Screen for Medical Patients manual.* London, England: Psychological Corporation.

Benedict, R. H. B., Fishman, I., McClellan, M. M., Bakshi, R., & Weinstock-Guttman, B. (2003). Validity of the Beck Depression Inventory—Fast Screen in multiple sclerosis. *Multiple Sclerosis, 9,* 393–396. http://dx.doi.org/10.1191/1352458503ms902oa

Brandt, J. (1991). The Hopkins Verbal Learning Test: Development of a new memory test with six equivalent forms. *The Clinical Neuropsychologist, 5,* 125–142.

Busch, C. R., & Alpern, H. P. (1998). Depression after mild traumatic brain injury: A review of current research. *Neuropsychology Review, 8,* 95–108. http://dx.doi.org/10.1023/A:1025661200911

Chen, J. K., Johnston, K. M., Petrides, M., & Ptito, A. (2008). Neural substrates of symptoms of depression following concussion in male athletes with persisting postconcussion symptoms. *Archives of General Psychiatry, 65,* 81–89. http://dx.doi.org/10.1001/archgenpsychiatry.2007.8

Chrisman, S. P., & Richardson, L. P. (2014). Prevalence of diagnosed depression in adolescents with history of concussion. *Journal of Adolescent Health, 54,* 582–586. http://dx.doi.org/10.1016/j.jadohealth.2013.10.006

Covassin, T., Crutcher, B., Bleecker, A., Heiden, E. O., Dailey, A., & Yang, J. (2014). Postinjury anxiety and social support among collegiate athletes: A comparison between orthopaedic injuries and concussions. *Journal of Athletic Training, 49,* 462–468. http://dx.doi.org/10.4085/1062-6059-49.2.03

Ellis, M. J., Ritchie, L. J., Koltek, M., Hosain, S., Cordingley, D., Chu, S., . . . Russell, K. (2015). Psychiatric outcomes after pediatric sports-related concussion. *Journal of Neurosurgery: Pediatrics, 16,* 709–718. http://dx.doi.org/10.3171/2015.5.PEDS15220

Erlanger, D., Feldman, D., Kutner, K., Kaushik, T., Kroger, H., Festa, J., . . . Broshek, D. (2003). Development and validation of a web-based neuropsychological test protocol for sports-related return-to-play decision-making. *Archives of Clinical Neuropsychology, 18,* 293–316.

Eysenck, M. W. (2013). Anxiety and cognitive performance. In C. Mohiyeddini, M. W. Eysenck, & S. Bauer (Eds.), *Handbook of psychology of emotions: Vol. 1. Recent theoretical perspectives and novel empirical findings* (pp. 336–353). Hauppauge, NY: Nova Science.

Hamilton, M. (1967). Development of a rating scale for primary depressive illness. *British Journal of Social and Clinical Psychology, 6,* 278–296.

Hutchison, M., Mainwaring, L. M., Comper, P., Richards, D. W., & Bisschop, S. M. (2009). Differential emotional responses of varsity athletes to concussion and musculoskeletal injuries. *Clinical Journal of Sport Medicine, 19,* 13–19. http://dx.doi.org/10.1097/JSM.0b013e318190ba06

Iverson, G. L., & Lange, R. T. (2011). Post-concussion syndrome. In M. R. Schoenberg & J. G. Scott (Eds.), *The little black book of neuropsychology* (pp. 745–763). New York, NY: Springer.

Jorge, R., & Robinson, R. G. (2002). Mood disorders after traumatic brain injury. *NeuroRehabilitation, 17*, 311–324.

Kerr, Z. Y., Marshall, S. W., Harding, H. P., Jr., & Guskiewicz, K. M. (2012). Nine-year risk of depression diagnosis increases with increasing self-reported concussions in retired professional football players. *The American Journal of Sports Medicine, 40*, 2206–2212. http://dx.doi.org/10.1177/0363546512456193

Kontos, A. P., Covassin, T., Elbin, R. J., & Parker, T. (2012). Depression and neuro-cognitive performance after concussion among male and female high school and collegiate athletes. *Archives of Physical Medicine and Rehabilitation, 93*, 1751–1756. http://dx.doi.org/10.1016/j.apmr.2012.03.032

Kontos, A. P., Deitrick, J. M., & Reynolds, E. (2016). Mental health implications and consequences following sport-related concussion. *British Journal of Sports Medicine, 50*, 139–140. http://dx.doi.org/10.1136/bjsports-2015-095564

Kontos, A. P., Elbin, R. J., Schatz, P., Covassin, T., Henry, L., Pardini, J., & Collins, M. W. (2012). A revised factor structure for the post-concussion symptom scale: Baseline and postconcussion factors. *The American Journal of Sports Medicine, 40*, 2375–2384. http://dx.doi.org/10.1177/0363546512455400

Lovell, M. (2007). *Immediate Post-Concussion Assessment Testing (ImPACT) Test: Clinical Interpretive manual*. Pittsburgh, PA: ImPACT Applications.

Maier, W., Buller, R., Philipp, M., & Heuser, I. (1988). The Hamilton Anxiety Scale: Reliability, validity and sensitivity to change in anxiety and depressive disorders. *Journal of Affective Disorders, 14*, 61–68.

Mainwaring, L. M., Hutchison, M., Bisschop, S. M., Comper, P., & Richards, D. W. (2010). Emotional response to sport concussion compared to ACL injury. *Brain Injury, 24*, 589–597. http://dx.doi.org/10.3109/02699051003610508

McCrory, P., Meeuwisse, W., Dvořák, J., Aubry, M., Bailes, J., Broglio, S., . . . Vos, P. E. (2017). Consensus statement on concussion in sport—The 5th international conference on concussion in sport held in Berlin, October 2016. *British Journal of Sports Medicine, 51*, 838–847.

McCrory, P., Meeuwisse, W. H., Kutcher, J. S., Jordan, B. D., & Gardner, A. (2013). What is the evidence for chronic concussion-related changes in retired athletes: Behavioural, pathological and clinical outcomes? *British Journal of Sports Medicine, 47*, 327–330. http://dx.doi.org/10.1136/bjsports-2013-092248

McNair, D. M., Lorr, M., & Droppleman, L. F. (1971). *Manual for the Profile of Mood States*. San Diego, CA: Educational and Industrial Testing Services.

Meares, S., Shores, E. A., Taylor, A. J., Batchelor, J., Bryant, R. A., Baguley, I. J., . . . Marosszeky, J. E. (2011). The prospective course of postconcussion syndrome: The role of mild traumatic brain injury. *Neuropsychology, 25*, 454–465. http://dx.doi.org/10.1037/a0022580

Meier, T. B., Bellgowan, P. S. F., Singh, R., Kuplicki, R., Polanski, D. W., & Mayer, A. R. (2015). Recovery of cerebral blood flow following sports-related concussion. *JAMA Neurology, 72*, 530–538. http://dx.doi.org/10.1001/jamaneurol.2014.4778

Merritt, V. C., & Arnett, P. A. (2014). Premorbid predictors of postconcussion symptoms in collegiate athletes. *Journal of Clinical and Experimental Neuropsychology, 36*, 1098–1111. http://dx.doi.org/10.1080/13803395.2014.983463

Merritt, V. C., Bradson, M. L., Meyer, J. E., & Arnett, P. A. (2018). Evaluating the test–retest reliability of symptom indices associated with the ImPACT Post-Concussion Symptom Scale (PCSS). *Journal of Clinical and Experimental Neuropsychology, 40*, 377–388. http://dx.doi.org/10.1080/13803395.2017.1353590

Meyer, J., & Arnett, P. (2017, February). *Post-concussion depression and cognitive functioning in collegiate athletes.* Paper presented at the International Neuropsychological Society, New Orleans, LA.

Meyer, J. E., & Arnett, P. A. (2015). Validation of the Affective Word List as a measure of verbal learning and memory. *Journal of Clinical and Experimental Neuropsychology, 37*, 316–324. http://dx.doi.org/10.1080/13803395.2015.1012486

Pardini, D., Stump, J., Lovell, M., Collins, M., Moritz, K., & Fu, F. (2004). The Post Concussion Symptom Scale (PCSS): A factor analysis. *British Journal of Sports Medicine, 38*, 661–662.

Ponsford, J., Cameron, P., Fitzgerald, M., Grant, M., Mikocka-Walus, A., & Schönberger, M. (2012). Predictors of postconcussive symptoms 3 months after mild traumatic brain injury. *Neuropsychology, 26*, 304–313. http://dx.doi.org/10.1037/a0027888

Rabinowitz, A. R., & Arnett, P. A. (2013). Intraindividual cognitive variability before and after sports-related concussion. *Neuropsychology, 27*, 481–490. http://dx.doi.org/10.1037/a0033023

Radloff, L. S. (1977). The CES-D Scale: A self-report depression scale for research in the general population. *Applied Psychological Measurement, 1*, 385–401.

Ramanathan, D. M., Rabinowitz, A. R., Barwick, F. H., & Arnett, P. A. (2012). Validity of affect measurements in evaluating symptom reporting in athletes. *Journal of the International Neuropsychological Society, 18*, 101–107. http://dx.doi.org/10.1017/S1355617711001457

Rapoport, M. J., Kiss, A., & Feinstein, A. (2006). The impact of major depression on outcome following mild-to-moderate traumatic brain injury in older adults. *Journal of Affective Disorders, 92*, 273–276. http://dx.doi.org/10.1016/j.jad.2005.05.022

Roiger, T., Weidauer, L., & Kern, B. (2015). A longitudinal pilot study of depressive symptoms in concussed and injured/nonconcussed National Collegiate Athletic Association Division I student-athletes. *Journal of Athletic Training, 50*, 256–261. http://dx.doi.org/10.4085/1062-6050-49.3.83

Sarason, I. G., Levine, H. M., Basham, R. B., & Sarason, B. R. (1983). Assessing social support: The Social Support Questionnaire. *Journal of Personality and Social Psychology, 44*, 127–139.

Schatz, P., & Glatts, C. (2013). "Sandbagging" baseline test performance on ImPACT, without detection, is more difficult than it appears. *Archives of Clinical Neuropsychology, 28*, 236–244. http://dx.doi.org/10.1093/arclin/act009

Spielberger, C. D. (1983). *State–Trait Anxiety Inventory (Form Y)*. Redwood City, CA: Mind Garden.

Spielberger, C. D., Gorsuch, R. L., Lushene, R., Vagg, P. R., & Jacobs, G. A. (1983). *Manual for the State–Trait Anxiety Inventory*. Palo Alto, CA: Consulting Psychologists Press.

Strain, J., Didehbani, N., Cullum, C. M., Mansinghani, S., Conover, H., Kraut, M. A., . . . Womack, K. B. (2013). Depressive symptoms and white matter dysfunction in retired NFL players with concussion history. *Neurology, 81*, 25–32. http://dx.doi.org/10.1212/WNL.0b013e318299ccf8

Strober, L. B., & Arnett, P. A. (2015). Depression in multiple sclerosis: The utility of common self-report instruments and development of a disease-specific measure. *Journal of Clinical and Experimental Neuropsychology, 37*, 722–732. http://dx.doi.org/10.1080/13803395.2015.1063591

Vargas, G. A., Rabinowitz, A. R., Meyer, J. E., & Arnett, P. A. (2015). Predictors and prevalence of postconcussion depression symptoms in collegiate athletes. *Journal of Athletic Training, 50*, 250–255. http://dx.doi.org/10.4085/1062-6050-50.3.02

Yang, J., Peek-Asa, C., Covassin, T., & Torner, J. C. (2015). Post-concussion symptoms of depression and anxiety in division I collegiate athletes. *Developmental Neuropsychology, 40*, 18–23. http://dx.doi.org/10.1080/87565641.2014.973499

II

BIOLOGICAL UNDERPINNINGS AND CONSEQUENCES

4

INTEGRATION OF GENETIC FACTORS WITH NEUROPSYCHOLOGICAL VARIABLES IN PREDICTING SPORTS CONCUSSION OUTCOME

VICTORIA C. MERRITT AND PETER A. ARNETT

The exploration of genetic factors within the context of sports concussion is a relatively new area of study that has received minimal research attention. However, provided that there has been a widespread interest in understanding the effects of concussion on acute functioning and long-term well-being, it may be advantageous to go beyond solely examining environmental factors and also develop an understanding of how genetic factors influence concussion outcome and recovery processes. Furthermore, given the heterogeneity in outcomes that are often observed after concussion, it seems that there are many factors that contribute to the clinical presentation of the concussed athlete. This not only raises questions of the role of genetics in concussion outcome but also leads to the inquiry of gene × environment interactions that may influence response to injury.

http://dx.doi.org/10.1037/0000114-005

Neuropsychology of Sports-Related Concussion, P. A. Arnett (Editor)

In this chapter, we review the research that has been conducted on genetic factors and sports concussion outcome and examine the broader traumatic brain injury (TBI) literature to highlight relationships that have been established with respect to specific genotypes and TBI. The primary focus of this chapter is to review how various genes have been linked to both broad and specific outcomes after brain injury, and to then consider the clinical implications of this research within the context of sports concussion. We also present a case study highlighting how a specific gene may influence outcome after concussion in college athletes, offer ideas for future research, and include a few clinical take-home points.

THE SUBJECTIVE AND OBJECTIVE EXPERIENCE
OF THE CONCUSSED ATHLETE

To date, many research efforts have been made to study not only the immediate consequences of sports-related concussion but also to more specifically understand the nature and course of recovery following such brain injuries. By definition, concussions are considered "mild" TBIs, yet it is well understood that a variety of clinically meaningful sequelae develop after concussion. Thus, evaluation of subjective complaints and objective functioning is critical in the assessment of sports concussion.

With respect to subjective complaints, it is common for concussed athletes to report physical symptoms, such as headache, dizziness, and visual disturbance, as well as cognitive symptoms, such as feeling mentally foggy, having difficulty concentrating, and trouble remembering (Guskiewicz, Weaver, Padua, & Garrett, 2000; Kontos et al., 2012; Lovell et al., 2006; Merritt, Rabinowitz, & Arnett, 2015). Additional symptoms that may be reported by athletes who have been concussed include irritability, nervousness, fatigue, and difficulty sleeping (Kontos et al., 2012; Lovell et al., 2006). Although this is not an exhaustive list of symptoms, it provides a picture of the symptom profile that may accompany concussion.

With respect to objective functioning, neuropsychological assessments conducted on athletes with brain injuries reveal a range of cognitive performance deficits. For example, impairments or deficits in learning and memory, attention and processing speed, and on tasks of executive functioning have been documented (Covassin, Elbin, Harris, Parker, & Kontos, 2012; Echemendia, Putukian, Mackin, Julian, & Shoss, 2001; McClincy, Lovell, Pardini, Collins, & Spore, 2006). When considering the subjective and objective experience of the concussed athlete, it is reasonable to hypothesize that environmental factors and genetic factors likely influence response to, and recovery from, brain injury. However, we currently are only in the beginning stages of understanding how genetics influence postconcussion sequelae.

SETTING THE STAGE FOR GENETICS RESEARCH WITHIN SPORTS CONCUSSION

Although it is common for concussed athletes to return to baseline levels of cognitive functioning and experience symptom resolution within 1 to 2 weeks postinjury (Iverson, Brooks, Collins, & Lovell, 2006; McClincy et al., 2006; McCrea et al., 2003), other athletes experience ongoing cognitive deficits and remain symptomatic for several weeks or even months after their injury (Lau, Collins, & Lovell, 2011, 2012; Meehan, d'Hemecourt, & Comstock, 2010). Many studies within and outside of the sports concussion literature have hypothesized a variety of possibilities to explain the heterogeneity in recovery rates and outcome after concussion. Demographic factors such as age, biological sex, and history of concussion (Broshek et al., 2005; Field, Collins, Lovell, & Maroon, 2003; Guskiewicz et al., 2003; Pellman, Lovell, Viano, & Casson, 2006; Ponsford et al., 2000), as well as premorbid or preinjury factors such as cognitive functioning, psychological and emotional well-being, and personality characteristics (Cicerone & Kalmar, 1997; Merritt & Arnett, 2014; Ponsford et al., 2000, 2012), have been examined as predictors of postconcussion outcomes. Furthermore, injury-specific factors such as the mechanism of injury, the nature or force of the impact and biomechanics of the injury, and the presence and duration of loss of consciousness and retrograde or anterograde amnesia (Lange et al., 2013; Lau, Kontos, Collins, Mucha, & Lovell, 2011; McCrea et al., 2013; Merritt et al., 2015) have also been evaluated as potential contributors to recovery and outcomes following brain injury. Yet despite these numerous pursuits, there remain unanswered questions regarding the phenomenon of disparate outcomes after what seem to be similar concussive injuries.

Examining the role of genetics may hold promise for better understanding the heterogeneity in recovery patterns after concussion or brain injury. McAllister (2009) proposed that there are several ways in which genes affect response to neurotrauma; these include influencing (a) the extent of the injury, (b) the repair or recovery processes after injury, (c) premorbid functioning, and (d) the existence or development of neurobehavioral disorders. Although our current understanding of how genetics affect each of these domains is still in its infancy, a growing body of literature has started to examine specific genes that may be involved in the repair and recovery process after brain injury. Additionally, researchers have begun to examine how genes may influence premorbid functioning before neurological insult such as TBI. In the present chapter, we focus primarily on a gene affecting the repair and recovery process following neurotrauma, as well as on a gene implicated in premorbid functioning, but we also recognize other genes that may be important in TBI outcome and recovery.

TBI CANDIDATE GENES

To date, the apolipoprotein E (APOE) gene has been the most widely studied gene with regard to its role in recovery and outcome following TBI (Dardiotis et al., 2010; Jordan, 2007). However, the majority of research on the APOE gene thus far has focused on patients with more severe brain injuries, and a primary emphasis has been on examining global outcomes as opposed to more specific sequelae of brain injury. Furthermore, much of the published work on the APOE gene and TBI has been within the context of military or civilian TBI as opposed to sports-related concussion. In addition to APOE, other genes that have been linked to the repair and recovery process after TBI include brain-derived neurotrophic factor (BDNF) and the serotonin transporter gene (5-HTT; McAllister, 2009).

With respect to the genes implicated in premorbid functioning, a potential candidate gene that has emerged in recent years is the catechol-o-methyltransferase (COMT) gene. The COMT gene is involved in the production of the COMT enzyme, which is responsible for the metabolic degradation of catecholamines such as dopamine (Dickinson & Elvevåg, 2009; Savitz, Solms, & Ramesar, 2006; Weinberger et al., 2001). It is well understood that dopamine plays an integral role in modulating cognitive functioning, especially processes that are mediated by the frontal cortex (Cools & D'Esposito, 2011; Cropley, Fujita, Innis, & Nathan, 2006). At present, however, the COMT gene has not been widely studied in brain injured populations, but a considerable amount of research has examined the role of the gene on neuropsychological outcome in patients with schizophrenia (Diaz-Asper et al., 2008; Egan et al., 2001; Goldberg et al., 2003), as well as healthy populations (Aguilera et al., 2008; Malhotra et al., 2002). Because similar cognitive processes (i.e., frontal-executive cognitive functions) are affected as a result of brain injury, COMT may be an important gene to explore in the context of TBI and concussion. Additional genes associated with premorbid functioning are the dopamine D2 receptor (DRD2), the dopamine transporter gene (DAT), the norepinephrine transporter gene (NET), and the dopamine beta hydroxylase gene (DBH; McAllister, 2009; Wilson & Montgomery, 2007). These genes have also not been extensively examined within the TBI literature, but each has been proposed as a promising candidate gene from which we may be able to further understand the relationship between genetic factors and TBI.

GENE FUNCTIONS AND
NEUROPSYCHOLOGICAL OUTCOMES

The following section is arranged according to candidate gene. *APOE* is discussed first, followed by *COMT*. The main function(s) of each gene are reviewed, followed by a discussion of how the gene has been examined within the context of sports concussion or the greater TBI literature.

APOE Gene

Function

As noted earlier, the *APOE* gene has been the most widely studied gene with respect to concussion susceptibility and outcome. *APOE* has several functions within the central nervous system (CNS), including the maintenance and integrity of neuronal membranes, and it is involved in the restoration of neurons following brain injury or insult (Dardiotis et al., 2010; Mahley, Weisgraber, & Huang, 2006; Wilson & Montgomery, 2007). The gene, located on chromosome 19, comprises three primary alleles—ε2, ε3, and ε4—and each allele has been found to differentially affect the process through which neurons are repaired and restored following injury. When compared with the ε2 and ε3 alleles, the ε4 allele exerts adverse pathological functions on the CNS and has thus been implicated as a risk factor for neuropathology (Mahley et al., 2006).

The frequency of the *APOE* alleles differs by ethnicity (Eichner et al., 2002). Within Caucasian populations, the frequency of having an ε2 allele is 4% to 8%, an ε3 allele is 75% to 83%, and an ε4 allele is 10% to 19% (Eichner et al., 2002; Farrer et al., 1997; Roses, 1996). Within African American populations, the frequency of having an ε2 allele is 13%, an ε3 allele is 67%, and an ε4 allele is 20% (Eichner et al., 2002).

Susceptibility to Brain Injury

Only a limited amount of research has examined the question of whether having an ε4 allele predisposes an individual to sustaining a brain injury. At present, there is not a conclusive answer to this question, but data from the sports concussion literature suggest that there is not a strong association between the possession of an ε4 allele and the occurrence of concussion. Terrell and colleagues (2008) examined the relationship between *APOE* genotypes and history of concussion in athletes and found no association between having an ε4 allele and having had previous concussions. Kristman et al. (2008) reported similar findings. In another study, Tierney et al. (2010) found no association between having an ε4 allele and history of concussion but did report a relationship between history of concussion and possessing an ϵ2 and ϵ4 allele, along with the *APOE* promoter *219 G/T* allele (a gene variant that occurs in the promoter region of the *APOE* locus).

Global Functional Outcomes

Although there are various ways to evaluate outcome following concussion or TBI, a relatively straightforward method that has frequently been used is to characterize outcome according to the Glasgow Outcome Scale (GOS) score. The GOS is a global measure comprising a 5-point rating scale that assesses functional outcome after a brain injury (Jennett & Bond, 1975). The GOS categories include (a) death, (b) persistent vegetative state, (c) severe disability, (d) moderate disability, and (e) good recovery. Given that the GOS is such a broad tool, this measure is rarely used within the context of sports concussion and is typically reserved for assessing outcome after moderate or severe TBI.

Using this approach, several studies evaluating primarily moderate and severe TBI have concluded that patients with a brain injury who possess at least one ϵ4 allele are more likely to have an adverse outcome (as defined by a GOS rating of 1, 2, or 3 in most studies) at 6 months postinjury compared with those without the ϵ4 allele (Chiang, Chang, & Hu, 2003; Friedman et al., 1999; Liaquat, Dunn, Nicoll, Teasdale, & Norrie, 2002; Teasdale, Murray, & Nicoll, 2005; Teasdale, Nicoll, Murray, & Fiddes, 1997). Relatedly, a study by Alexander et al. (2007) examined recovery rates (as assessed by the GOS) after severe TBI among those with and without the ϵ4 allele and found that participants with an ϵ4 allele recovered more slowly than participants who did not possess an ϵ4 allele. In contrast to these positive findings, however, some studies have reported no differences in GOS outcome between TBI patients with and without the ϵ4 allele (Millar, Nicoll, Thornhill, Murray, & Teasdale, 2003; Nathoo, Chetty, van Dellen, Connolly, & Naidoo, 2003; Willemse-van Son, Ribbers, Hop, van Duijn, & Stam, 2008). These reported discrepancies may be attributable to a number of factors related to the samples studied, including differences in age, injury severity, and timing of assessment postinjury.

Neuropsychological Outcomes

When bearing in mind how the *APOE* gene may influence neuropsychological functioning, it is important to consider the influence of genotype on symptoms, as well as objective neurocognitive performance. With respect to symptoms, recent work in our lab examined the effects of the ϵ4 allele on global symptom reporting in a sample of concussed college athletes (Merritt & Arnett, 2016). In this study, college athletes were tested within 3 months after their injury, with the majority of the sample tested within the first week. Athletes were divided into two groups based on the presence or absence of the $\epsilon4$ allele. Concussed athletes with an $\epsilon4$ allele ($\epsilon4+$ group) reported a greater total symptom score on the Post-Concussion Symptom Scale (PCSS) than concussed athletes without an $\epsilon4$ allele ($\epsilon4-$group). When dividing the PCSS into symptom clusters, *physical* and *cognitive* symptoms were significantly different between the allele groups, with $\epsilon4+$ athletes reporting greater symptoms than $\epsilon4-$athletes. These results suggest that the detrimental effects of the $\epsilon4$ allele may be specific to the development of certain symptoms and may lead to differential symptom profiles among concussed athletes.

In another study conducted in our lab, we explored whether the *APOE* $\epsilon4$ allele affects both the presence and severity of headache symptoms in a concussed and nonconcussed sample of collegiate athletes (Merritt, Ukueberuwa, & Arnett, 2016). The results of this study showed that in the concussed sample (when evaluated within 3 months postinjury), having an $\epsilon4$ allele was associated with the presence of headache symptoms, as well as greater headache severity. Conversely, within the nonconcussed athlete sample, no relationship was identified between the $\epsilon4$ allele and headache presence and severity, suggesting that there may be a meaningful interaction between having an $\epsilon4$ allele and sustaining a concussion. Stated differently, the results from this study suggest that in the absence of a concussion, having an $\epsilon4$ allele has little influence on the development of headache symptoms; however, when an athlete sustains a concussion and has an $\epsilon4$ allele, headache symptoms are more likely to be reported and experienced at a greater severity level.

Other studies outside of the sports concussion literature have also found a detrimental influence of the $\epsilon4$ allele on postconcussion symptoms. Ariza et al. (2006) examined postconcussion symptoms using the Neurobehavioral Rating Scale—Revised in a sample of patients with moderate to severe TBI. Ariza and colleagues (2006) reported that compared with patients without the $\epsilon4$ allele, patients with the $\epsilon4$ allele endorsed a greater amount of symptoms across all symptom domains, including executive/cognition, positive symptoms, negative symptoms, mood/affect, and oral- and motor-related symptoms 6 months after sustaining a TBI.

In contrast to the preceding studies, others have concluded that there is not a link between the $\epsilon4$ allele and postconcussion symptoms. Chamelian, Reis, and Feinstein (2004) examined a range of outcome variables at 6 months postinjury, including self-reported symptoms as assessed by the Rivermead Post-Concussion Symptoms Questionnaire, in a sample of patients with mild to moderate TBI. Their group found no differences in symptom reporting between $\epsilon4+$ and $\epsilon4-$participants, concluding that the $\epsilon4$ allele does not appear to influence outcome after TBI. In a study examining children (aged 8–15 years) with mild TBI, Moran et al. (2009) reported no differences in symptom reporting at 3 and 12 months postinjury when comparing ε4+ and ε4–participants. In this study, symptoms were evaluated using the Post-Concussive Symptom Interview and the Health Behavior Inventory, and both child and parent ratings of symptoms were obtained. It is likely that the disparate findings may be a function of the heterogeneity in the samples studied.

With respect to *APOE* and neurocognitive outcomes after concussion or TBI, the majority of published studies have examined whether there are differences between ε4+ and ε4–participants with respect to mean level cognitive performance. In a study examining patients with moderate to severe TBI 6 months postinjury, Ariza et al. (2006) reported that those with the ε4 allele performed more poorly on tests of learning, memory, and executive functioning than patients without the ε4 allele. Others have found similar effects of the ε4 allele when evaluating cognitive performance between 3 and 8 weeks postinjury (Crawford et al., 2002; Liberman, Stewart, Wesnes, & Troncoso, 2002). Sundström et al. (2004) evaluated within-person change by comparing TBI patients' pre- and postinjury neurocognitive scores. Their results showed that ε4+ patients showed significantly poorer postinjury performance compared to preinjury performance, whereas ε4–patients did not demonstrate significant changes between pre- and postinjury assessments. Aside from these studies, however, many others have found no relationship between having an ε4 allele and neurocognitive performance following TBI at various time points following injury (Chamelian et al., 2004; Millar et al., 2003; Padgett, Summers, Vickers, McCormack, & Skilbeck, 2016; Ponsford, Rudzki, Bailey, & Ng, 2007), and in fact, two studies demonstrated that having an ε4 allele was associated with *better* neurocognitive performance on at least one measure following brain injury (Han et al., 2007; Moran et al., 2009).

Within the sports-concussion literature, Kutner, Erlanger, Tsai, Jordan, and Relkin (2000) examined professional football players of varying ages with and without the ε4 allele and reported that ε4+ athletes performed worse on cognitive measures than ε4–athletes. Additionally, the study showed that older athletes with the ε4 allele performed worse on the cognitive measures than younger players of any genotype (Kutner et al., 2000). Importantly, however, this study did not examine recently concussed athletes but instead studied professional football players who may have had a history of concussion.

To our knowledge, the only other published study examining the *APOE* gene in the context of sports concussion was conducted in our lab. We specifically sought to examine the relationship between ε4 genotype and neurocognitive outcomes by assessing whether ε4+ and ε4–athletes differ in their cognitive performance following concussion (Merritt, Rabinowitz, & Arnett, 2018). In addition to examining mean level performance between allele groups, we also assessed the number of impaired scores obtained on cognitive testing following concussion. Our results showed that although there was no association between having an ε4 allele and mean neurocognitive performance, athletes with an ε4 allele were more likely than athletes without an ε4 allele to have at least three impaired scores postconcussion. Finally, we evaluated neurocognitive performance variability following concussion and our results indicated that ε4+ athletes exhibited greater performance variability than ε4–athletes (Merritt et al., 2018). These findings suggest that those with an ε4 allele, compared with those without an ε4 allele, may exhibit less efficient cognitive processing following concussion.

COMT Gene

Function

One potential candidate gene that has been extensively studied in healthy populations and has been linked to cognition is the COMT gene, which has more recently begun to receive attention in the TBI literature. The COMT gene is involved in the production of the COMT enzyme, which is responsible for the metabolic breakdown of catecholamines such as dopamine (Dickinson & Elvevåg, 2009; Savitz et al., 2006; Weinberger et al., 2001). The COMT gene is located on the long arm of chromosome 22, and a single nucleotide polymorphism of this gene exists where valine (*Val*) is substituted for methionine (*Met*); the result is three functional polymorphisms: *Val/Val, Val/Met,* and *Met/Met* (Savitz et al., 2006; Weinberger et al., 2001). The *Val* and *Met* alleles differentially affect cortical dopamine metabolism; the *Val* allele is associated with high enzymatic activity, resulting in reduced cortical dopamine, and the *Met* allele is associated with low enzymatic activity, resulting in greater availability of cortical dopamine (Dickinson & Elvevåg, 2009; Jordan, 2007). Given the interplay between dopamine and prefrontal cognitive functioning, it has been proposed that the COMT gene may have a unique influence on cognitive tasks mediated by this region—that is, executive functions (Egan et al., 2001; Meyer-Lindenberg & Weinberger, 2006).

Neuropsychological Outcomes

Although the COMT gene has been well studied in healthy populations, exploring the influence of the COMT gene on cognitive functioning following concussion and TBI is a relatively new area of investigation. To our knowledge, only three published TBI studies have examined this relationship, with varying results. Lipsky et al. (2005) studied a group of 113 military service members who had sustained mild, moderate, or severe TBIs and were evaluated via neuropsychological testing within 1 year after injury. The authors evaluated several measures of executive functioning, including the Wisconsin Card Sorting Test (WCST), Stroop, Trail Making Test (TMT) A and B, Controlled Oral Word Association Test (COWAT), and Animal Naming, to determine whether the COMT genotype was differentially related to cognitive performance. Lipsky et al. (2005) reported that the number of perseverative responses on the WCST yielded a significant difference between genotype groups, with those homozygous for Val demonstrating the greatest number of errors and those homozygous for Met demonstrating the fewest number of errors.

Flashman, Saykin, Rhodes, and McAllister (2004) investigated a group of 39 mild-to-moderate TBI patients and 27 healthy control participants. Similar to Lipsky et al. (2005), several measures of executive function were administered to determine whether there were genetic differences between COMT Val and Met allele carriers. The authors reported that compared with healthy control participants, patients with TBI demonstrated worse executive functioning, but moreover, participants with the Val allele performed more poorly on the reaction time component of the Continuous Performance Test than participants with the Met allele (Flashman et al., 2004).

Most recently, Willmott, Withiel, Ponsford, and Burke (2014) examined 223 patients with moderate to severe TBI and evaluated whether the COMT gene differentially affected neuropsychological performance in the acute recovery period following TBI. Outcome measures included tests of executive functioning, attention, working memory, processing speed, and learning and memory. The authors also sought to determine whether the COMT gene had any influence on longer term functional outcomes post-TBI as determined by the Extended GOS. In contrast to the foregoing studies, Willmott et al. (2014) reported no significant differences between Val and Met allele carriers on any of the neuropsychological measures evaluated acutely (on average, participants were tested 29 days postinjury), nor did they find any differences on functional outcomes at 12 and 24 months postinjury. The authors concluded that there was insufficient evidence in their study to show that the COMT genotype is related to cognitive outcomes following brain injury.

Importantly, the studies reviewed here did not focus exclusively on mild TBI and instead included participants with moderate to severe TBI in their analyses. This caveat needs to be considered when interpreting the findings. To more fully understand the effects of the COMT gene on neuropsychological performance following TBI and concussion, it will be necessary for more research to be conducted. At present, no published studies have examined COMT in the sports concussion literature, but recent work in our lab has started to explore such relationships. As more investigators examine the COMT gene and its association with concussion outcomes, we will begin to develop a more complete understanding of what role the COMT gene plays in postconcussion neuropsychological performance.

Other Potential Candidate Genes

As noted earlier, several other genes or gene variants have been hypothesized to be associated with outcome following TBI. These include *BDNF*, *5-HTT*, *DRD2*, *DAT*, *NET*, and *DBH*. Not surprisingly, these genes have not been examined within the context of sports-related concussion, and only a limited number of studies have examined the relationship between these genes and outcome post-TBI. Discussion of these studies goes beyond the scope of this chapter, but the interested reader can refer to Dardiotis et al. (2010) and McAllister (2009) for more information.

CONCLUSIONS AND FUTURE DIRECTIONS

When considering the current state of the literature on the relationship between genetic factors and neuropsychological outcomes following sports concussion, it is evident that this is an area of research in need of further development. Even when considering the broader TBI literature, our understanding of genetic influences on neuropsychological variables is limited. Among the genes that have been studied, the *APOE* gene has received the most attention. Although the literature is somewhat mixed, there does appear to be some evidence to suggest that the ε4 allele of the *APOE* gene plays an important role in neuropsychological outcomes postconcussion.

One of the most compelling findings that resulted from the studies that have been conducted within the sports concussion literature is that the ε4 allele appears to influence neuropsychological outcomes only *after* a concussion is sustained, suggesting that there is an interdependent relationship between the ε4 allele and the presence of neurological insult (i.e., concussion). Furthermore, when considering the range of symptoms that are often endorsed after concussion, this review suggests that the symptoms most influenced by the ε4 allele are physical and cognitive-related symptoms. Given these findings, it is conceivable that those who are ε4+ may be more susceptible to experiencing symptoms that are a direct result of the "neurometabolic cascade" that ensues following concussion (Giza & Hovda, 2001, 2014) and that a hierarchy of symptoms exists whereby some symptoms (i.e., physical and cognitive symptoms) are a direct result of the concussive hit, and other symptoms (i.e., affective and sleep symptoms) develop as secondary factors. If this is true, studying genetic factors could bring about important implications for understanding the origin and development of the controversial "postconcussion syndrome" and could help improve diagnostic classification criteria.

Furthermore, when evaluating the relationship between the *APOE* gene and neurocognitive performance in concussed athletes, the findings suggest that assessing impaired scores, as well as performance variability, may be a more sensitive method for detecting genetic influences on neurocognitive functioning. Specifically, results from our lab indicate that the ε4 allele may globally affect CNS functioning and thereby interfere with efficient cognitive processing, resulting in more impairment and increased intraindividual variability across tests. Of course, these findings will need to be replicated, but the present data suggest that an important relationship exists between the ε4 allele of the *APOE* gene and neurocognitive performance after sports-related concussion.

Although the sports concussion literature is currently limited when it comes to examining genetic factors, it is anticipated that this area of research will significantly increase in the near future. The present data suggest that continuing to explore genetic factors within the context of brain injury is a worthy endeavor, especially within the domain of sports concussion. Future research should not only continue to examine the *APOE* gene within the context of collegiate athletes, but it would be beneficial to expand this research to both older and younger athlete samples. Furthermore, it will be necessary to expand our understanding of the *COMT* gene and its relationship to brain injury outcome because evidence suggests that this gene likely influences postconcussion neuropsychological functioning. Beyond the *APOE* and *COMT* genotypes, we would benefit from a greater understanding of how other genes may play a role in concussion outcome (*BDNT, 5-HTT, COMT, DAT*, etc.), and it would be advantageous to eventually examine the effects of gene × gene interactions on neuropsychological outcomes. The exploration of genetic factors is a promising area of research and has important clinical implications for those susceptible to brain injury. By continuing this line of research, it seems promising that we may be able to make more informed decisions about concussion management and may be able to better inform return to play decisions after sports concussion.

CASE STUDY

For the purpose of illustrating how genetics may influence neuropsychological outcome following brain injury, we have outlined in this section the neuropsychological profile of two concussed college athletes: one athlete with two *APOE* ε4 alleles and another without any *APOE* ε4 alleles. Of note, both athletes were administered the same neuropsychological test battery.

Note. Some of the original details of these cases have been changed to protect the confidentiality of the individual tested.

Case 1: Female Soccer Athlete

APOE Genotype: ε4, ε4

At the time this 20-year-old woman was tested, she was approximately 5 days postinjury. She sustained her injury when she experienced a head-to-head hit with an opposing player. She denied loss of consciousness and any anterograde or retrograde amnesia. Before this injury, she had a history of one concussion that occurred when she was 19 years old.

At the time of her concussion, the athlete recalled experiencing the following symptoms rated on a scale of 0 to 6, where 0 is *none* and 6 is *severe*: disorientation (3), dizziness (2), balance problems (4), mental fogginess (4), and problems with attention and concentration (4). By 30 minutes postinjury, she reported nausea (2), balance problems (2), sensitivity to light (2), continued mental fogginess and problems with sustained attention and concentration (both 4), and headache (2). At the time of our testing, this athlete reported a number of continuing mild problems with many of these symptoms. She also reported the emergence of sleep problems that were characterized by trouble falling asleep, then waking up at night and having difficulty falling back to sleep due to worry and rumination. The athlete denied significant physical exertion since her injury but noted that when she was walking around, she experienced increased headache and mental fogginess.

For the neuropsychological testing, the athlete scored significantly below baseline on six indices of sustained attention and information processing speed (Vigil Commission Errors, Symbol Digit Modalities Test, Comprehensive Trail-Making Test—2, Digit Span—Forward, Stroop—Word Test, and Pennsylvania State University Cancellation Task), and two indices of verbal memory (Rivermead Behavioral Memory Test—Story—Delayed Recall, Hopkins Verbal Learning Test—Revised—Delayed Recall). Her PCSS score also increased from 0 at baseline to 18 postconcussion. This athlete also reported mild depression symptoms, an increase over her report of no depression at baseline. An objective measure of effort suggested that she put forth good effort toward testing at both time points.

It was recommended that this athlete attend some short-term counseling to help address her worries and mild depression and normalize her postconcussional experience, as well as provide reasonable expectations for a timeline of recovery. It was felt that such treatment to reduce worry would help her sleep better, something that would likely facilitate a more rapid recovery from her concussion. It was also recommended that she be referred back for testing when her PCSS score was closer to her baseline.

Case 2: Female Soccer Athlete

APOE Genotype: ε3, ε3

At the time this 18-year-old woman was tested, she was 3 days postinjury. She sustained her injury from a head-to-head hit with an opponent during a soccer match. She denied loss of consciousness or any anterograde amnesia but reported about 5 minutes of retrograde amnesia. She reported mild to moderate postconcussion symptoms immediately after the impact, including dizziness (4 out of 6 where 0 is *none* and 6 is *severe*), visual disturbance (3), pressure in the head (5), problems with attention (2), and headache (2). At the time of our testing, this athlete reported only continued sensitivity to noise (3), and headache (2). The athlete denied significant physical exertion since her injury. Before this injury, she had never had a concussion.

For the neuropsychological testing, the athlete displayed significant declines from baseline on two indices of sustained attention (Vigil Commission Errors and Digit Span—Backward). She reported some current postconcussion symptoms, but this report of symptoms (PCSS = 4) was actually lower than what she had reported at baseline (PCSS = 20). Relatedly, although she reported mild depression at baseline, she denied significant depression at the time of our testing. The athlete displayed adequate effort on testing at baseline and at the time of our current testing, so performance on testing was thought to be an accurate representation of her cognitive abilities. Given that the base rate of decline on our neurocognitive test battery is two or fewer tests, we determined that this athlete was back to her neurocognitive baseline.

When interpreting the preceding neuropsychological profiles, it is evident that there are clear differences between the two athletes with respect to their overall symptom scores and cognitive performance. The athlete who is homozygous for the ε4 allele demonstrated a greater symptom burden than the athlete who did not possess any ε4 alleles. Additionally, the athlete with two ε4 alleles exhibited poorer postinjury cognitive performance compared with the athlete without any ε4 alleles. These case examples are consistent with some of the research reported earlier in the chapter and suggest that having an ε4 allele may predispose individuals to poorer neuropsychological functioning after a brain injury. With all this said, these case comparisons are complicated by the fact that the athlete without any ε4 alleles reported a high level of symptoms on the PCSS at baseline, as well as mild depression. Thus, it is possible that she performed better cognitively postconcussion because any distress or depression she may have experienced at baseline had now resolved. In addition to illustrating the possible importance of allele status in relation to postconcussion outcomes, then, these cases show that possible genetic influences can be potentially confounded by other factors.

CLINICAL TAKE-HOME POINTS

1. *The APOE gene appears to have an influence on neuropsychological outcomes, at least within the acute injury period, after sports concussion.* If this finding continues to be replicated, this may have important implications for athletes' safety and well-being.
2. *The need for individually targeted treatments may be necessary.* It is possible that athletes possessing "risk-factor" genes may benefit from more immediate treatments and psychoeducation regarding concussion recovery.
3. *The ethical implications associated with this research will need to be considered at length, should the current findings be consistently replicated in larger samples.* In particular, it will be necessary to consider how "risk-factor" genes may be associated with concussion susceptibility, prolonged recovery, and later life degeneration.

KEY QUESTIONS TO BE ADDRESSED IN THE NEXT 5 YEARS

1. *How does the APOE gene influence postconcussion neuropsychological outcomes across development (youth/adolescent athletes, college athletes, professional athletes)?* Future research should not only continue to examine the *APOE* gene within the context of collegiate athletes, but it would be beneficial to expand this research to both older and younger athlete samples. Also necessary will be to conduct genetic studies using much larger sample sizes.
2. *How is the COMT gene, as well as other target genes discussed (e.g., BDNF, 5-HTT, DAT), related to neuropsychological performance in concussed athletes?* Given the proposed mechanism and function of these genes, it is plausible that they may modify or influence symptom development and cognitive processing within the context of concussion. Learning more about the extent to which each gene influences neuropsychological performance will enhance our broader understanding of the multitude of factors that influence concussion outcome.
3. *How can gene × gene interactions, as well as gene × environmental interactions, help us to develop a more complete understanding of the extent to which genes influence outcome after concussion?* After developing a better understanding of the

specific genes that affect postconcussion neuropsychological performance, it would be advantageous to examine how these relevant genes interact with one another, as well as with pertinent environmental factors.

REFERENCES

Aguilera, M., Barrantes-Vidal, N., Arias, B., Moya, J., Villa, H., Ibáñez, M. I., . . . Fañanás, L. (2008). Putative role of the COMT gene polymorphism (Val158Met) on verbal working memory functioning in a healthy population. *American Journal of Medical Genetics: Part B. Neuropsychiatric Genetics, 147B*, 898–902. http://dx.doi.org/10.1002/ajmg.b.30705

Alexander, S., Kerr, M. E., Kim, Y., Kamboh, M. I., Beers, S. R., & Conley, Y. P. (2007). Apolipoprotein E4 allele presence and functional outcome after severe traumatic brain injury. *Journal of Neurotrauma, 24*, 790–797. http://dx.doi.org/10.1089/neu.2006.0133

Ariza, M., Pueyo, R., Matarín, M. M., Junqué, C., Mataró, M., Clemente, I., . . . Sahuquillo, J. (2006). Influence of APOE polymorphism on cognitive and behavioural outcome in moderate and severe traumatic brain injury. *Journal of Neurology, Neurosurgery & Psychiatry, 77*, 1191–1193. http://dx.doi.org/10.1136/jnnp.2005.085167

Broshek, D. K., Kaushik, T., Freeman, J. R., Erlanger, D., Webbe, F., & Barth, J. T. (2005). Sex differences in outcome following sports-related concussion. *Journal of Neurosurgery, 102*, 856–863. http://dx.doi.org/10.3171/jns.2005.102.5.0856

Chamelian, L., Reis, M., & Feinstein, A. (2004). Six-month recovery from mild to moderate traumatic brain injury: The role of APOE-ε4 allele. *Brain: A Journal of Neurology, 127*, 2621–2628. http://dx.doi.org/10.1093/brain/awh296

Chiang, M.-F., Chang, J.-G., & Hu, C.-J. (2003). Association between apolipoprotein E genotype and outcome of traumatic brain injury. *Acta Neurochirurgica, 145*, 649–653. http://dx.doi.org/10.1007/s00701-003-0069-3

Cicerone, K. D., & Kalmar, K. (1997). Does premorbid depression influence postconcussive symptoms and neuropsychological functioning? *Brain Injury, 11*, 643–648. http://dx.doi.org/10.1080/026990597123197

Cools, R., & D'Esposito, M. (2011). Inverted-U-shaped dopamine actions on human working memory and cognitive control. *Biological Psychiatry, 69*, e113–e125. http://dx.doi.org/10.1016/j.biopsych.2011.03.028

Covassin, T., Elbin, R. J., Harris, W., Parker, T., & Kontos, A. (2012). The role of age and sex in symptoms, neurocognitive performance, and postural stability in athletes after concussion. *The American Journal of Sports Medicine, 40*, 1303–1312. http://dx.doi.org/10.1177/0363546512444554

Crawford, F. C., Vanderploeg, R. D., Freeman, M. J., Singh, S., Waisman, M., Michaels, L., . . . Mullan, M. J. (2002). APOE genotype influences acquisition and recall following traumatic brain injury. *Neurology, 58,* 1115–1118. http://dx.doi.org/10.1212/WNL.58.7.1115

Cropley, V. L., Fujita, M., Innis, R. B., & Nathan, P. J. (2006). Molecular imaging of the dopaminergic system and its association with human cognitive function. *Biological Psychiatry, 59,* 898–907. http://dx.doi.org/10.1016/j.biopsych.2006.03.004

Dardiotis, E., Fountas, K. N., Dardioti, M., Xiromerisiou, G., Kapsalaki, E., Tasiou, A., & Hadjigeorgiou, G. M. (2010). Genetic association studies in patients with traumatic brain injury. *Neurosurgical Focus, 28,* E9.

Diaz-Asper, C. M., Goldberg, T. E., Kolachana, B. S., Straub, R. E., Egan, M. F., & Weinberger, D. R. (2008). Genetic variation in catechol-O-methyltransferase: Effects on working memory in schizophrenic patients, their siblings, and healthy controls. *Biological Psychiatry, 63,* 72–79. http://dx.doi.org/10.1016/j.biopsych.2007.03.031

Dickinson, D., & Elvevåg, B. (2009). Genes, cognition and brain through a COMT lens. *Neuroscience, 164,* 72–87. http://dx.doi.org/10.1016/j.neuroscience.2009.05.014

Echemendia, R. J., Putukian, M., Mackin, R. S., Julian, L., & Shoss, N. (2001). Neuropsychological test performance prior to and following sports-related mild traumatic brain injury. *Clinical Journal of Sport Medicine, 11,* 23–31. http://dx.doi.org/10.1097/00042752-200101000-00005

Egan, M. F., Goldberg, T. E., Kolachana, B. S., Callicott, J. H., Mazzanti, C. M., Straub, R. E., . . . Weinberger, D. R. (2001). Effect of COMT Val108/158 Met genotype on frontal lobe function and risk for schizophrenia. *Proceedings of the National Academy of Sciences of the United States of America, 98,* 6917–6922. http://dx.doi.org/10.1073/pnas.111134598

Eichner, J. E., Dunn, S. T., Perveen, G., Thompson, D. M., Stewart, K. E., & Stroehla, B. C. (2002). Apolipoprotein E polymorphism and cardiovascular disease: A HuGE review. *American Journal of Epidemiology, 155,* 487–495. http://dx.doi.org/10.1093/aje/155.6.487

Farrer, L. A., Cupples, L. A., Haines, J. L., Hyman, B., Kukull, W. A., Mayeux, R., . . . van Duijn, C. M. (1997). Effects of age, sex, and ethnicity on the association between apolipoprotein E genotype and Alzheimer disease: A meta-analysis. *JAMA, 278,* 1349–1356. http://dx.doi.org/10.1001/jama.1997.03550160069041

Field, M., Collins, M. W., Lovell, M. R., & Maroon, J. (2003). Does age play a role in recovery from sports-related concussion? A comparison of high school and collegiate athletes. *The Journal of Pediatrics, 142,* 546–553. http://dx.doi.org/10.1067/mpd.2003.190

Flashman, L. A., Saykin, A. J., Rhodes, C. H., & McAllister, T. W. (2004). Effect of COMT Val/Met genotype on frontal lobe functioning in traumatic brain injury. *The Journal of Neuropsychiatry and Clinical Neurosciences, 16,* 238–239.

Friedman, G., Froom, P., Sazbon, L., Grinblatt, I., Shochina, M., Tsenter, J., . . . Groswasser, Z. (1999). Apolipoprotein E-ε4 genotype predicts a poor outcome in survivors of traumatic brain injury. *Neurology, 52,* 244–248. http://dx.doi.org/10.1212/WNL.52.2.244

Giza, C. C., & Hovda, D. A. (2001). The neurometabolic cascade of concussion. *Journal of Athletic Training, 36,* 228–235.

Giza, C. C., & Hovda, D. A. (2014). The new neurometabolic cascade of concussion. *Neurosurgery, 75,* S24–S33.

Goldberg, T. E., Egan, M. F., Gscheidle, T., Coppola, R., Weickert, T., Kolachana, B. S., . . . Weinberger, D. R. (2003). Executive subprocesses in working memory: Relationship to catechol-O-methyltransferase Val158Met genotype and schizophrenia. *Archives of General Psychiatry, 60,* 889–896. http://dx.doi.org/10.1001/archpsyc.60.9.889

Guskiewicz, K. M., McCrea, M., Marshall, S. W., Cantu, R. C., Randolph, C., Barr, W., . . . Kelly, J. P. (2003). Cumulative effects associated with recurrent concussion in collegiate football players: The NCAA Concussion Study. *JAMA, 290,* 2549–2555. http://dx.doi.org/10.1001/jama.290.19.2549

Guskiewicz, K. M., Weaver, N. L., Padua, D. A., & Garrett, W. E., Jr. (2000). Epidemiology of concussion in collegiate and high school football players. *The American Journal of Sports Medicine, 28,* 643–650. http://dx.doi.org/10.1177/03635465000280050401

Han, S. D., Drake, A. I., Cessante, L. M., Jak, A. J., Houston, W. S., Delis, D. C., . . . Bondi, M. W. (2007). Apolipoprotein E and traumatic brain injury in a military population: Evidence of a neuropsychological compensatory mechanism? *Journal of Neurology, Neurosurgery & Psychiatry, 78,* 1103–1108. http://dx.doi.org/10.1136/jnnp.2006.108183

Iverson, G. L., Brooks, B. L., Collins, M. W., & Lovell, M. R. (2006). Tracking neuropsychological recovery following concussion in sport. *Brain Injury, 20,* 245–252. http://dx.doi.org/10.1080/02699050500487910

Jennett, B., & Bond, M. (1975). Assessment of outcome after severe brain damage. A practical scale. *The Lancet, 1,* 480–484. http://dx.doi.org/10.1016/S0140-6736(75)92830-5

Jordan, B. D. (2007). Genetic influences on outcome following traumatic brain injury. *Neurochemical Research, 32,* 905–915. http://dx.doi.org/10.1007/s11064-006-9251-3

Kontos, A. P., Elbin, R. J., Schatz, P., Covassin, T., Henry, L., Pardini, J., & Collins, M. W. (2012). A revised factor structure for the Post-Concussion Symptom Scale: Baseline and postconcussion factors. *The American Journal of Sports Medicine, 40,* 2375–2384. http://dx.doi.org/10.1177/0363546512455400

Kristman, V. L., Tator, C. H., Kreiger, N., Richards, D., Mainwaring, L., Jaglal, S., . . . Comper, P. (2008). Does the apolipoprotein ε4 allele predispose varsity athletes to concussion? A prospective cohort study. *Clinical Journal of Sport Medicine, 18,* 322–328. http://dx.doi.org/10.1097/JSM.0b013e31817e6f3e

Kutner, K. C., Erlanger, D. M., Tsai, J., Jordan, B., & Relkin, N. R. (2000). Lower cognitive performance of older football players possessing apolipoprotein E ε4. *Neurosurgery, 47*, 651–657. http://dx.doi.org/10.1097/00006123-200009000-00026

Lange, R. T., Brickell, T., French, L. M., Ivins, B., Bhagwat, A., Pancholi, S., & Iverson, G. L. (2013). Risk factors for postconcussion symptom reporting after traumatic brain injury in U.S. military service members. *Journal of Neurotrauma, 30*, 237–246. http://dx.doi.org/10.1089/neu.2012.2685

Lau, B. C., Collins, M. W., & Lovell, M. R. (2011). Sensitivity and specificity of subacute computerized neurocognitive testing and symptom evaluation in predicting outcomes after sports-related concussion. *The American Journal of Sports Medicine, 39*, 1209–1216. http://dx.doi.org/10.1177/0363546510392016

Lau, B. C., Collins, M. W., & Lovell, M. R. (2012). Cutoff scores in neurocognitive testing and symptom clusters that predict protracted recovery from concussions in high school athletes. *Neurosurgery, 70*, 371–379. http://dx.doi.org/10.1227/NEU.0b013e31823150f0

Lau, B. C., Kontos, A. P., Collins, M. W., Mucha, A., & Lovell, M. R. (2011). Which on-field signs/symptoms predict protracted recovery from sport-related concussion among high school football players? *The American Journal of Sports Medicine, 39*, 2311–2318. http://dx.doi.org/10.1177/0363546511410655

Liaquat, I., Dunn, L. T., Nicoll, J. A. R., Teasdale, G. M., & Norrie, J. D. (2002). Effect of apolipoprotein E genotype on hematoma volume after trauma. *Journal of Neurosurgery, 96*, 90–96. http://dx.doi.org/10.3171/jns.2002.96.1.0090

Liberman, J. N., Stewart, W. F., Wesnes, K., & Troncoso, J. (2002). Apolipoprotein E ε4 and short-term recovery from predominantly mild brain injury. *Neurology, 58*, 1038–1044. http://dx.doi.org/10.1212/WNL.58.7.1038

Lipsky, R. H., Sparling, M. B., Ryan, L. M., Xu, K., Salazar, A. M., Goldman, D., & Warden, D. L. (2005). Association of COMT Val158Met genotype with executive functioning following traumatic brain injury. *The Journal of Neuropsychiatry and Clinical Neurosciences, 17*, 465–471. http://dx.doi.org/10.1176/jnp.17.4.465

Lovell, M. R., Iverson, G. L., Collins, M. W., Podell, K., Johnston, K. M., Pardini, D., . . . Maroon, J. C. (2006). Measurement of symptoms following sports-related concussion: Reliability and normative data for the post-concussion scale. *Applied Neuropsychology, 13*, 166–174. http://dx.doi.org/10.1207/s15324826an1303_4

Mahley, R. W., Weisgraber, K. H., & Huang, Y. (2006). Apolipoprotein E4: A causative factor and therapeutic target in neuropathology, including Alzheimer's disease. *Proceedings of the National Academy of Sciences of the United States of America, 103*, 5644–5651. http://dx.doi.org/10.1073/pnas.0600549103

Malhotra, A. K., Kestler, L. J., Mazzanti, C., Bates, J. A., Goldberg, T., & Goldman, D. (2002). A functional polymorphism in the COMT gene and performance on a test of prefrontal cognition. *The American Journal of Psychiatry, 159*, 652–654. http://dx.doi.org/10.1176/appi.ajp.159.4.652

McAllister, T. W. (2009). Genetic factors. In J. M. Silver, T. W. McAllister, & S. C. Yudofsky (Eds.), *Textbook of traumatic brain injury* (2nd ed., pp. 37–54). Arlington, VA: American Psychiatric Publishing.

McClincy, M. P., Lovell, M. R., Pardini, J., Collins, M. W., & Spore, M. K. (2006). Recovery from sports concussion in high school and collegiate athletes. *Brain Injury, 20,* 33–39. http://dx.doi.org/10.1080/02699050500309817

McCrea, M., Guskiewicz, K. M., Marshall, S. W., Barr, W., Randolph, C., Cantu, R. C., . . . Kelly, J. P. (2003). Acute effects and recovery time following concussion in collegiate football players: The NCAA Concussion Study. *JAMA, 290,* 2556–2563. http://dx.doi.org/10.1001/jama.290.19.2556

McCrea, M., Guskiewicz, K., Randolph, C., Barr, W. B., Hammeke, T. A., Marshall, S. W., . . . Kelly, J. P. (2013). Incidence, clinical course, and predictors of prolonged recovery time following sport-related concussion in high school and college athletes. *Journal of the International Neuropsychological Society, 19,* 22–33. http://dx.doi.org/10.1017/S1355617712000872

Meehan, W. P., III, d'Hemecourt, P., & Comstock, R. D. (2010). High school concussions in the 2008–2009 academic year: Mechanism, symptoms, and management. *The American Journal of Sports Medicine, 38,* 2405–2409. http://dx.doi.org/10.1177/0363546510376737

Merritt, V. C., & Arnett, P. A. (2014). Premorbid predictors of postconcussion symptoms in collegiate athletes. *Journal of Clinical and Experimental Neuropsychology, 36,* 1098–1111. http://dx.doi.org/10.1080/13803395.2014.983463

Merritt, V. C., & Arnett, P. A. (2016). Apolipoprotein E (APOE) ε4 allele is associated with increased symptom reporting following sports concussion. *Journal of the International Neuropsychological Society, 22,* 89–94. http://dx.doi.org/10.1017/S1355617715001022

Merritt, V. C., Rabinowitz, A. R., & Arnett, P. A. (2015). Injury-related predictors of symptom severity following sports-related concussion. *Journal of Clinical and Experimental Neuropsychology, 37,* 265–275. http://dx.doi.org/10.1080/13803395.2015.1004303

Merritt, V. C., Rabinowitz, A. R., & Arnett, P. A. (2018). The influence of the apolipoprotein E (APOE) gene on subacute post-concussion neurocognitive performance in college athletes. *Archives of Clinical Neuropsychology, 33,* 36–46. http://dx.doi.org/10.1093/arclin/acx051

Merritt, V. C., Ukueberuwa, D. M., & Arnett, P. A. (2016). Relationship between the apolipoprotein E gene and headache following sports-related concussion. *Journal of Clinical and Experimental Neuropsychology, 38,* 941–949. http://dx.doi.org/10.1080/13803395.2016.1177491

Meyer-Lindenberg, A., & Weinberger, D. R. (2006). Intermediate phenotypes and genetic mechanisms of psychiatric disorders. *Nature Reviews Neuroscience, 7,* 818–827. http://dx.doi.org/10.1038/nrn1993

Millar, K., Nicoll, J. A. R., Thornhill, S., Murray, G. D., & Teasdale, G. M. (2003). Long term neuropsychological outcome after head injury: Relation to APOE genotype. *Journal of Neurology, Neurosurgery & Psychiatry, 74*, 1047–1052. http://dx.doi.org/10.1136/jnnp.74.8.1047

Moran, L. M., Taylor, H. G., Ganesalingam, K., Gastier-Foster, J. M., Frick, J., Bangert, B., . . . Yeates, K. O. (2009). Apolipoprotein E4 as a predictor of outcomes in pediatric mild traumatic brain injury. *Journal of Neurotrauma, 26*, 1489–1495. http://dx.doi.org/10.1089/neu.2008.0767

Nathoo, N., Chetty, R., van Dellen, J. R., Connolly, C., & Naidoo, R. (2003). Apolipoprotein E polymorphism and outcome after closed traumatic brain injury: Influence of ethnic and regional differences. *Journal of Neurosurgery, 98*, 302–306. http://dx.doi.org/10.3171/jns.2003.98.2.0302

Padgett, C. R., Summers, M. J., Vickers, J. C., McCormack, G. H., & Skilbeck, C. E. (2016). Exploring the effect of the apolipoprotein E (APOE) gene on executive function, working memory, and processing speed during the early recovery period following traumatic brain injury. *Journal of Clinical and Experimental Neuropsychology, 38*, 551–560. http://dx.doi.org/10.1080/13803395.2015.1137557

Pellman, E. J., Lovell, M. R., Viano, D. C., & Casson, I. R. (2006). Concussion in professional football: Recovery of NFL and high school athletes assessed by computerized neuropsychological testing—Part 12. *Neurosurgery, 58*, 263–274. http://dx.doi.org/10.1227/01.NEU.0000200272.56192.62

Ponsford, J., Cameron, P., Fitzgerald, M., Grant, M., Mikocka-Walus, A., & Schönberger, M. (2012). Predictors of postconcussive symptoms 3 months after mild traumatic brain injury. *Neuropsychology, 26*, 304–313. http://dx.doi.org/10.1037/a0027888

Ponsford, J., Rudzki, D., Bailey, K., & Ng, K. T. (2007). Impact of apolipoprotein gene on cognitive impairment and recovery after traumatic brain injury. *Neurology, 68*, 619–620. http://dx.doi.org/10.1212/01.wnl.0000254609.04330.9d

Ponsford, J., Willmott, C., Rothwell, A., Cameron, P., Kelly, A. M., Nelms, R., . . . Ng, K. (2000). Factors influencing outcome following mild traumatic brain injury in adults. *Journal of the International Neuropsychological Society, 6*, 568–579. http://dx.doi.org/10.1017/S1355617700655066

Roses, A. D. (1996). Apolipoprotein E alleles as risk factors in Alzheimer's disease. *Annual Review of Medicine, 47*, 387–400. http://dx.doi.org/10.1146/annurev.med.47.1.387

Savitz, J., Solms, M., & Ramesar, R. (2006). The molecular genetics of cognition: Dopamine, COMT and BDNF. *Genes, Brain & Behavior, 5*, 311–328. http://dx.doi.org/10.1111/j.1601-183X.2005.00163.x

Sundström, A., Marklund, P., Nilsson, L. G., Cruts, M., Adolfsson, R., Van Broeckhoven, C., & Nyberg, L. (2004). APOE influences on neuropsychological function after mild head injury: Within-person comparisons. *Neurology, 62*, 1963–1966. http://dx.doi.org/10.1212/01.WNL.0000129268.83927.A8

Teasdale, G. M., Murray, G. D., & Nicoll, J. A. R. (2005). The association between APOE ε4, age and outcome after head injury: A prospective cohort study. *Brain: A Journal of Neurology, 128*, 2556–2561. http://dx.doi.org/10.1093/brain/awh595

Teasdale, G. M., Nicoll, J. A. R., Murray, G., & Fiddes, M. (1997). Association of apolipoprotein E polymorphism with outcome after head injury. *The Lancet, 350*, 1069–1071. http://dx.doi.org/10.1016/S0140-6736(97)04318-3

Terrell, T. R., Bostick, R. M., Abramson, R., Xie, D., Barfield, W., Cantu, R., . . . Ewing, T. (2008). APOE, APOE promoter, and Tau genotypes and risk for concussion in college athletes. *Clinical Journal of Sport Medicine, 18*, 10–17. http://dx.doi.org/10.1097/JSM.0b013e31815c1d4c

Tierney, R. T., Mansell, J. L., Higgins, M., McDevitt, J. K., Toone, N., Gaughan, J. P., . . . Krynetskiy, E. (2010). Apolipoprotein E genotype and concussion in college athletes. *Clinical Journal of Sport Medicine, 20*, 464–468. http://dx.doi.org/10.1097/JSM.0b013e3181fc0a81

Weinberger, D. R., Egan, M. F., Bertolino, A., Callicott, J. H., Mattay, V. S., Lipska, B. K., . . . Goldberg, T. E. (2001). Prefrontal neurons and the genetics of schizophrenia. *Biological Psychiatry, 50*, 825–844. http://dx.doi.org/10.1016/S0006-3223(01)01252-5

Willemse-van Son, A. H. P., Ribbers, G. M., Hop, W. C. J., van Duijn, C. M., & Stam, H. J. (2008). Association between apolipoprotein-ε4 and long-term outcome after traumatic brain injury. *Journal of Neurology, Neurosurgery & Psychiatry, 79*, 426–430. http://dx.doi.org/10.1136/jnnp.2007.129460

Willmott, C., Withiel, T., Ponsford, J., & Burke, R. (2014). COMT Val158Met and cognitive and functional outcomes after traumatic brain injury. *Journal of Neurotrauma, 31*, 1507–1514. http://dx.doi.org/10.1089/neu.2013.3308

Wilson, M., & Montgomery, H. (2007). Impact of genetic factors on outcome from brain injury. *British Journal of Anaesthesia, 99*, 43–48. http://dx.doi.org/10.1093/bja/aem142

5

NEUROIMAGING AND SPORTS-RELATED CONCUSSION

EMILY C. GROSSNER, ANDREW R. MAYER,
AND FRANK G. HILLARY

Given the diagnostic and prognostic uncertainties associated with sports-related mild traumatic brain injury (mTBI or concussion, with these terms used interchangeably in this chapter), there has been recent emphasis on electrophysiological and neuroimaging methods to provide novel insights into the brain changes associated with it. The goal of this chapter is to describe the primary findings from the literature using advanced neuroimaging methods to understand the structural, functional, and metabolic brain changes occurring after sports-related concussion (SRC)—in particular, with respect to how those markers predict cognition and recovery. For our purposes, *functional* brain imaging refers to the study of dynamic cerebral processes, including magnetoencephalography and blood oxygen level–dependent functional magnetic resonance imaging (BOLD fMRI or fMRI; described subsequently). We also integrate these findings with a growing literature using diffusion

The figure in this chapter was inspired by Figure 4 in Eierud et al. (2014). We thank them for their assistance in creating this figure.

http://dx.doi.org/10.1037/0000114-006
Neuropsychology of Sports-Related Concussion, P. A. Arnett (Editor)

tensor imaging (DTI) and magnetic resonance spectroscopy (MRS) to examine brain structure and metabolism postinjury.

Traditional clinical structural imaging techniques, such as computed tomography (CT) or MRI, do not commonly detect subtle axonal abnormalities or neurochemical cascades occurring secondary to milder forms of TBI (Giza & Hovda, 2001; Shenton et al., 2012), instead have been more traditionally used to detect and track change in gross, macrostructural lesions (Bigler & Maxwell, 2012; Yuh et al., 2013). Functional brain imaging, including fMRI and proton MRS, was introduced as a possible diagnostic approach in mild cases of TBI due to the negative findings in traditional structural imaging (e.g., CT and T1-/T2-weighted MRI), which occur for the majority of patients. Recovery trajectories in SRC have proven particularly thorny. Functional imaging methods such as fMRI have offered unparalleled opportunities to examine the consequences of concussion noninvasively. Investigators have turned to other imaging methods to increase sensitivity in detecting the effects of mTBI. The first mTBI (mixed sports and non–sports-related) study using BOLD fMRI methods was performed in 1999 by McAllister and colleagues. In the nearly 20 years that followed, more than 100 studies have commonly confirmed that TBI results in functional brain alterations, but the nature of these functional brain alterations has varied—in particular, for studies of SRC, leaving investigators without a consistent physiological marker indicative of injury (for a review, see Mayer, Bellgowan, & Hanlon, 2015). It is a goal of this chapter to direct the reader to several common (even competing) themes in the literature and to provide future direction for the use of functional brain imaging to understand concussion-related brain changes.

CONCUSSION DEFINED

As noted elsewhere in this volume, concussion directly results from the application of external forces acting on the head and has a heterogeneous clinical presentation. In the context of functional brain imaging results, this heterogeneity is illustrated nicely in a study by Hutchison, Schweizer, Tam, Graham, and Comper (2014) that presents cases of two male athletes who sustained concussion. Each player was cleared to play in approximately the same amount of time based on normal neuropsychological testing results. Results from fMRI data analysis revealed different patterns of brain activation, with one player displaying greater and more diffuse BOLD activation during two tasks than the other player, regardless of similar symptom presentation and neuropsychological performance (Hutchison et al., 2014). This example highlights a critical limitation to functional brain imaging methods as the sole (or primary) method to identify a concussion biomarker sensitive and specific to injury between clinical cases. Although no specific concussion marker has emerged via functional neuroimaging methods to date, brain imaging methods have provided a number of novel hypotheses regarding how neural systems can adapt to disruption. We therefore focus on patterns of change and recovery in individuals following injury and offer future directions to constrain the hypotheses and methods for research in this area. We first discuss the early "activation" studies focused on deficits in cognitive functioning via task-based methods and then integrate more recent work examining the intrinsic functioning of distributed networks after concussion. Of note, the etiologies, demographics, and psychosocial histories are commonly quite distinct between concussion and non–sports-related mTBI literatures, so we have integrated studies of mTBI only in cases where the samples include concussed athletes (e.g., McAllister et al., 2001; Sours, George, Zhuo, Roys, & Gullapalli, 2015; Sours, Zhuo, Roys, Shanmuganathan, & Gullapalli, 2015). We offer reference to the broader mTBI and even moderate to severe TBI literatures only where relevant to provide context for concussion findings, but our focus in this chapter is on the sports concussion literature.

BRAIN ACTIVATION STUDIES

The earliest functional neuroimaging studies in TBI were in resting studies using positron emission tomography (PET) imaging (for reviews, see Byrnes et al., 2013; Ricker, Hillary, & DeLuca, 2001). However, in the early 1990s, fMRI methods emerged, providing a measurable surrogate for neural firing by capitalizing on the endogenous BOLD contrast, which is a combination of hemodynamic factors that includes blood flow and the relative changes in the ratio of oxyhemoglobin to de-oxyhemoglobin (Bandettini, Wong, Hinks, Tikofsky, & Hyde, 1992; Logothetis, 2008; Logothetis, Pauls, Augath, Trinath, & Oeltermann, 2001; Ogawa, Lee, Kay, & Tank, 1990). After the formative work by McAllister, Saykin, et al. (1999) and McAllister, Sparling, et al. (2001) that leveraged these methods to examine working memory in mTBI, the literature turned to focus on task-based perturbation studies for more than a decade.

Task-based studies offered the opportunity to examine the cognitive, motor, and sensory processes thought to be affected after TBI, and one of the largest of these literatures focused on working memory and processing speed deficits. Early adaptation of the N-back task, a common working memory rehearsal paradigm, to the fMRI environment offered the opportunity to examine working memory deficits in vivo. The N-back task requires participants to hold information in mind and rehearse small pieces of verbal or spatial information (more on the findings using this task follows) and has been used frequently in the SRC literature.

Early work using the N-back revealed that reliable patterns of brain activation could be elicited with this paradigm, including frontoparietal networks for attentional control and stimulus representation (Owen, McMillan, Laird, & Bullmore, 2005). One common finding in moderate and severe TBI and even other neurological disorders (Hillary, 2008; Hillary et al., 2006) is higher activation in the dorsolateral prefrontal cortex, anterior cingulate, and parietal systems associated with attentional-control when during working memory tasks. This finding was later recapitulated in mTBI and concussion (Dettwiler et al., 2014; McAllister et al., 2001; Slobounov, Gay, Johnson, & Zhang, 2012). This "recruitment" of additional neural resources during task processing has not been universally observed in concussion, however, with some examiners noting decreased signal during effortful task processing after concussion. For example, reduced activation associated with a working memory task has been demonstrated in areas such as the dorsal cingulate, ventrolateral prefrontal cortex, and prefrontal cortex (Chen, Johnston, Collie, McCrory, & Ptito, 2007). In a different sample, these same investigators found mixed results, which indicated that concussed individuals had more activation peaks than healthy control subjects, but overall less activation in the dorsolateral prefrontal cortex (Chen et al., 2004).

A review of this literature has revealed that some of these differences may be attributable to the type of task or task load, with greater cognitive control demand requiring increased prefrontal cortex resource use (for a review, see Bryer, Medaglia, Rostami, & Hillary, 2013). Table 5.1 provides a summary of these findings. The interpretation by Bryer and colleagues was supported empirically in a study using a modified N-back paradigm, which required variable cognitive and attentional demands by including conditions with capitalization of letter stimuli and differing spatial positioning (Dettwiler et al., 2014). This study demonstrated that mTBI participants showed higher activation in the left and right dorsolateral prefrontal cortex and left inferior parietal cortex during the 2-back condition than healthy controls (Dettwiler et al., 2014). These results were relatively consistent; prefrontal cortex recruitment was observable in participants with TBI at 2 days and 2 weeks postinjury. In fact, increased activation in the dorsolateral prefrontal cortical areas was relatively stable, persisting even at 2 months postinjury (Dettwiler et al., 2014).

Not all imaging work in concussion has focused on verbal working memory; using a virtual environment to examine spatial navigation and memory, examiners have created scenarios for testing memory dysfunction after mTBI that had greater ecological validity (Slobounov et al., 2010). When navigating through a virtual environment without a specific memorization goal, concussed individuals demonstrated greater BOLD response in the right hippocampus and higher activation in the left dorsolateral prefrontal cortex

TABLE 5.1
Sports-Related Concussion Activation Studies Using fMRI

Study	N		Gender		Mean age (in years)		Mean concussion-imaging time difference	Imaging modality
	Pt	Control	Pt	Control	Pt	Control		
Chen et al. (2004)	16	8	16 M	8 M	26.9 ± 7.2	27.6 ± 5.2	4.7 months	fMRI
Jantzen et al. (2004)	4	4	4 M	4 M	20	20	Unknown	fMRI
Lovell et al. (2007)	28	13	"Largely male"		18.3 ± 3.5	16.6 ± 2.4	Time 1: 6.6 ± 4.7 days; Time 2: 35.1 days	fMRI
Chen et al. (2007)	18	10	18 M	10 M	27.2 ± 5.5 30.8 ± 5.6	21.9 ± 1.6	6.4 ± 8.7; 4.0 ± 2.9 months	fMRI
Chen et al. (2008)	9	6	9 M	6 M	31.7 ± 5.4	20 ± 0.9	Time 1: 3 ± 2 months; Time 2: 14.7 ± 7.6 months	fMRI
Zhang et al. (2010)	15	15		21 M 9 F	20.8 ± 1.7	21.3 ± 1.5	"Within 30 days"	fMRI DTI
Slobounov et al. (2010)	15	15		21 M 9 F	20.8 ± 1.7	21.3 ± 1.5	"Within 30 days"	fMRI
Pardini et al. (2010)	16	NA	6 F, 10 M	NA	16.3	NA	6.5 days	fMRI
Terry et al. (2012)	20	20	20 M	20 M	20.3 ± 1.17	20.4 ± 1.6	19.6 months	fMRI
Hammeke et al. (2013)	12	12	12 M	12 M	16.5 ± 0.52	16.5 ± 0.52	13 hours; 49 days	fMRI
Ford et al. (2013)	27	14	17 M	14 M	63.4 ± 5.9	62.2 ± 6.3	Unknown	fMRI
Dettwiler et al. (2014)	15	15	3 F, 12 M	3 F, 12 M	19.8 ± 0.94	19.8 ± 1.73	2 days; 2 weeks; 2 months	fMRI
Dean et al. (2015)	16	9	9 F, 7 M	5 F, 4 M	26.9	21.9	6.1 years	fMRI DTI MRS

Note. Search terms for the studies in Table 5.1 input into PubMed included *fMRI* + concussion AND task activation. These results comprehensively included studies from prior reviews (Mayer et al., 2015). No studies were included if they did not specify that individuals sustained a concussion from playing a sport. Studies on youth and pediatric concussion were also excluded. DTI = diffusion tensor imaging; F = female; fMRI = functional magnetic resonance imaging; M = male; MRS = magnetic resonance spectroscopy; NA = not applicable; Pt = patient.

and cerebellum (Zhang et al., 2010). When explicitly instructed to encode specific routes within the virtual environment, concussed individuals displayed higher activation in the right dorsolateral prefrontal cortex and the left parietal cortex (Slobounov et al., 2010). Activation patterns were similar for healthy and concussed participants during the retrieval part of the task, thus emphasizing a brain response difference occurring at encoding more so than during retrieval of information. The increased activation in dorsolateral prefrontal cortex in a virtual reality environment mirrors the findings in controlled studies using the N-back, demonstrating increased neural recruitment after injury.

Conceptualizing Activation Patterns

The somewhat paradoxical finding from several studies suggesting that brain injury elicits increased localized brain response has prompted a number of explanations, including brain reorganization and compensatory hypotheses. Brain reorganization hypotheses generally claim that there are permanent changes in the network associated with goal-directed behavior after injury. Given the relatively nonspecific nature of the BOLD signal, these positions may have the least support to date. The most common explanation is that increased activation represents *neural compensation*, which maintains some similarities to brain reorganization, but the increased resource permits task completion without permanently changing the brain.

Others have argued (see Hillary, 2008; Hillary, Genova, Chiaravalloti, et al., 2006; Hillary, Genova, Medaglia, et al., 2010; Scheibel et al., 2003) that increased BOLD response to task after TBI might be a result of the increased role of cognitive control and attentional resources because task demands are more slowly processed. What separates all of these explanations is the role recruitment has for functioning and its relative permanence during moments of task engagement. Recruitment of the prefrontal cortex is now more commonly interpreted as slowed, effortful processing associated with diminished performance that is transient and performance dependent (Hillary et al., 2010; Medaglia et al., 2012). The possible secondary consequences of "hyperactivity" in the brain are addressed again later.

Postconcussive Symptoms and Subconcussive Hits

Functional brain imaging results in the absence of a behavioral reference point are difficult to interpret, so it has been important for investigators to draw specific links between behavioral consequences of concussion with functional imaging findings. Increased symptom severity, as measured by the Post-Concussive Symptom Scale (Lovell & Collins, 1998), has been shown to be associated with an increased BOLD response for the 2-back condition in the premotor cortex and posterior parietal cortex (Pardini et al., 2010). These findings were partially replicated in a separate study showing a relationship between poorer performance on the N-back, higher postconcussive symptom (PCS) scores, and higher activation in the left superior frontal gyrus, bilateral hippocampal gyrus, posterior cingulate gyrus, and precuneus (Smits et al., 2009). When testing memory for abstract words and drawings, a moderate PCS group was less accurate than low PCS and healthy control groups. The healthy control subjects demonstrated higher BOLD activation in the dorsal cingulate and dorsolateral prefrontal cortex and ventrolateral prefrontal cortex, which is consistent with what the authors expected for this type of working memory task (Chen et al., 2007). The low PCS group did not show activation in the dorsolateral prefrontal cortex and the moderate PCS group showed little activation in the frontal lobe overall and showed significant increased activation only in the dorsal cingulate. Additionally, the two concussion groups had increased activation in the left temporal lobe during the working memory task, and the healthy control group did not (Chen et al., 2007). Together, these results demonstrate that more severe symptoms after concussion are associated with decreased accuracy and may be predictive of greater brain response to task perturbation in frontal and temporal regions.

There is emerging evidence for distinct fMRI activation profiles in patients who have experienced subconcussive injuries. Other studies have shown different activation patterns in individuals with head injury when examining working memory. Interestingly, football athletes who were not diagnosed with a concussion but sustained high impact hits during the season and demonstrated decreased postseason neuropsychological test scores had decreased activation in the dorsolateral prefrontal cortex (Talavage et al., 2014). This difference in activation pattern could be due to these athletes more closely resembling healthy control subjects because any injury they sustained did not warrant a formal concussion diagnosis. For a review of activation studies on SRC, see Table 5.1.

FUNCTIONAL CONNECTIVITY STUDIES

The concept of functional connectivity was first introduced in a landmark paper in 1995 by Bharat Biswal (Biswal, Yetkin, Haughton, & Hyde, 1995). However, the concept of intrinsic brain activity was controversial, and the potential impact of these findings went relatively unnoticed in the functional brain imaging literature in favor of task-based paradigms for almost a decade. Resting-state functional connectivity (RSFC) examines the temporal coherence between spatially distinct regions when an individual is not performing an external task (Biswal et al., 2010). RSFC is now at the center of the cognitive neurosciences with focus on understanding the interrelationships between multiple subnetworks communicating within the brain (Fox et al., 2005; Raichle et al., 2001; van den Heuvel & Hulshoff Pol, 2010).

Research using functional connectivity to examine SRC has focused on connectivity to a targeted region of interest (e.g., seed based), as well as approaches that allow whole-brain surveillance of connectivities, or global connectivity (e.g., independent component analyses, voxelwise approaches). Global metrics have been shown to be sensitive to large-scale neurological disruption in other disorders, such as moderate–severe TBI (see Caeyenberghs et al., 2012; Nakamura, Hillary, & Biswal, 2009) and Alzheimer's disease (see Sheline & Raichle, 2013; Tijms et al., 2013). However, in a recent study, global connectivity measures did not produce any significant differences between healthy control participants and concussed athletes, but concussed individuals did demonstrate an increase in regional homogeneity at 1 week and 1 month postinjury in multiple brain areas, including the bilateral postcentral gyrus, bilateral motor areas, right lingual and fusiform gyri, and right middle and superior temporal gyri (Meier, Bellgowan, & Mayer, 2017). These data suggest that global metrics may not have sensitivity to the more subtle effects of concussion, creating a need for analyses with greater nuance considering the symptom severity and time since injury.

Within the RSFC literature several robust subnetworks have been identified to demonstrate synchronous activity across distinct situational demands, for example, task and rest (Bassett, Meyer-Lindenberg, Achard, Duke, & Bullmore, 2006; Salvador et al., 2005; Stam, 2004). These networks provide more targeted analyses of brain disruption after injury, including the widely studied default mode (DMN), the executive control (ECN), and the salience (SN) networks. The DMN has been observed to operate in "anticorrelated" fashion with the ECN as individuals shift in and out of goal-directed behavior (Liang et al., 2013; van den Heuvel & Hulshoff Pol, 2010). The DMN has received significant attention for purported roles in monitoring internal states and semantic processing (e.g., hubs = posterior cingulate cortex and medial frontal cortex; Liang et al., 2013). The ECN includes those subnetworks involved in active task processing (e.g., hubs = lateral prefrontal cortex and inferior parietal lobe).

Functional Connectivity in Concussion

Much like studies focused on localized effects in signal amplitude (i.e., task-induced activation), studies examining functional brain connectivity have not converged at a consistent set of findings. In general, studies reveal regional changes reflecting increases and decreases in functional connections between brain regions after injury (i.e., hyperconnectivity or hypoconnectivity, respectively; for a review, see Chong & Schwedt, 2015). Some studies have demonstrated primarily hyperconnectivity (Abbas et al., 2014; Bharath et al., 2015; Czerniak et al., 2015; Militana et al., 2016), others have shown primarily hypoconnectivity (Mayer et al., 2011; Slobounov et al., 2011; Zhang et al., 2012), but most studies report both findings depending on the regions of interest (Borich, Babul, Yuan, Boyd, & Virji-Babul, 2015; Johnson, Neuberger, et al., 2014; Johnson, Zhang, et al., 2012; Messé et al., 2013; Zhou et al., 2012). For example, in studies demonstrating hyperconnectivity, a group of concussed collegiate athletes who had sustained a concussion during the previous 6 months demonstrated stronger connectivity between the anterior cingulate cortex and the left superior parietal lobe and multiple areas in the frontal lobe (Czerniak et al., 2015). There was also higher connectivity between right and left dorsolateral prefrontal cortex to multiple areas, including temporal structures (Czerniak et al., 2015). Others have shown increased functional connectivity to areas of the DMN, including the anterior and posterior cingulate, hippocampus, precuneus, and ventromedial prefrontal cortex (Borich et al., 2015; Johnson, Zhang, et al., 2012; Militana et al., 2016). These results are consistent with previous findings of increased connectivity in mixed samples of sports-related and non–sports-related mTBI and concussion (Messé et al., 2013; Sours, George, et al., 2015; Sours, Zhuo, et al., 2015). Borich and colleagues' (2015) findings in concussed high school athletes were mixed, including higher connectivity in the posterior cingulate cortex, the right frontal pole, and left frontal operculum cortex, but lower connectivity in the frontal and parietal cortices. Despite the differences in functional connectivity between concussed participants and healthy control subjects, there were no observed significant differences in neuropsychological test performance, indicating that these network adjustments may be subclinical or that they are related to unmeasured cognitive or emotional factors (Czerniak et al., 2015; Militana et al., 2016).

By contrast, Johnson, Zhang, and colleagues (2012) reported primarily decreased connectivity in the frontoparietal areas for athletes who had sustained a greater number of concussions but found increased number and strength of connections in the medial prefrontal cortex. Additionally, others have found decreased connectivity within the medial prefrontal cortical regions of the DMN at 1-month postconcussion (for reviews, see Chong & Schwedt, 2015; Zhou et al., 2012). Zhang and colleagues (2012) reported weaker connections between the posterior cingulate cortex and the medial prefrontal cortex, as well as between the posterior cingulate cortex and the left lateral parietal cortex for concussed athletes who had completed an exercise program. Overall the findings examining neural network changes postconcussion have been mixed (for a review, see Slobounov et al., 2012). Ultimately, the neural network response following injury is likely dependent on several factors, including time postinjury and prior exposure to concussion, as well as the specific regions of interest that are under examination. The lack of consistency may reflect the distinct methods and samples under study in the literature to date. It will be increasingly important for investigators to replicate findings and identify common methods and metrics of analysis so that greater convergence may be achieved.

Interestingly, resting-state fMRI has also revealed differences in connectivity for concussed individuals who were asymptomatic or athletes who played a collision sport but had never been diagnosed with a concussion. Asymptomatic athletes, who had been returned to play 24 hours before the scan, demonstrated overall fewer and weaker connections. They had fewer connections from the posterior cingulate cortex to the dorsolateral prefrontal cortex and the parahippocampal gyrus relative to healthy control subjects. The asymptomatic group demonstrated fewer and weaker connections in the bilateral parietal cortex but had increased and stronger connections in the medial prefrontal cortex than the control group (Johnson, Zhang, et al., 2012). Conversely, football players with no current diagnosed concussion demonstrated significant hyperconnectivity over healthy control subjects and specifically had a greater number of connections during pre- and postseason, as well as months 2 and 3 of the season (Abbas et al., 2014). Johnson and colleagues (2014) demonstrated mixed findings of athletes who sustained subconcussive hits, reporting increased connectivity between orbitofrontal cortices and the left supramarginal gyrus and decreased connectivity between the right retrosplenial cingulate cortex and the right dorsal posterior cingulate cortex. Athletes with a history of previous concussions had overall decreased connectivity, and those with no past concussion had increased connectivity from pre- to postgame (Johnson et al., 2014). These results suggest that there may be alterations in brain network connectivity that persist after players are determined to be symptom-free or in the absence of a formal concussion diagnosis.

The evolution of changes in brain connectivity over time after concussion remains unclear, but this small group of studies indicates that it may take a nonlinear path from regional hypoconnectivity and later hyperconnectivity over the course of the first 6 months postinjury. One summary of the literature is that hyperconnectivity may be more likely to occur in frontal areas after concussion and reduced connectivity is observed in posterior regions of the brain (Chong & Schwedt, 2015). This profile of altered network connectivity converges with the literature in more severe TBI, where the findings have been much more consistent (for empirical work, see Bernier et al., 2017; Caeyenberghs et al., 2012; Hillary, Medaglia, et al., 2011; Hillary, Rajtmajer, et al., 2014; Roy et al., 2017; Palacios et al., 2011; Sharp et al., 2011; Venkatesan et al., 2015; and for a critical review, see Caeyenberghs, Verhelst, Clemente, & Wilson, 2017).

What remains to be determined is the direct link between the evolution of the connectivity response and symptom report; current findings are mixed.

One critical issue for clinical professionals making decisions about early recovery after concussion relates to physical exertion. There is growing evidence that significant physical exertion early after injury results in increased symptom reporting (Slobounov et al., 2011). One study that administered a stress test to athletes and then used RSFC methods to examine network changes revealed less interhemispheric connectivity for the concussed athlete group than the healthy control subjects at all phases of exercise (rest, stress, and recovery; Slobounov et al., 2011). In the hippocampal network, concussed athletes demonstrated reduced connectivity between left and right hippocampus at rest, but this increased during stress and recovery. Both the concussed group and the healthy control subjects demonstrated increased connectivity to the precuneus after stress, but the two groups did not differ in terms of overall connectivity. In the dorsolateral prefrontal cortex, the TBI group had decreased interhemispheric connectivity compared with the healthy control subjects and less connectivity between the dorsolateral prefrontal cortex and the supramarginal gyrus and the bilateral right dorsal frontal cortex (Slobounov et al., 2011). The authors concluded that the reduced interhemispheric connectivity was attributable to damage to the corpus callosum during injury. Consistent with Meier and colleagues (2017), these findings reveal that global changes may be subtle and indicative of connectivity loss, which is not consistent with the regional affects observed in other studies (see Borich et al., 2015; Czerniak et al., 2015; Militana et al., 2016), indicating that if neural systems adapt to injury through enhanced signaling, the effects may be more evident locally. A summary of the studies using fMRI to examine brain related changes post-concussion is available in Table 5.2.

Interpreting Hyperconnectivity and Its Possible Consequences

Overall, investigators have observed increased resource use (hyper-activation–hyperconnectivity), loss of focal and integrated network responses (hypoactivation–hypoconnectivity) in SRC, or, commonly, both of these results (for a review, see Caeyenberghs et al., 2017). These findings are well aligned with the two goals within this literature: (a) to identify loss of brain function due to the physiological (blood flow) or structural/white matter changes after injury, and (b) to determine the brain response to injury (i.e., compensation). The former approach is reminiscent of the "lesion-model," which has dominated the neurological sciences for two centuries and represents the foundation of the cognitive neuropsychology model, pairing specific injury consequences with behavioral outcomes (for reviews, see

TABLE 5.2
Sports-Related Concussion Connectivity Studies Using fMRI

Study	N		Gender		Mean age (in years)		Mean concussion-imaging time difference	Imaging modality
	Pt	Control	Pt	Control	Pt	Control		
Slobounov et al. (2011, 2012)	17	17	35% F, 65% M		21.3 ± 1.5	20.8 ± 1.7	fMRI	fMRI
Johnson, Zhang, et al. (2012)	14	15	9 F, 5 M	8 F, 7 M	20.6 ± 1.2	20.4 ± 0.8	10 days	fMRI
Abbas et al. (2014)	22	10	22 M	10 M	16.7	16.7	NA	fMRI
Czerniak et al. (2015)	9	12	2 F, 7 M	6 F, 5 M	20.3 ± 0.4	20 ± 0.4	112 days	fMRI
Zhu et al. (2015)	8	11	8 M	11 M	20 ± 1.3	20.5 ± 1.8	24 hours; 7 ± 1 day; 30 ± 1 days	fMRI DTI MRS
List et al. (2015)	20	21	2 F, 18 M	2 F, 18 M	25.5 ± 5.3	25.7 ± 5.2	Unknown	fMRI DTI
Meier et al. (2017)	43	51	9 F, 34 M	16 F, 35 M	20.29 ± 1.31	20.26 ± 1.44	1 day; 1 week; 1 month	fMRI

Note. Search terms for the studies in Table 5.2 input into PubMed included *fMRI* + concussion AND connectivity. These results comprehensively included studies from prior reviews (Mayer et al., 2015). No studies were included if they did not specify that individuals sustained a concussion from playing a sport. Studies on youth and pediatric concussion were also excluded. DTI = diffusion tensor imaging; F = female; fMRI = functional magnetic resonance imaging; M = male; MRS = magnetic resonance spectroscopy; NA = not applicable; Pt = patient.

Catani & ffytche, 2005; Geschwind, 1965a, 1965b). One reason for mixed success using a lesion model to understand concussion is that the results of concussion are diffuse and relatively subtle with few identifiable relationships between disruption and behavioral outcome, leaving investigators to speculate about the mechanism for observable brain changes (e.g., diffuse axonal injury). Therefore, a perspective that focuses solely on mapping specific lesions to functional loss scenarios focuses on the functional loss and does not address how the system has adapted to disruption.

If we focus for a moment on the finding that SRC induces local increases in brain activity and even distributed increases in network connections, there are two important additional caveats that one must consider. The first has to do with interpretation. The most common interpretation of additional neural resources, either locally during system perturbation (i.e., task activation) or increased network involvement by hubs, is that this response represents "compensation." Unfortunately, neural compensation as an explanation for a brain response after TBI does not constrain theory or offer testable hypotheses because it is often defined in a way that represents little more than a restatement of the observed effect; that is, due to neurological compromise, more resources are being used (for a history of this problem, see Davis, Dennis, Daselaar, Fleck, & Cabeza, 2008; Dennis & Cabeza, 2011; Hillary, 2008; Medaglia et al., 2012). Moreover, the same explanation is used to describe likely dissociable responses by brain regions, with possibly divergent behavioral consequences. Hyperconnectivity in one network substrate cannot be presumed to have any "compensatory" action without understanding the varied substrates within the subnetwork that are similarly connected. To address the role of increased resource use after mTBI, there must be targeted and serial analysis of specified brain regions after injury tracking change against cognitive or functional changes (or both). For brain connectivity analyses to ultimately be the basis for a biomarker in concussion, more refined hypotheses must be developed regarding the nature of brain responses to injury with specific ties to behavioral outcomes.

A second consideration for increased neural resource use after concussion is that such a response may place increased stress on metabolic resources. Evidence that elevated brain metabolism is associated with unwanted consequences has been intensifying across separate literatures for some time. The brain's most highly connected networks (e.g., DMN) contain nodes with disproportionately high deposition of amyloid beta (Aβ; Buckner et al., 2005), a marker for neurodegeneration. Research in animals (Bero et al., 2012; Busche et al., 2012; Cirrito et al., 2005) and humans (de Haan, Mott, van Straaten, Scheltens, & Stam, 2012; Myers et al., 2014; Vlassenko et al., 2010) has more directly demonstrated that regions with the highest metabolism during normal brain functioning show enhanced Aβ deposition. Corroborating these findings, recent network simulations using a neural mass model reveal that transient increases in activity preceded gradual declines and these effects are disproportionately evident in hub regions (de Haan et al., 2012). Given that TBI has been linked to increased Aβ deposition (see Brody et al., 2008; Scott et al., 2016) and these effects may be predicted by the amount of time that has elapsed since injury in more severe forms of TBI (Scott et al., 2016), the long-term influences of hyperconnectivity after SRC must be examined with a critical eye in particular in individuals with genetic risk for neurodegeneration later in life (for a review of this argument, see Hillary & Grafman, 2017).

DTI STUDIES

DTI is a structural imaging method that examines the movement of water, diffusing in different directions, which can provide information about brain tissue and white matter fiber tracts in the brain (Basser, Mattiello, & LeBihan, 1994). The size and shape of the water diffusion is measured to examine these small structural aspects of the brain tissue and matter. Fractional anisotropy (FA) and mean diffusivity (MD) are two common measurements of the anisotropy and magnitude of the diffusion, respectively. Radial diffusivity (RD) and axial diffusivity (AD) are two additional measurements used in DTI that putatively measure more focal pathology in axons, myelin, and the extracellular environment. DTI is a helpful tool for understanding the effects of concussion on white matter because it is able to detect minute axonal injuries, which might contribute to long-lasting postconcussive symptoms (Shenton et al., 2012).

When used to examine large white matter tracts, such as the genu of the corpus callosum, DTI studies of individuals who have sustained a concussion or mTBI present different findings depending on imaging time postinjury. Several studies using DTI in mTBI samples have demonstrated lower fractional anisotropy in brain areas such as the corpus callosum, internal capsule, and centrum semiovale (Shenton et al., 2012), especially when considered during the chronic phase (see Inglese et al., 2005; Miles et al., 2008). However, findings from the acute to subacute injury stage are mixed, with equal number of studies reporting increased as well as decreased FA (Dodd et al., 2014). A study of non–sports-related mTBI reported opposite findings of higher fractional anisotropy in the corpus callosum (Bazarian et al., 2007). Additionally, Murugavel and colleagues (2014) examined a sample of concussed athletes that demonstrated increased RD at 2 days postinjury in areas of the internal capsule, sagittal striatum, and anterior thalamic radiation, with resolution of these effects by 2 weeks postinjury. Contrary to RD, FA values were increased at 2 weeks postinjury, compared with 2 days. Of note, those findings were within the concussed group sample, and at 2 weeks, there were no significant differences found between concussed athletes and healthy control subjects (Murugavel et al., 2014). Further examining acute and chronic injuries, Henry and colleagues (2011) tested athletes at 5 days postconcussion and again 6 months later. At both time periods, concussed athletes demonstrated increased FA and AD, as well as decreased MD values in the corticospinal tracts and the corpus callosum. Similarly, Meier and colleagues (2017) recently observed increased FA during the acute as well as subacute (up to 1 month) postinjury phases. The data thus far indicate possibly nonlinear relationships between diffusion metrics of white matter and time postinjury as an important consideration when attempting to generalize findings.

Additional studies have found that individuals with mTBI have more brain areas with increased RD than healthy participants (Panenka et al., 2015), but the timing may influence findings. For example, in examining participants with mTBI 8 days postinjury, there were variations in FA in the left cingulum bundle (Panenka et al., 2015). Some have shown a decrease in FA or increase in MD during the chronic phases of injury, as opposed to opposite findings during the acute phase (Slobounov et al., 2012). Additionally, at least one study has failed to demonstrate differences in FA between mTBI and healthy control participants at 30 days postinjury, although there was higher variability in FA values within concussed individuals (Zhang et al., 2010).

Factors such as subconcussive hits, repetitive head impacts, and prior history of concussion can also produce differing results. RD has been shown to be a sensitive measure of subconcussive hits (Murugavel et al., 2014). Soccer players with no diagnosed concussion displayed higher RD in areas such as the corpus callosum, orbitofrontal cortex, superior frontal gyrus, internal and external capsules, as well as other association fibers (Murugavel et al., 2014). AD in the corpus callosum was also higher in the soccer players than the control swimmer athletes (Koerte et al., 2015). Additionally, football players who sustained multiple repetitive head impacts, but no formal concussion diagnosis, were examined preseason, postseason, and again after 6 months of no contact sports. The athletes had greater changes in FA and MD from pre- to postseason, as well as from preseason to 6 months later (Bazarian et al., 2014). Specifically, reduced FA and increased MD in the corpus callosum was found from pre- to postseason in athletes and these differences persisted 6 months after the end of the season. These findings are aligned with the growing awareness of the importance of assessing repetitive subconcussive events, revealing possible long-standing changes in white matter. Of note, increased FA from preseason to the 6-month follow-up correlated with higher verbal memory scores and decreased FA from preseason to the follow-up was associated with lower impulse control scores (Bazarian et al., 2014). Expansion of the relationship between these imaging findings and long-term behavioral consequences is warranted.

Lastly, a prior history of concussions has been shown to change DTI results. Hockey players with and without a history of concussion were assessed at the end of the season. The prior concussion group revealed increased FA in the corona radiata, internal capsule, and frontal and temporal areas. This group also demonstrated increased AD in the corona radiata. The concussed group had decreased RD in the corpus callosum, corona radiata, areas of the internal and external capsule, and areas in the orbitofrontal and temporal white matter (Sasaki et al., 2014). This is consistent with prior findings of concussed individuals, even though athletes in this concussion group were not currently suffering from a concussion. For more studies using DTI as a means of examining damage following concussion, see Table 5.3.

Dean and colleagues (2015) combined the use of fMRI, DTI, and MRS to investigate the changes in the brain following concussion at 1-year post-injury, finding that decreased structural integrity was associated with higher activation in task-relevant areas and lower activation in areas not associated with the task (Dean et al., 2015). This also suggests that both structural and functional deficits can persist long after concussion (greater than 1 year), and these deficits may be ideally assessed using combined imaging metrics (i.e., DTI or fMRI).

MRS STUDIES

MRS can be used to noninvasively measure changes in the chemistry of the brain after injury, which may indicate neuronal damage of diffuse axonal injury (Shenton et al., 2012). This technique uses magnetic signals from nuclei and measures the main metabolites of N-acetylaspartate (NAA), choline (Cho), myo-inositol, lactate, creatine (Cr), and phospho-creatine (Belanger, Vanderploeg, Curtiss, & Warden, 2007). These metabolites provide information regarding neuronal integrity, membrane damage, glial activation, ischemia and hypoxia, and energy metabolism, respectively (Toth, 2015). Newer sequences also include a measure of glutamate/glutamine and GABA, which indicate excitatory and inhibitory neurotransmission (Tremblay et al., 2014). In addition, localized correlated spectroscopy has been used to improve on the one-dimensional MRS technique to identify multiple molecules at a time, compared with measuring only one molecule with traditional MRS (Lin et al., 2015).

A review of nine studies found that the most significant finding across studies was a decrease in NAA associated with concussion, particularly during the month after the concussion (Gardner, Iverson, & Stanwell, 2014).

TABLE 5.3
Sports-Related Concussion Studies Using DTI and MRS

Study	N Pt	N Control	Gender Pt	Gender Control	Mean age (in years) Pt	Mean age (in years) Control	Mean concussion-imaging time difference	Imaging modality
Vagnozzi et al. (2008)	14	5	9 M	Unknown	27 ± 4.8		3, 4, 7, 15, 20, and 45 days	MRS
Henry et al. (2010)	12	12	Unknown	Unknown	22.1 ± 0.8	32 ± 0.7	3.4 ± 1.9 days	MRS
Zhang et al. (2010)	15	15	21 M, 9 F	21 M, 9 F	20.8 ± 1.7	21.3 ± 1.5	"Within 30 days"	fMRI, DTI
Bazarian et al. (2012)	9 (1 with concuss)	6	9 M	6 M	Unknown	Unknown	72 hours post-concuss; 1–3 months for non	DTI
Cubon et al. (2011)	10	10	5 F, 5 M	5 F, 5 M	19.7 ± 1.6	20.4 ± 1.8	115 days	DTI
Chamard et al. (2013)	10	10	10 F	10 F	21.7 ± 2.06	21 ± 1.33	18.9 months	MRS, DTI
Murugavel et al. (2014)	21	16	21 M	16 M	20.2 ± 1.0	19.9 ± 1.7	2 days, 2 weeks, 2 months	DTI
Dean et al. (2015)	16	9	9 F, 7 M	5 F, 4 M	26.9	21.9	6.1 years	fMRI, DTI, MRS
Zhu et al. (2015)	8	11	8 M	11 M	20 ± 1.3	20.5 ± 1.8	24 hours; 7 ± 1 day; 30 ± 1 days	fMRI, DTI

Note. Search terms for the studies in Table 5.3 input into PubMed included *diffusion tensor* + *concussion* for DTI studies and *concussion* + spectroscopy. These results comprehensively included studies from prior reviews (Pulsipher et al., 2011). No studies were included if they did not specify that individuals sustained a concussion from playing a sport. Studies on youth and pediatric concussion were also excluded. DTI = diffusion tensor imaging; F = female; fMRI = functional magnetic resonance imaging; M = male; MRS = magnetic resonance spectroscopy; Pt = patient.

Other common findings in this population include an increase in choline levels (Slobounov et al., 2012) and an increase in glutamate/glutamine (Tremblay et al., 2014). Conversely, a study using proton MRS in an emergency department sample found that participants who had sustained mTBIs had alterations in Cr/phosphocreatine, glutamine/glutamate, and glutamate, but not NAA and Cho, which tend to be more associated with cellular energetics rather than overall dysfunction from mTBI (Gasparovic et al., 2009). A follow-up study with a larger cohort (Yeo et al., 2011) indicated a negative correlation between NAA and days postinjury, suggesting a more dynamic recovery curve for NAA (see also Vagnozzi et al., 2010). Considering other factors associated with concussion, such as time postinjury and severity of injury, might clarify the differences between some of these metabolic findings.

In work examining more acute injuries, concussed athletes who were scanned 1 to 6 days postconcussion had lower levels of glutamate and NAA in the primary motor cortex, as well as lower levels of glutamate in the dorsolateral prefrontal cortex (Henry et al., 2010). Interestingly, the concussed athletes and healthy control subjects did not differ on neuropsychological measures, but levels of NAA/Cr and glutamate/Cr in the primary motor cortex did negatively correlate with the symptoms reported by the concussed group (Henry et al., 2010). In another study from Johnson and colleagues, metabolite ratios were examined for athletes with differing history of prior concussions (one, two, or three or more concussions). These athletes were examined during the subacute phase of injury and were all scanned within 30 days postconcussion. In the genu of the corpus callosum, the NAA/Cho and the NAA/Cr ratios were decreased for the concussed group compared with the healthy control subjects for all individuals with any previous number of concussions. Interestingly, the number of prior concussions did not intensify the decreased levels of metabolites (Johnson, Gay, et al., 2012). There were similar decreased metabolite ratios for athletes who had sustained only one concussion or more than three concussions. Finally, when examining concussed athletes at 3, 15, 22, and 30 days after injury, NAA/Cr and NAA/Cho ratios were lower compared with control subjects at 3, 15, and 22 days, with levels increasing at each time point. By 30 days, these metabolite ratios were no longer different from than those of the control group (Vagnozzi et al., 2010). The difference between these concussed athletes and those in Johnson, Gay, and colleagues' (2012) study is that these athletes reported being symptom-free by 30 days, which may explain the differing findings.

Athletes with prior history of concussion, as well as those with repetitive head trauma and no concussions, also demonstrate neurometabolic disruption. In retired contact-sport athletes, repeated brain trauma was found to yield significantly higher levels of glutamine/glutamate, Cho, fucosylated molecules, and phenylalanine than healthy control participants (Lin et al.,

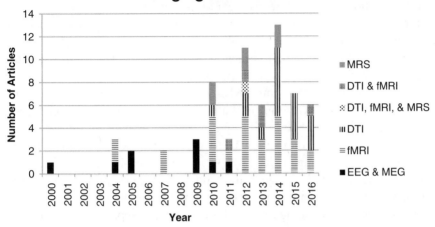

Figure 5.1. Sports-related concussion articles using different imaging modalities from 2000 through 2016. Studies included in this figure are all empirically based, comprised only adult participants, and did not include comorbid conditions (e.g., depression, posttraumatic stress disorder).

2015). These findings were seen despite no structural brain abnormalities and no recent concussion. Other studies have reported changes in NAA in a sample of mixed martial artists over a 1-year period (Mayer et al., 2015). In soccer players with a history of heading the ball but not diagnosed concussion, there were higher levels of Cho and myo-inositol (Koerte et al., 2015). These findings indicate that neurometabolic changes persist long after sustaining a concussion, and even in the absence of a formal concussion diagnosis. For more studies using MRS as a means of examining the neurometabolic changes that occur after SRC, see Table 5.3.

Figure 5.1 visually depicts the rise in imaging studies of SRC over the past 16 years.

SUMMARY

SRC presents diagnostic and prognostic challenges for a number of reasons, including distinct injury profiles and grades of injury and severity, as well as heterogeneity in symptom presentation. The physiological, metabolic, and structural effects of concussion are invisible to traditional structural neuroimaging measures, such as MRI or CT scans. In the past 2 decades, researchers have been using advanced imaging measures, such as fMRI, DTI, and MRS, in attempts to develop a biomarker that identifies concussion and its effects including brain markers for symptoms and their resolution. Although some consistent findings have emerged (e.g., reduced FA in anterior corpus callosum in chronic mTBI patients), the outcome of the functional, structural, and metabolic imaging to date has fallen short of a reliable biomarker of concussion. Use of functional brain imaging has provided novel insights into the brain systems affected postconcussion, but there is a growing consensus that a marker for SRC will not be composed of a single functional imaging task result or functional connectivity metric. Future success in using functional brain imaging to understand SRC will require nuanced hypotheses and methods that constrain interpretation, allowing for greater specificity beyond "compensation" (Hillary & Grafman, 2017), as well as integration of additional methods including metabolic imaging and studies of changes in physiology such as blood–brain barrier and brain perfusion. We have offered several possible future directions for imaging to contribute to the development of a biomarker (see Key Questions to Be Addressed in the Next 5 Years).

CASE STUDY

This case is modified from Hutchison and colleagues' (2014) description of two college athletes who sustained an SRC. Both of these athletes sustained a concussion from a hit in a team sport (hockey and volleyball, respectively). They each reported no loss of consciousness or posttraumatic amnesia after the injuries but felt confused and "foggy," had a headache, and displayed photophobia. A sports medicine physician evaluated the athletes by performing standard physical and neurological examinations. The athletes also underwent a neuropsychological examination, similar to the one received at baseline, as per the university's athletic policy. Both athletes did not demonstrate any significant decline in this neuropsychological evaluation compared with their baseline evaluations. The athletes also received an fMRI scan for nondiagnostic research purposes at the university to explore changes in brain activation after a concussion diagnosis.

The fMRI procedure comprised several tasks, including one measuring attention and reaction time, another involving spatial reasoning skills, and a third demanding working memory performance. BOLD signals were compared for each athlete. The first athlete demonstrated increased activation in areas of the brain typically associated with these tasks, whereas the second athlete demonstrated decreased activation in the same brain regions. These differences occurred in the context of similar neuropsychological performance and symptom reporting. These two cases exemplify the heterogeneity in outcomes after concussion and how imaging measures such as fMRI provide additional information about abnormalities that would not have been evident by self-report or neuropsychological assessment alone. Although fMRI may be sensitive to these individual differences, its utility in mTBI diagnostics requires establishing the specificity of the BOLD response, linking symptoms and functional brain changes.

CLINICAL TAKE-HOME POINTS

1. *Clinicians should be aware that functional neuroimaging measures have not been validated for diagnostic purposes.* Because of the mixed findings reported in the literature, there are no neuroimaging biomarkers that can be used to diagnose sports-related concussion.
2. *A multifaceted approach to diagnosing concussion remains the standard practice, including self-reported symptoms and neuropsychological measures of cognitive, motor, sensory, and vestibular functioning.* The addition of neuroimaging measures may help to further characterize the nature of deficit based on structural or functional abnormalities.
3. *Traditional structural neuroimaging measures, such as MRI or CT, often do not show abnormalities following a sports-related concussion.* Advanced imaging measures such as fMRI, DTI, and MRS have shown some sensitivity to brain changes after concussion.

KEY QUESTIONS TO BE ADDRESSED IN THE NEXT 5 YEARS

1. *Brain imaging methods have provided novel insights regarding regional and systemic changes associated with sports-related concussion, but much remains unknown about the timing of brain changes and the direct links to outcome.*
2. *After much investigation, the diagnostic use of functional brain imaging diagnostically has not resulted in identification of a "biomarker."* Efforts to do so require reconceptualization of how imaging can inform concussion diagnostics.
3. *The ideal timing for the use of metabolic and functional imaging to isolate concussion effects remains undetermined.*
4. *The role of serial imaging in substantiating the subtle effects of subconcussive events requires investigation.* Ultimately combining estimates of premorbid functioning, genetics, and imaging may improve prognostication.

REFERENCES

Abbas, K., Shenk, T. E., Poole, V. N., Breedlove, E. L., Leverenz, L. J., Nauman, E. A., . . . Robinson, M. E. (2014). Alteration of default mode network in high school football athletes due to repetitive subconcussive mild traumatic brain injury: A resting-state functional magnetic resonance imaging study. *Brain Connectivity, 5,* 91–101. http://dx.doi.org/10.1089/brain.2014.0279

Bandettini, P. A., Wong, E. C., Hinks, R. S., Tikofsky, R. S., & Hyde, J. S. (1992). Time course EPI of human brain function during task activation. *Magnetic Resonance in Medicine, 25,* 390–397. http://dx.doi.org/10.1002/mrm.1910250220

Basser, P. J., Mattiello, J., & LeBihan, D. (1994). MR diffusion tensor spectroscopy and imaging. *Journal of Biophysiology, 66,* 259–267.

Bassett, D. S., Meyer-Lindenberg, A., Achard, S., Duke, T., & Bullmore, E. (2006). Adaptive reconfiguration of fractal small-world human brain functional networks. *Proceedings of the National Academy of Sciences of the United States of America, 103,* 19518–19523. http://dx.doi.org/10.1073/pnas.0606005103

Bazarian, J. J., Zhong, J., Blyth, B., Zhu, T., Kavcic, V., & Peterson, D. (2007). Diffusion tensor imaging detects clinically important axonal damage after mild traumatic brain injury: A pilot study. *Journal of Neurotrauma, 24,* 1447–1459. http://dx.doi.org/10.1089/neu.2007.0241

Bazarian, J. J., Zhu, T., Blyth, B., Borrino, A., & Zhong, J. (2012). Subject-specific changes in brain white matter on diffusion tensor imaging after sports-related concussion. *Magnetic Resonance Imaging, 30,* 171–180.

Bazarian, J. J., Zhu, T., Zhong, J., Janigro, D., Rozen, E., Roberts, A., . . . Blackman, E. G. (2014). Persistent, long-term cerebral white matter changes after sports-related repetitive head impacts. *PLoS One, 9,* e94734. http://dx.doi.org/10.1371/journal.pone.0094734

Belanger, H. G., Vanderploeg, R. D., Curtiss, G., & Warden, D. L. (2007). Recent neuroimaging techniques in mild traumatic brain injury. *The Journal of Neuropsychiatry and Clinical Neurosciences, 19,* 5–20. http://dx.doi.org/10.1176/jnp.2007.19.1.5

Bernier, R. A., Roy, A., Venkatesan, U. M., Grossner, E. C., Brenner, E. K., & Hillary, F. G. (2017). Dedifferentiation does not account for hyperconnectivity after traumatic brain injury. *Frontiers in Neurology, 8,* 1–11. http://dx.doi.org/10.3389/fneur.2017.00297

Bero, A. W., Bauer, A. Q., Stewart, F. R., White, B. R., Cirrito, J. R., Raichle, M. E., . . . Holtzman, D. M. (2012). Bidirectional relationship between functional connectivity and amyloid-β deposition in mouse brain. *The Journal of Neuroscience, 32,* 4334–4340. http://dx.doi.org/10.1523/JNEUROSCI.5845-11.2012

Bharath, R. D., Munivenkatappa, A., Gohel, S., Panda, R., Saini, J., Rajeswaran, J., . . . Biswal, B. B. (2015). Recovery of resting brain connectivity ensuing mild traumatic brain injury. *Frontiers in Human Neuroscience, 9,* 513. http://dx.doi.org/10.3389/fnhum.2015.00513

Bigler, E. D., & Maxwell, W. L. (2012). Neuropathology of mild traumatic brain injury: Relationship to neuroimaging findings. *Brain Imaging and Behavior, 6,* 108–136. http://dx.doi.org/10.1007/s11682-011-9145-0

Biswal, B. B., Mennes, M., Zuo, X. N., Gohel, S., Kelly, C., Smith, S. M., . . . Milham, M. P. (2010). Toward discovery science of human brain function. *Proceedings of the National Academy of Sciences of the United States of America, 107,* 4734–4739. http://dx.doi.org/10.1073/pnas.0911855107

Biswal, B., Yetkin, F. Z., Haughton, V. M., & Hyde, J. S. (1995). Functional connectivity in the motor cortex of resting human brain using echo-planar MRI. *Magnetic Resonance in Medicine, 34,* 537–541. http://dx.doi.org/10.1002/mrm.1910340409

Borich, M., Babul, A.-N., Yuan, P. H., Boyd, L., & Virji-Babul, N. (2015). Alterations in resting-state brain networks in concussed adolescent athletes. *Journal of Neurotrauma, 32,* 265–271. http://dx.doi.org/10.1089/neu.2013.3269

Brody, D. L., Magnoni, S., Schwetye, K. E., Spinner, M. L., Esparza, T. J., Stocchetti, N., . . . Holtzman, D. M. (2008). Amyloid-β dynamics correlate with neurological status in the injured human brain. *Science, 321,* 1221–1224. http://dx.doi.org/10.1126/science.1161591

Bryer, E. J., Medaglia, J. D., Rostami, S., & Hillary, F. G. (2013). Neural recruitment after mild traumatic brain injury is task dependent: A meta-analysis. *Journal of the International Neuropsychological Society, 19,* 751–762. http://dx.doi.org/10.1017/S1355617713000490

Buckner, R. L., Snyder, A. Z., Shannon, B. J., LaRossa, G., Sachs, R., Fotenos, A. F., . . . Mintun, M. A. (2005). Molecular, structural, and functional characterization of Alzheimer's disease: Evidence for a relationship between default activity, amyloid, and memory. *The Journal of Neuroscience, 25,* 7709–7717. http://dx.doi.org/10.1523/JNEUROSCI.2177-05.2005

Busche, M. A., Chen, X., Henning, H. A., Reichwald, J., Staufenbiel, M., Sakmann, B., & Konnerth, A. (2012). Critical role of soluble amyloid-β for early hippocampal hyperactivity in a mouse model of Alzheimer's disease. *Proceedings of the National Academy of Sciences of the United States of America, 109,* 8740–8745. http://dx.doi.org/10.1073/pnas.1206171109

Byrnes, K. R., Wilson, C. M., Brabazon, F., von Leden, R., Jurgens, J. S., Oakes, T. R., & Selwyn, R. G. (2013). FDG-PET imaging in mild traumatic brain injury: A critical review. *Frontiers in Neuroenergetics, 5*(13), 1–24.

Caeyenberghs, K., Leemans, A., Heitger, M. H., Leunissen, I., Dhollander, T., Sunaert, S., . . . Swinnen, S. P. (2012). Graph analysis of functional brain networks for cognitive control of action in traumatic brain injury. *Brain, 135,* 1293–1307. http://dx.doi.org/10.1093/brain/aws048

Caeyenberghs, K., Verhelst, H., Clemente, A., & Wilson, P. H. (2017). Mapping the functional connectome in traumatic brain injury: What can graph metrics tell us? *NeuroImage, 160,* 113–123. http://dx.doi.org/10.1016/j.neuroimage.2016.12.003

Catani, M., & ffytche, D. H. (2005). The rises and falls of disconnection syndromes. *Brain, 128,* 2224–2239. http://dx.doi.org/10.1093/brain/awh622

Chamard, E., Lassonde, M., Henry, L., Tremblay, J., Boulanger, Y., De Beaumont, L., & Théoret, H. (2013). Neurometabolic and microstructural alterations following a sports-related concussion in female athletes. *Brain Injury, 27,* 1038–1046.

Chen, J. K., Johnston, K. M., Collie, A., McCrory, P., & Ptito, A. (2007). A validation of the post concussion symptom scale in the assessment of complex concussion using cognitive testing and functional MRI. *Journal of Neurology, Neurosurgery, and Psychiatry, 78,* 1231–1238. http://dx.doi.org/10.1136/jnnp.2006.110395

Chen, J. K., Johnston, K. M., Frey, S., Petrides, M., Worsley, K., & Ptito, A. (2004). Functional abnormalities in symptomatic concussed athletes: An fMRI study. *NeuroImage, 22,* 68–82. http://dx.doi.org/10.1016/j.neuroimage.2003.12.032

Chen, J. K., Johnston, K. M., Petrides, M., & Ptito, A. (2008). Recovery from mild head injury in sports: Evidence from serial functioning magnetic resonance imaging studies in male athletes. *Clinical Journal of Sport Medicine, 18,* 241–247.

Chong, C. D., & Schwedt, T. J. (2015). White matter damage and brain network alterations in concussed patients: A review of recent diffusion tensor imaging and resting-state functional connectivity data. *Current Pain and Headache Reports, 19,* 485. http://dx.doi.org/10.1007/s11916-015-0485-0

Cirrito, J. R., Yamada, K. A., Finn, M. B., Sloviter, R. S., Bales, K. R., May, P. C., . . . Holtzman, D. M. (2005). Synaptic activity regulates interstitial fluid amyloid-β levels in vivo. *Neuron, 48,* 913–922. http://dx.doi.org/10.1016/j.neuron.2005.10.028

Cubon, V. A., Putukian, M., Boyer, C., & Dettwiler, A. (2011). A diffusion tensor imaging study on the white matter skeleton in individuals with sports-related concussion. *Journal of Neurotrauma, 28,* 189–201.

Czerniak, S. M., Sikoglu, E. M., Navarro, A. A. L., McCafferty, J., Eisenstock, J., Stevenson, J. H., . . . Moore, C. M. (2015). A resting state functional magnetic resonance imaging study of concussion in collegiate athletes. *Brain Imaging and Behavior, 9,* 323–332.

Davis, S. W., Dennis, N. A., Daselaar, S. M., Fleck, M. S., & Cabeza, R. (2008). Que PASA? The posterior–anterior shift in aging. *Cerebral Cortex, 18,* 1201–1209. http://dx.doi.org/10.1093/cercor/bhm155

de Haan, W., Mott, K., van Straaten, E. C., Scheltens, P., & Stam, C. J. (2012). Activity dependent degeneration explains hub vulnerability in Alzheimer's disease. *PLoS Computational Biology, 8,* e1002582. http://dx.doi.org/10.1371/journal.pcbi.1002582

Dean, P. J. A., Sato, J. R., Vieira, G., McNamara, A., & Sterr, A. (2015). Multimodal imaging of mild traumatic brain injury and persistent postconcussion syndrome. *Brain and Behavior, 5,* 45–61.

Dennis, N. A., & Cabeza, R. (2011). Age-related dedifferentiation of learning systems: An fMRI study of implicit and explicit learning. *Neurobiology of Aging, 32,* 2318.e17–2318.e30. http://dx.doi.org/10.1016/j.neurobiolaging.2010.04.004

Dettwiler, A., Murugavel, M., Putukian, M., Cubon, V., Furtado, J., & Osherson, D. (2014). Persistent differences in patterns of brain activation after sports-related concussion: A longitudinal functional magnetic resonance imaging study. *Journal of Neurotrauma, 31,* 180–188. http://dx.doi.org/10.1089/neu.2013.2983

Dodd, A. B., Epstein, K., Ling, J. M., & Mayer, A. R. (2014). Diffusion tensor imaging findings in semi-acute mild traumatic brain injury. *Journal of Neurotrauma, 31,* 1235–1248. http://dx.doi.org/10.1089/neu.2014.3337

Eierud, C., Craddock, R. C., Fletcher, S., Aulakh, M., King-Casas, B., Kuehl, D., & LaConte, S. M. (2014). Neuroimaging after mild traumatic brain injury: Review and meta-analysis. *NeuroImage: Clinical, 4,* 283–294. http://dx.doi.org/10.1016/j.nicl.2013.12.009

Ford, J. H., Giovanello, K. S., & Guskiewicz, K. M. (2013). Episodic memory in former professional football players with a history of concussion: An event-related functional neuroimaging study. *Journal of Neurotrauma, 30,* 1683–1701.

Fox, M. D., Snyder, A. Z., Vincent, J. L., Corbetta, M., Van Essen, D. C., & Raichle, M. E. (2005). The human brain is intrinsically organized into dynamic, anticorrelated functional networks. *Proceedings of the National Academy of Sciences of the United States of America, 102,* 9673–9678. http://dx.doi.org/10.1073/pnas.0504136102

Gardner, A., Iverson, G. L., & Stanwell, P. (2014). A systematic review of proton magnetic resonance spectroscopy findings in sport-related concussion. *Journal of Neurotrauma, 31,* 1–18. http://dx.doi.org/10.1089/neu.2013.3079

Gasparovic, C., Yeo, R., Mannell, M., Ling, J., Elgie, R., Phillips, J., . . . Mayer, A. R. (2009). Neurometabolite concentrations in gray and white matter in mild traumatic brain injury: An 1H-magnetic resonance spectroscopy study. *Journal of Neurotrauma, 26,* 1635–1643. http://dx.doi.org/10.1089/neu.2009.0896

Geschwind, N. (1965a). Disconnexion syndromes in animals and man. I. *Brain, 88,* 237–294. http://dx.doi.org/10.1093/brain/88.2.237

Geschwind, N. (1965b). Disconnexion syndromes in animals and man. II. *Brain, 88,* 585–644. http://dx.doi.org/10.1093/brain/88.3.585

Giza, C. C., & Hovda, D. A. (2001). The neurometabolic cascade of concussion. *Journal of Athletic Training, 36,* 228–235.

Hammeke, T. A., McCrea, M., Coats, S. M., Verber, M. D., Durgerian, S., Flora, K., . . . Rao, S. M. (2013). Acute and subacute changes in neural activation during the recovery from sport-related concussion. *Journal of the International Neuropsychological Society, 19,* 863–872.

Henry, L. C., Tremblay, J., Tremblay, S., Lee, A., Brun, C., Lepore, N., . . . Lassonde, M. (2011). Acute and chronic changes in diffusivity measures after

sports concussion. *Journal of Neurotrauma, 28,* 2049–2059. http://dx.doi.org/
10.1089/neu.2011.1836

Henry, L. C., Tremblay, S., Boulanger, Y., Ellemberg, D., & Lassonde, M. (2010). Neurometabolic changes in the acute phase after sports concussions correlate with symptom severity. *Journal of Neurotrauma, 27,* 65–76. http://dx.doi.org/10.1089/neu.2009.0962

Hillary, F. G. (2008). Neuroimaging of working memory dysfunction and the dilemma with brain reorganization hypotheses. *Journal of the International Neuro-psychological Society, 14,* 526–534. http://dx.doi.org/10.1017/S1355617708080788

Hillary, F. G., Genova, H. M., Chiaravalloti, N. D., Rypma, B., & DeLuca, J. (2006). Prefrontal modulation of working memory performance in brain injury and disease. *Human Brain Mapping, 27,* 837–847. http://dx.doi.org/10.1002/hbm.20226

Hillary, F. G., Genova, H. M., Medaglia, J. D., Fitzpatrick, N. M., Chiou, K. S., Wardecker, B. M., . . . DeLuca, J. (2010). The nature of processing speed deficits in traumatic brain injury: Is less brain more? *Brain Imaging and Behavior, 4,* 141–154. http://dx.doi.org/10.1007/s11682-010-9094-z

Hillary, F. G., & Grafman, J. H. (2017). Injured brains and adaptive networks: The benefits and costs of hyperconnectivity. *Trends in Cognitive Sciences, 21,* 385–401. http://dx.doi.org/10.1016/j.tics.2017.03.003

Hillary, F. G., Medaglia, J. D., Gates, K., Molenaar, P. C., Slocomb, J., Peechatka, A., & Good, D. C. (2011). Examining working memory task acquisition in a disrupted neural network. *Brain, 134,* 1555–1570.

Hillary, F. G., Rajtmajer, S. M., Roman, C. A., Medaglia, J. D., Slocomb-Dluzen, J. E., Calhoun, V. D., . . . Wylie, G. R. (2014). The rich get richer: Brain injury elicits hyperconnectivity in core subnetworks. *PLoS One, 9,* e104021. http://dx.doi.org/10.1371/journal.pone.0104021

Hutchison, M. G., Schweizer, T. A., Tam, F., Graham, S. J., & Comper, P. (2014). FMRI and brain activation after sport concussion: A tale of two cases. *Frontiers in Neurology, 5,* 46. http://dx.doi.org/10.3389/fneur.2014.00046

Inglese, M., Makani, S., Johnson, G., Cohen, B. A., Silver, J. A., Gonen, O., & Grossman, R. I. (2005). Diffuse axonal injury in mild traumatic brain injury: A diffusion tensor imaging study. *Journal of Neurosurgery, 103,* 298–303. http://dx.doi.org/10.3171/jns.2005.103.2.0298

Jantzen, K. J., Anderson, B., Steinberg, F. L., & Kelso, J. S. (2004). A prospective functional MR imaging study of mild traumatic brain injury in college football players. *American Journal of Neuroradiology, 25,* 738–745.

Johnson, B., Gay, M., Zhang, K., Neuberger, T., Horovitz, S. G., Hallett, M., . . . Slobounov, S. (2012). The use of magnetic resonance spectroscopy in the sub-acute evaluation of athletes recovering from single and multiple mild traumatic brain injury. *Journal of Neurotrauma, 29,* 2297–2304. http://dx.doi.org/10.1089/neu.2011.2294

Johnson, B., Neuberger, T., Gay, M., Hallett, M., & Slobounov, S. (2014). Effects of subconcussive head trauma on the default mode network of the brain. *Journal of Neurotrauma, 31*, 1907–1913.

Johnson, B., Zhang, K., Gay, M., Horovitz, S., Hallett, M., Sebastianelli, W., & Slobounov, S. (2012). Alteration of brain default network in subacute phase of injury in concussed individuals: Resting-state fMRI study. *NeuroImage, 59*, 511–518. http://dx.doi.org/10.1016/j.neuroimage.2011.07.081

Koerte, I. K., Lin, A. P., Muehlmann, M., Merugumala, S., Liao, H., Starr, T., . . . Shenton, M. E. (2015). Altered neurochemistry in former professional soccer players without a history of concussion. *Journal of Neurotrauma, 32*, 1287–1293. http://dx.doi.org/10.1089/neu.2014.3715

Liang, X., Zou, Q., He, Y., & Yang, Y. (2013). Coupling of functional connectivity and regional cerebral blood flow reveals a physiological basis for network hubs of the human brain. *Proceedings of the National Academy of Sciences of the United States of America, 110*, 1929–1934. http://dx.doi.org/10.1073/pnas.1214900110

Lin, A. P., Ramadan, S., Stern, R. A., Box, H. C., Nowinski, C. J., Ross, B. D., & Mountford, C. E. (2015). Changes in the neurochemistry of athletes with repetitive brain trauma: Preliminary results using localized correlated spectroscopy. *Alzheimer's Research & Therapy, 7*, 13. http://dx.doi.org/10.1186/s13195-015-0094-5

List, J., Ott, S., Bukowski, M., Lindenberg, R., & Flöel, A. (2015). Cognitive function and brain structure after recurrent mild traumatic brain injuries in young-to-middle-aged adults. *Frontiers in Human Neuroscience, 9*, 228. http://dx.doi.org/10.3389/fnhum.2015.00228

Logothetis, N. K. (2008). What we can do and what we cannot do with fMRI. *Nature, 453*, 869–878. http://dx.doi.org/10.1038/nature06976

Logothetis, N. K., Pauls, J., Augath, M., Trinath, T., & Oeltermann, A. (2001). Neurophysiological investigation of the basis of the fMRI signal. *Nature, 412*, 150–157. http://dx.doi.org/10.1038/35084005

Lovell, M. R., & Collins, M. W. (1998). Neuropsychological assessment of the college football player. *The Journal of Head Trauma Rehabilitation, 13*, 9–26. http://dx.doi.org/10.1097/00001199-199804000-00004

Lovell, M. R., Pardini, J. E., Welling, J., Collings, M. W., Bakal, J., Lazar, N., . . . Becker, J. T. (2007). Functional brain abnormalities are related to clinical recovery and time to return-to-play in athletes. *Neurosurgery, 61*, 352–360.

Mayer, A. R., Bellgowan, P. S. F., & Hanlon, F. M. (2015). Functional magnetic resonance imaging of mild traumatic brain injury. *Neuroscience and Biobehavioral Reviews, 49*, 8–18. http://dx.doi.org/10.1016/j.neubiorev.2014.11.016

Mayer, A. R., Mannell, M. V., Ling, J., Gasparovic, C., & Yeo, R. A. (2011). Functional connectivity in mild traumatic brain injury. *Human Brain Mapping, 32*, 1825–1835. http://dx.doi.org/10.1002/hbm.21151

McAllister, T. W., Saykin, A. J., Flashman, L. A., Sparling, M. B., Johnson, S. C., Guerin, S. J., . . . Yanofsky, N. (1999). Brain activation during working memory 1 month after mild traumatic brain injury: A functional MRI study. *Neurology*, *53*, 1300–1308. http://dx.doi.org/10.1212/WNL.53.6.1300

McAllister, T. W., Sparling, M. B., Flashman, L. A., Guerin, S. J., Mamourian, A. C., & Saykin, A. J. (2001). Differential working memory load effects after mild traumatic brain injury. *Neurology*, *14*, 1004–1012. http://dx.doi.org/10.1006/nimg.2001.0899

Medaglia, J. D., Chiou, K. S., Slocomb, J., Fitzpatrick, N. M., Wardecker, B. M., Ramanathan, D., . . . Hillary, F. G. (2012). The less BOLD, the wiser: Support for the latent resource hypothesis after traumatic brain injury. *Human Brain Mapping*, *33*, 979–993. http://dx.doi.org/10.1002/hbm.21264

Meier, T. B., Bellgowan, P. S. F., & Mayer, A. R. (2017). Longitudinal assessment of local and global functional connectivity following sports-related concussion. *Brain Imaging and Behavior*, *11*, 129–140. http://dx.doi.org/10.1007/s11682-016-9520-y

Messé, A., Caplain, S., Pélégrini-Issac, M., Blancho, S., Lévy, R., Aghakhani, N., . . . Lehéricy, S. (2013). Specific and evolving resting-state network alterations in post-concussion syndrome following mild traumatic brain injury. *PLoS One*, *8*, 1–10. http://dx.doi.org/10.1371/journal.pone.0065470

Miles, L., Grossman, R. I., Johnson, G., Babb, J. S., Diller, L., & Inglese, M. (2008). Short-term DTI predictors of cognitive dysfunction in mild traumatic brain injury. *Brain Injury*, *22*, 115–122. http://dx.doi.org/10.1080/02699050801888816

Militana, A. R., Donahue, M. J., Sills, A. K., Solomon, G. S., Gregory, A. J., Strother, M. K., & Morgan, V. L. (2016). Alterations in default-mode network connectivity may be influenced by cerebrovascular changes within 1 week of sports related concussion in college varsity athletes: A pilot study. *Brain Imaging and Behavior*, *10*, 559–568. http://dx.doi.org/10.1007/s11682-015-9407-3

Murugavel, M., Cubon, V., Putukian, M., Echemendia, R., Cabrera, J., Osherson, D., & Dettwiler, A. (2014). A longitudinal diffusion tensor imaging study assessing white matter fiber tracts after sports-related concussion. *Journal of Neurotrauma*, *31*, 1860–1871. http://dx.doi.org/10.1089/neu.2014.3368

Myers, N., Pasquini, L., Göttler, J., Grimmer, T., Koch, K., Ortner, M., . . . Sorg, C. (2014). Within-patient correspondence of amyloid-β and intrinsic network connectivity in Alzheimer's disease. *Brain: A Journal of Neurology*, *137*, 2052–2064. http://dx.doi.org/10.1093/brain/awu103

Nakamura, T., Hillary, F. G., & Biswal, B. B. (2009). Resting network plasticity following brain injury. *PLoS ONE*, *4*, e8220. http://dx.doi.org/10.1371/journal.pone.0008220

Ogawa, S., Lee, T. M., Kay, A. R., & Tank, D. W. (1990). Brain magnetic resonance imaging with contrast dependent on blood oxygenation. *Proceedings of the National Academy of Sciences of the United States of America*, *87*, 9868–9872. http://dx.doi.org/10.1073/pnas.87.24.9868

Owen, A. M., McMillan, K. M., Laird, A. R., & Bullmore, E. (2005). N-back working memory paradigm: A meta-analysis of normative functional neuroimaging studies. *Human Brain Mapping, 25*, 46–59. http://dx.doi.org/10.1002/hbm.20131

Palacios, E. M., Fernandez-Espejo, D., Junque, C., Sanchez-Carrion, R., Roig, T., Tormos, J. M., . . . Vendrell, P. (2011). Diffusion tensor imaging differences relate to memory deficits in diffuse traumatic brain injury. *BMC Neurology, 11*, 24.

Panenka, W. J., Lange, R. T., Bouix, S., Shewchuk, J. R., Heran, M. K. S., Brubacher, J. R., . . . Iverson, G. L. (2015). Neuropsychological outcome and diffusion tensor imaging in complicated versus uncomplicated mild traumatic brain injury. *PLoS ONE, 10*, e0122746. http://dx.doi.org/10.1371/journal.pone.0122746

Pardini, J. E., Pardini, D. A., Becker, J. T., Dunfee, K. L., Eddy, W. F., Lovell, M. R., & Welling, J. S. (2010). Postconcussive symptoms are associated with compensatory cortical recruitment during a working memory task. *Neurosurgery, 67*, 1020–1027. http://dx.doi.org/10.1227/NEU.0b013e3181ee33e2

Pulsipher, D. T., Campbell, R. A., Thoma, R., & King, J. H. (2011). A critical review of neuroimaging applications in sports concussion. *Head and Neurologic Conditions, 10*, 14–20. http://dx.doi.org/10.1249/JSR.0b013e31820711b8

Raichle, M. E., MacLeod, A. M., Snyder, A. Z., Powers, W. J., Gusnard, D. A., & Shulman, G. L. (2001). A default mode of brain function. *Proceedings of the National Academy of Sciences of the United States of America, 98*, 676–682. http://dx.doi.org/10.1073/pnas.98.2.676

Ricker, J. H., Hillary, F. G., & DeLuca, J. (2001). Functionally activated brain imaging (O-15 PET and fMRI) in the study of learning and memory after traumatic brain injury. *The Journal of Head Trauma Rehabilitation, 16*, 191–205. http://dx.doi.org/10.1097/00001199-200104000-00007

Roy, A., Bernier, R. A., Wang, J., Benson, M., French, J. J., Jr., Good, D. C., & Hillary, F. G. (2017). The evolution of cost-efficiency in neural networks during recovery from traumatic brain injury. *PLoS ONE, 12*, e0170541. http://dx.doi.org/10.1371/journal.pone.0170541

Salvador, R., Suckling, J., Coleman, M. R., Pickard, J. D., Menon, D., & Bullmore, E. (2005). Neurophysiological architecture of functional magnetic resonance images of human brain. *Cerebral Cortex, 15*, 1332–1342. http://dx.doi.org/10.1093/cercor/bhi016

Sasaki, T., Pasternak, O., Mayinger, M., Muehlmann, M., Savadjiev, P., Bouix, S., . . . Koerte, I. K. (2014). Hockey Concussion Education Project, Part 3. White matter microstructure in ice hockey players with a history of concussion: A diffusion tensor imaging study. *Journal of Neurosurgery, 120*, 882–890. http://dx.doi.org/10.3171/2013.12.JNS132092

Scheibel, R. S., Pearson, D. A., Faria, L. P., Kotrla, K. J., Aylward, E., Bachevalier, J., & Levin, H. S. (2003). An fMRI study of executive functioning after severe diffuse TBI. *Brain Injury, 17*, 919–930.

Scott, G., Ramlackhansingh, A. F., Edison, P., Hellyer, P., Cole, J., Veronese, M., . . . Sharp, D. J. (2016). Amyloid pathology and axonal injury after brain trauma. *Neurology, 86*, 821–828. http://dx.doi.org/10.1212/WNL.0000000000002413

Sharp, D. J., Beckmann, C. F., Greenwood, R., Kinnunen, K. M., Bonnelle, V., De Boissezon, X., . . . Leech, R. (2011). Default mode network functional and structural connectivity after traumatic brain injury. *Brain, 134*, 2233–2247. http://dx.doi.org/10.1093/brain/awr175

Sheline, Y. I., & Raichle, M. E. (2013). Resting state functional connectivity in pre-clinical Alzheimer's disease. *Biological Psychiatry, 74*, 340–347. http://dx.doi.org/10.1016/j.biopsych.2012.11.028

Shenton, M. E., Hamoda, H. M., Schneiderman, J. S., Bouix, S., Pasternak, O., Rathi, Y., . . . Zafonte, R. (2012). A review of magnetic resonance imaging and diffusion tensor imaging findings in mild traumatic brain injury. *Brain Imaging and Behavior, 6*, 137–192. http://dx.doi.org/10.1007/s11682-012-9156-5

Slobounov, S., Gay, M., Johnson, B., & Zhang, K. (2012). Concussion in athletics: Ongoing clinical and brain imaging research controversies. *Brain Imaging and Behavior, 6*, 223–243. http://dx.doi.org/10.1007/s11682-012-9167-2

Slobounov, S. M., Gay, M., Zhang, K., Johnson, B., Pennell, D., Sebastianelli, W., . . . Hallett, M. (2011). Alteration of brain functional network at rest and in response to YMCA physical stress test in concussed athletes: RsFMRI study. *Neuro-Image, 55*, 1716–1727. http://dx.doi.org/10.1016/j.neuroimage.2011.01.024

Slobounov, S. M., Zhang, K., Pennell, D., Ray, W., Johnson, B., & Sebastianelli, W. (2010). Functional abnormalities in normally appearing athletes following mild traumatic brain injury: A functional MRI study. *Experimental Brain Research, 202*, 341–354. http://dx.doi.org/10.1007/s00221-009-2141-6

Smits, M., Dippel, D. W. J., Houston, G. C., Wielopolski, P. A., Koudstaal, P. J., Hunink, M. G. M., & van der Lugt, A. (2009). Postconcussion syndrome after minor head injury: Brain activation of working memory and attention. *Human Brain Mapping, 30*, 2789–2803. http://dx.doi.org/10.1002/hbm.20709

Sours, C., George, E. O., Zhuo, J., Roys, S., & Gullapalli, R. P. (2015). Hyper-connectivity of the thalamus during early stages following mild traumatic brain injury. *Brain Imaging and Behavior, 9*, 550–563. http://dx.doi.org/10.1007/s11682-015-9424-2

Sours, C., Zhuo, J., Roys, S., Shanmuganathan, K., & Gullapalli, R. P. (2015). Disruptions in resting state functional connectivity and cerebral blood flow in mild traumatic brain injury patients. *PLoS ONE, 10*, e0134019. http://dx.doi.org/10.1371/journal.pone.0134019

Stam, C. J. (2004). Functional connectivity patterns of human magnetoencephalographic recordings: A "small-world" network? *Neuroscience Letters, 355*, 25–28. http://dx.doi.org/10.1016/j.neulet.2003.10.063

Talavage, T. M., Nauman, E. A., Breedlove, E. L., Yoruk, U., Dye, A. E., Morigaki, K. E., . . . Leverenz, L. J. (2014). Functionally-detected cognitive impairment in high school football players without clinically-diagnosed concussion. *Journal of Neurotrauma, 31*, 327–338. http://dx.doi.org/10.1089/neu.2010.1512

Terry, D. P., Faraco, C. C., Smith, D., Diddams, M. J., Puente, A. N., & Miller, L. S. (2012). Lack of long-term fMRI differences after multiple sports-related concussions. *Brain Injury, 26*, 1684–1696. http://dx.doi.org/10.3109/02699052.2012.722259

Tijms, B. M., Wink, A. M., de Haan, W., van der Flier, W. M., Stam, C. J., Scheltens, P., & Barkhof, F. (2013). Alzheimer's disease: Connecting findings from graph theoretical studies of brain networks. *Neurobiology of Aging, 34*, 2023–2036. http://dx.doi.org/10.1016/j.neurobiolaging.2013.02.020

Toth, A. (2015). Magnetic resonance imaging application in the area of mild and acute traumatic brain injury: Implications for diagnostic markers? In F. H. Kobeissy (Ed.), *Brain neurotrauma: Molecular, neuropsychological, and rehabilitation aspects* (pp. 329–340). Boca Raton, FL: CRC Press/Taylor & Francis.

Tremblay, S., Beaulé, V., Proulx, S., Tremblay, S., Marjanska, M., Doyon, J., . . . Théoret, H. (2014). Multimodal assessment of primary motor cortex integrity following sport concussion in asymptomatic athletes. *Clinical Neurophysiology, 125*, 1371–1379. http://dx.doi.org/10.1016/j.clinph.2013.11.040

Vagnozzi, R., Signoretti, S., Cristofori, L., Alessandrini, F., Floris, R., Isgrò, E., . . . Lazzarino, G. (2010). Assessment of metabolic brain damage and recovery following mild traumatic brain injury: A multicentre, proton magnetic resonance spectroscopic study in concussed patients. *Brain, 133*, 3232–3242. http://dx.doi.org/10.1093/brain/awq200

Vagnozzi, R., Signoretti, S., Tavazzi, B., Floris, R., Ludovici, A., Marziali, S., . . . Lazzarino, G. (2008). Temporal window of metabolic brain vulnerability to concussion: A pilot 1H-magnetic resonance spectroscopic study in concussed athletes—Part III. *Neurosurgery, 62*, 1286–1296.

van den Heuvel, M. P., & Hulshoff Pol, H. E. (2010). Exploring the brain network: A review on resting-state fMRI functional connectivity. *European Neuropsychopharmacology, 20*, 519–534. http://dx.doi.org/10.1016/j.euroneuro.2010.03.008

Venkatesan, U. M., Dennis, N. A., & Hillary, F. G. (2015). Chronology and chronicity of altered resting-state functional connectivity after traumatic brain injury. *Journal of Neurotrauma, 32*, 252–264. http://dx.doi.org/10.1089/neu.2013.3318

Vlassenko, A. G., Vaishnavi, S. N., Couture, L., Sacco, D., Shannon, B. J., Mach, R. H., . . . Mintun, M. A. (2010). Spatial correlation between brain aerobic glycolysis and amyloid-β (Aβ) deposition. *Proceedings of the National Academy of Sciences of the United States of America, 107*, 17763–17767. http://dx.doi.org/10.1073/pnas.1010461107

Yeo, R. A., Gasparovic, C., Merideth, F., Ruhl, D., Doezema, D., & Mayer, A. R. (2011). A longitudinal proton magnetic resonance spectroscopy study of mild traumatic brain injury. *Journal of Neurotrauma, 28*, 1–11. http://dx.doi.org/10.1089/neu.2010.1578

Yuh, E. L., Mukherjee, P., Lingsma, H. F., Yue, J. K., Ferguson, A. R., Gordon, W. A., . . . TRACK-TBI Investigators. (2013). Magnetic resonance imaging improves 3-month outcome prediction in mild traumatic brain injury. *Annals of Neurology, 73*, 224–235. http://dx.doi.org/10.1002/ana.23783

Zhang, K., Johnson, B., Gay, M., Horovitz, S. G., Hallett, M., Sebastianelli, W., & Slobounov, S. (2012). Default mode network in concussed individuals in response to the YMCA physical stress test. *Journal of Neurotrauma, 29*, 756–765.

Zhang, K., Johnson, B., Pennell, D., Ray, W., Sebastianelli, W., & Slobounov, S. (2010). Are functional deficits in concussed individuals consistent with white matter structural alterations: Combined FMRI & DTI study. *Experimental Brain Research, 204*, 57–70. http://dx.doi.org/10.1007/s00221-010-2294-3

Zhou, Y., Milham, M. P., Lui, Y. W., Miles, L., Reaume, J., Sodickson, D. K., . . . Ge, Y. (2012). Default-mode network disruption in mild traumatic brain injury. *Radiology, 265*, 882–892. http://dx.doi.org/10.1148/radiol.12120748

Zhu, D. C., Covassin, T., Nogle, S., Doyle, S., Russell, D., Rearson, R. L., . . . Kaufman, D. I. (2015). A potential biomarker in sports-related concussion: Brain functional connectivity alteration of the default-mode network measured with longitudinal resting-state fMRI over thirty days. *Journal of Neurotrauma, 32*, 327–341.

6

CHRONIC TRAUMATIC ENCEPHALOPATHY AND THE LONG-TERM CONSEQUENCES OF REPETITIVE HEAD IMPACTS IN SPORTS

MICHAEL L. ALOSCO, ROSE C. HEALY, AND ROBERT A. STERN

This chapter focuses on the long-term consequences of sports-related repetitive head impacts (RHI), including impacts resulting in symptomatic concussions as well as subconcussive trauma. In concussion, there is a transfer of mechanical energy to the brain from a direct or indirect force to the head that results in neuronal injury and a wide range of associated symptoms and signs (Giza & Hovda, 2014; McCrory et al., 2017). In contrast, subconcussive head trauma is believed to involve similar, though of lesser magnitude, mechanical forces and neuronal injury, but not to result in the immediate symptoms and signs of concussion (Broglio, Eckner, Paulson, & Kutcher, 2012). Subconcussive head trauma often occurs in the setting of contact sports, particularly American football. Helmet accelerometer studies have shown that high school football players can average 600 subconcussive impacts per season, and this can increase to over 1,000 at the collegiate level (Broglio et al., 2011; Crisco et al., 2010; Gysland et al., 2012). Exposure to

http://dx.doi.org/10.1037/0000114-007
Neuropsychology of Sports-Related Concussion, P. A. Arnett (Editor)

RHI is currently at the cornerstone of clinical research due to its association with long-term neuropsychological, neuropsychiatric, and neurological sequelae, including those from chronic traumatic encephalopathy (CTE; Bieniek et al., 2015; McKee, Cairns, et al., 2016; McKee, Stein, et al., 2013). CTE is a neurodegenerative disease caused, in part, by exposure to RHI, and can currently only be diagnosed postmortem (McKee et al., 2016). CTE has the potential to affect millions, given the estimated 1.6 to 3.8 million sport- and recreational-related concussions that occur in the United States each year (Langlois, Rutland-Brown, & Wald, 2006), and the even more frequent subconcussive head trauma (Broglio et al., 2011; Crisco et al., 2010; Gysland et al., 2012).

Our understanding of the long-term neurological consequences of RHI exposure and CTE has improved over the last decade, but it remains an emerging field and many knowledge gaps remain, despite what is portrayed by the media. The objective of this chapter is to review the current literature examining later-life clinical and neurological outcomes associated with RHI exposure with a focus on CTE. We describe the long-term neuropsychological, neuropsychiatric, and neurological sequelae of RHI exposure. The neuropathological and clinical presentation of CTE are presented, followed by an illustrative case study of a clinically exemplar autopsy-confirmed case of CTE. The chapter concludes with directions for future research.

REPETITIVE HEAD IMPACTS: LONG-TERM NEUROPSYCHOLOGICAL, NEUROPSYCHIATRIC, AND NEUROLOGICAL SEQUELAE

Research in active contact sport athletes has shown that exposure to RHI is associated with short-term (e.g., following a single season of play) impairments in cognitive function (McAllister et al., 2012) and mood (Roiger, Weidauer, & Kern, 2015), as well as macro- and microscopic brain alterations (Adams, Adler, Jarvis, DelBello, & Strakowski, 2007; Bahrami et al., 2016; Bazarian et al., 2014; Koerte, Ertl-Wagner, Reiser, Zafonte, & Shenton, 2012). However, we review the later-life clinical sequelae from RHI exposure to facilitate comparisons to and conclusions for CTE. The long-term neuropsychological, neuropsychiatric, and neurological sequelae of RHI exposure has largely been studied in former contact sport athletes, most commonly former professional American football players. Former professional American football players have a high level of RHI exposure history, and CTE has been well documented in this cohort (McKee et al., 2013). For these reasons, research in former professional American football players is emphasized.

An objective of the Boston University (BU) Alzheimer's Disease (AD) and CTE Center (BU ADCTEC) is to characterize the later-life clinical phenotypes associated with exposure to RHI. The BU ADCTEC is home to the largest longitudinal research registry of living contact and noncontact sport athletes in the country, known as the Longitudinal Examination to Gather Evidence of Neurodegenerative Disease (LEGEND) study. In 2011, a National Institutes of Health (NIH)-funded grant was funded for a study referred to as Diagnosing and Evaluating Traumatic Encephalopathy using Clinical Tests (DETECT; principal investigator: Robert Stern; NS078337). The purpose of DETECT was to examine the later-life clinical presentation of former National Football League (NFL) players at high risk for CTE, and to begin to develop *in vivo* biomarkers for CTE. The DETECT study concluded in 2015 and recruited a total of 96 symptomatic former NFL players and 28 same-age asymptomatic controls without head trauma history. Published findings from LEGEND and DETECT have led to improved understanding on RHI exposure and later-life clinical outcomes.

In an initial study from LEGEND, executive functioning, measured by the Behavior Rating Inventory of Executive Function, adult version (BRIEF–A), was examined in a sample of 64 active and former college and professional American football players (Seichepine et al., 2013). Compared with age-corrected normative scores for healthy adults, football players reported significantly worse executive difficulties, which were most severe in football players aged 40 years and older. A more recent study from LEGEND addressed the lack of reliable and valid methods to quantify RHI exposure retrospectively. BU ADCTEC investigators developed the cumulative head impact index (CHII; Montenigro et al., 2017) using a sample of 93 former high school and college American football players from LEGEND. The CHII is an estimate of the total number of football-related head impacts received and is calculated from an algorithm based on the number of seasons played, position(s) played, levels played (youth, high school, college), and estimated head impact frequencies from published helmet accelerometer studies. There was a significant dose–response relationship between the CHII and risk for later-life clinically meaningful cognitive impairment, depression, apathy, and behavioral dysregulation. In the LEGEND cohort of amateur tackle football players, the CHII outperformed other metrics of RHI exposure (e.g., number of lifetime concussions, years of football played, and age of first exposure [AFE] to football) in the prediction of later-life clinical impairment.

Findings from DETECT have provided further insight into the relationship between RHI exposure and long-term clinical sequelae. AFE to tackle football was examined as a potential modifier of RHI-related cognitive impairment in a subset of former NFL players from DETECT. The premise for this study was that RHI exposure during critical periods of neurodevelopment may increase vulnerability to clinical impairment in later life, particularly in the context of ongoing RHI exposure. Those who began playing tackle football before the age of 12, a time period when many aspects of neurodevelopment are at their peak (Caviness, Kennedy, Richelme, Rademacher, & Filipek, 1996; Epstein, 1999; Giedd, 2008), exhibited greater impairments on tests of verbal memory and executive function in middle age, compared with those who began playing at 12 or older, controlling for many potential confounding variables, including total years of playing football (Stamm, Bourlas, et al., 2015). More recent findings from DETECT have shown that RHI exposure affects clinical domains beyond the realm of cognitive function. Former NFL players were observed to exhibit lower scores on a test of olfactory function (Brief Smell Identification Test [B-SIT]), relative to same-age controls. Lower scores on the B-SIT correlated with greater impairments in behavior/mood and psychomotor speed/executive function (Alosco, Jarnagin, et al., 2017).

RHI exposure may result in long-term neuropsychological and neuropsychiatric dysfunction through its association with structural, functional, and molecular brain alterations. AFE to tackle football was previously discussed to potentially increase vulnerability to later-life cognitive impairment (Stamm, Bourlas, et al., 2015). Additional findings indicate that AFE to football is associated with altered microstructural integrity of white matter. In that study, 20 pairs of former NFL players ($n = 40$) from DETECT were matched by age; one member of each pair began playing football before age 12 and one began at 12 or older (Stamm, Koerte, et al., 2015). Subjects underwent magnetic resonance imaging (MRI) with diffusion tensor imaging (DTI); former NFL players who began playing football before age 12 were found to have significantly lower fractional anisotropy (FA; a metric of white matter integrity) and higher radial diffusivity in the anterior corpus callosum at middle age, compared with those who began playing football at age 12 or older. The CHII has been calculated for all former NFL players in the DETECT sample, with the limitation of using helmet accelerometer statistics published in college football players, because there are no published helmet accelerometer studies in professional football players. It is likely, however, that the application of CHII in former professional football players would likely underestimate exposure to RHI. Greater exposure to RHI, using the CHII, has correlated with possible biomarkers of CTE in the DETECT sample (described further below), including levels of plasma tau (Alosco, Tripodis, Jarnagin, et al., 2017), and altered cellular energy metabolism, as measured through magnetic resonance spectroscopy (MRS; Alosco, Tripodis, Rowland, et al., 2017). Further, greater years playing tackle football has been linked with reduced thalamic volume in the DETECT subjects (Shultz et al., 2018).

Research independent of the ADCTEC corroborates the association between RHI exposure and long-term neurological changes. A recent study developed an index of RHI exposure in a sample of former NFL players, based on concussion frequency, severity, and timeframe, as well as cognitive reserve (Wright et al., 2016). This index predicted later-life cognitive function; however, a large proportion of the predictive variance of the index was accounted for by cognitive reserve, as measured by the American version of the National Adult Reading Test (AMNART), occupational status, and academic achievement. The index did not predict depression. Other research in former NFL players has shown increasing number of self-reported concussions corresponds with increased odds for being clinically diagnosed with mild cognitive impairment, in addition to greater subjective memory impairments (Guskiewicz et al., 2005). There is additional evidence of an association between number of reported concussions and depression risk in former NFL players (Didehbani, Munro Cullum, Mansinghani, Conover, & Hart, 2013; Guskiewicz et al., 2007; Kerr, Marshall, Harding, & Guskiewicz, 2012). Concussion history in former NFL players also predicts reduced hippocampal volume (Strain et al., 2015), as well as medial temporal and inferior parietal lobe functional activity and functional alterations in relational memory networks (as measured by functional MRI; Ford, Giovanello, & Guskiewicz, 2013).

CHRONIC TRAUMATIC ENCEPHALOPATHY

The in vivo literature provides support for exposure to RHI as a likely risk factor for later-life alterations in clinical function and brain structure and function. Postmortem studies provide evidence that RHI exposure is a primary precipitating factor of CTE. In this section, we discuss the history, neuropathology, and clinical presentation of CTE.

History

The historical origins of CTE dates back to 1928, when the term "punch drunk" was coined by Harrison Martland (Martland, 1928) to describe a syndrome of clinical features that Martland observed in prize fighters, which included behavioral disturbances and cognitive impairments. Following Martland's 1928 paper, many different terms emerged to describe a combination of behavior, mood, cognitive, and motor symptoms and signs in boxers, including the well-known term "dementia pugilistica" in 1937 (Millspaugh, 1937). In 1940, "chronic traumatic encephalopathy" was designated in reference to symptomatic boxers (Bowman & Blau, 1940). Postmortem studies in the 1950s and 1970s began to associate boxing with abnormal brain pathology (Brandenburg & Hallervorden, 1954; Corsellis, Bruton, & Freeman-Browne,

1973), including widespread hyperphosphorylated tau (p-tau) in the cerebrum and brain stem in 15 retired boxers (Corsellis et al., 1973).

CTE began to receive greater lay and scientific attention in 2005, when neuropathological changes of CTE were first described in a former NFL player. Mike Webster played as a lineman for the Pittsburgh Steelers and Kansas City Chiefs. He experienced depression and memory problems after football retirement, and he was demented before his cardiac-related death in 2002 at the age of 50. Pathologist Bennet Omalu and colleagues conducted a postmortem examination of his brain. The brain was macroscopically normal, but there was microscopic evidence of p-tau abnormalities, consistent with previous descriptions of CTE in boxers. This was published as a case study in *Neurosurgery* in 2005 (Omalu et al., 2005). Since that case, neuropathological evidence of CTE has been reported in over 100 deceased American professional football players and other contact sport athletes (e.g., ice hockey, soccer, boxing, rugby), as well as military veterans (Goldstein et al., 2012; McKee et al., 2013). There has been evidence of CTE in young adults (e.g., teens, 20s; McKee et al., 2013). CTE has received extensive media attention, in part, because of the deaths of high profile former NFL players (e.g., Dave Duerson, Junior Seau) who were diagnosed with CTE following death. However, because of the association between RHI exposure and CTE, and because of the millions of active and former contact sport athletes and military personnel and veterans, CTE may become a major societal and public health concern.

Neuropathological Features of CTE

Bennet Omalu continued to characterize the neuropathology of CTE through a series of published case reports (Omalu, Bailes, et al., 2011; Omalu, Bailes, Hammers, & Fitzsimmons, 2010; Omalu, DeKosky, et al., 2006; Omalu, Fitzsimmons, Hammers, & Bailes, 2010; Omalu, Hamilton, Kamboh, DeKosky, & Bailes, 2010; Omalu, Hammers, et al., 2011). It is the extensive and ongoing research by McKee and colleagues at the BU ADCTEC and Veterans Administration-BU-Concussion Legacy Foundation (VA-BU-CLF) brain bank that has led to significant refinement of the neuropathology of CTE. As part of a National Institute of Neurological Disorders and Stroke (NINDS)-funded study, known as Understanding Neurologic Injury in Traumatic Encephalopathy (UNITE; principal investigator: Ann McKee; Mez et al., 2015), a NINDS and National Institute of Biomedical Imaging and Bioengineering (NIBIB)–sponsored conference was convened to evaluate McKee and colleagues' (2013) proposed neuropathological diagnostic criteria for CTE (McKee et al., 2016). The consensus conference included a panel of seven independent neuropathologists with specific expertise in neurodegenerative tauopathies. The panel evaluated 25 selected cases of various tauopathies. The selected CTE cases were representative of the disease and were of at least moderate disease severity. There was good agreement among the panel for overall neuropathological diagnoses (kappa = 0.67), and it was even stronger for CTE (kappa = 0.78). The agreed upon consensus from this conference was that the pathognomonic lesion of CTE is the irregular deposition of p-tau around small blood vessels at the base of the cortical sulci. This pattern of p-tau was agreed to be distinct from any other neurodegenerative tauopathy, including AD and frontotemporal lobar degeneration (FTLD). In a convenience sample of 202 tackle football players, CTE was neuropathologically diagnosed in 177 participants using the McKee et al. NINDS/NIBIB neuropathological diagnostic criteria (Mez et al., 2017). CTE was diagnosed in 110 of 111 NFL players, seven of eight Canadian Football League players, nine of 14 who played semiprofessional football, 48 of 53 college football players, and three of 14 who played only high school football. This is the largest and most rigorous neuropathological case series of individuals diagnosed with CTE. The findings emphasize the link between participation in tackle football and CTE, and provide further evidence for CTE as a major public health concern.

McKee et al. (2013) proposed a four-stage classification schema to grade the pathological severity and progression of p-tau in CTE. This staging classification of CTE is currently being refined and validated. Gross pathology is unremarkable in Stage I. As the disease advances, there is cortical atrophy that progresses to the white matter, MTL, corpus callosum, mammillary bodies, thalamus, and hypothalamus. Other macroscopic pathologies include dilatation of the lateral and third ventricles, septal abnormalities (e.g., cavum septum, septal perforations), and pallor of the locus coeruleus and substantia nigra.

Regarding microscopic pathology, there are focal perivascular p-tau neurofibrillary tangles (NFT) and astrocytic tangles at the depths of cortical sulci in Stage I, typically in the superior, dorsolateral, and inferior frontal cortices. The p-tau NFT disperse throughout the cortex, extend into the superficial layers of the cortex, and appear in the MTL, olfactory bulb, mammillary bodies, diencephalon, brainstem, and spinal cord in Stage III. By Stage IV, the p-tau is widely dispersed throughout the cortex and subcortex, as well as the brainstem and spinal cord. Throughout the four stages of disease, there is progressively worsening axonal degeneration, fiber loss, and white matter atrophy. Most cases of CTE have evidence of TAR DNA-binding protein 43 (TDP-43), which becomes widespread in Stage IV, affecting the cerebrum, MTL, brainstem, diencephalon, basal ganglia, and to a lesser extent, the spinal cord. Unlike AD (Hyman et al., 2012), beta-amyloid peptide deposits have been present in only half of cases with CTE and, when present, are diffuse plaques and associated with older age and the *APOE ε4* allele (Stein, Montenigro, et al., 2015). That said, CTE is commonly comorbid with AD, among other neurodegenerative diseases, including Lewy body disease (LBD), motor neuron disease (MND), and FTLD (McKee et al., 2013). Argyrophilic grain disease and Parkinson's disease have also been implicated as possible common comorbidities with CTE (Armstrong, McKee, Stein, Alvarez, & Cairns, 2017).

RHI Exposure and CTE

Not all individuals exposed to RHI develop CTE and not all symptoms observed in individuals with CTE are from CTE p-tau pathology. The clinical and neuropathological presentation of CTE is likely influenced by various factors including: demographic (e.g., age), head trauma exposure (e.g., extent, nature, duration), medical (e.g., cardiovascular disease), genetic (e.g., *APOE ε4*, microtubule-associated protein tau [MAPT] gene), and lifestyle (e.g., physical and mental activity, substance use, diet).

Subconcussive head impacts appear to play a prominent role in the pathogenesis of CTE. Recent research found that 16% of neuropathologically confirmed cases of CTE with exposure to repetitive subconcussive head impacts had no reported history of clinical concussion (Stein, Alvarez, & McKee, 2015). In the 68 cases with neuropathologically diagnosed CTE reported on by McKee and colleagues (McKee et al., 2013), family-estimated number of concussions was unrelated to CTE neuropathological stage. Of this sample, 64 had a history of repetitive subconcussive head impacts from participation in contact sports, including American football ($n = 50$), ice hockey ($n = 5$), boxing ($n = 8$), and professional wrestling ($n = 1$). The remaining four cases with CTE were military veterans ($n = 3$), and one individual with a history of self-injurious head banging. Among the American football players, longer duration of football play correlated with worse CTE disease severity. There was no evidence of CTE neuropathology in the 18 age- and gender-matched controls without a history of exposure to RHI.

A methodological limitation of the existing neuropathological CTE research is ascertainment bias due to recruitment of subjects with suspected CTE who agreed to brain donation. The objective of postmortem CTE research is to neuropathologically define the disease, not to determine epidemiology. Research from other neurodegenerative disease brain banks without recruitment bias corroborate findings form McKee et al. regarding the association between RHI and CTE. Bieniek et al. (2015) reviewed the medical charts of >1,700 brain donation cases from the Mayo Clinic brain bank to determine history of contact sport participation. A total of 66 male brain donors were identified to have played contact sports at the high school or college level, and 34 of the 66 played American football. The authors neuropathologically examined each of these 66 brains for evidence of CTE neuropathology, and 21 of the 66 former contact sport athletes exhibited the diagnostic lesion of CTE, that is, perivascular p-tau at the depths of the cortical sulci (McKee et al., 2016). There was no evidence of CTE neuropathology in 198 age- and disease-matched men and women without a history of exposure to contact sports. Of these 198 individuals without evidence of CTE, 33 had a history of a single nonathletic TBI, suggesting that an isolated TBI is not sufficient for the development of CTE. A recent report from England of deceased former soccer players with clinical dementia prior to death found that four of six brains examined had clear CTE pathology (Ling et al., 2017). The authors note that only one of the four former soccer players with CTE had a known history of concussion (and that subject only had a single concussion), suggesting that it is routine play and heading of the ball that may lead to CTE.

The mechanisms underlying the association between RHI exposure and CTE are unknown and speculative at this time. Theories, however, have been proposed. The linear rotational forces from acute concussion result in shearing and tearing of axons and blood vessels to cause diffuse axonal injury and a cascade of other neurometabolic disturbances (e.g., ionic flux and glutamate release, neuroinflammation; Giza & Hovda, 2014; Maxwell, Povlishock, & Graham, 1997; Medana & Esiri, 2003). Perivascular regions and the cortical sulci may represent focal stress points susceptible to the acceleration and deceleration forces that occur during head trauma (Blumbergs et al., 1994; Cloots, Gervaise, van Dommelen, & Geers, 2008; Cloots, van Dommelen, Nyberg, Kleiven, & Geers, 2011; Gaetz, 2004; McKee, Daneshvar, Alvarez, & Stein, 2014; Oppenheimer, 1968; Povlishock, 1993; Smith et al., 1999). Axonal injury from recurrent head trauma may initiate misfolding, phosphorylation, and aggregation of the tau protein to lead to neuronal death (McKee, Daneshvar, et al., 2014; McKee, Stein, Kiernan, & Alvarez, 2015; McKee, Stein, Nowinski, et al., 2013; Mouzon et al., 2014). Although the pathophysiological disturbances of a single concussion are short-lived, recurrent head trauma may prolong or preclude recovery. Blaylock and Maroon (2011) theorized that recurrent head injuries result in hyperactivity of microglia, leading to extensive releases of cytokines and excitotoxin neurochemicals, such as glutamate. Simultaneous to glutamate release from microglia activation, there is glutamate accumulation from gliosis and chronic astrocytosis. The prolonged and extensive release of glutamate with each head injury may result in chronic immunoexcitotoxicity to trigger neural degeneration. A recent study sought to test the relationships among RHI exposure, neuroinflammation, and p-tau in a sample of 66 former American football players who donated their brains to the VA-BU-CLF and were neuropathologically diagnosed with *only* CTE (Cherry et al., 2016).

The results showed that increased neuroinflammation (i.e., increased CD68 cell density and enhanced microglia reactivity) predicted worse p-tau neuropathology in the dorsolateral frontal cortex of subjects with CTE. Duration of RHI exposure (i.e., years of football play) had a direct effect on p-tau burden, as well as an indirect effect via neuroinflammation. More recently, Tagge et al. showed that experimental head injury in mice resulted in a host of CNS pathology, including axonopathy, blood–brain barrier disruption, astrocytosis, microgliosis, monocyte infiltration, and phosphorylated tau that was subjacent to the impact (Tagge et al., 2018). The phosphorylated tau spread into the cerebral cortex by 5.5 months after the injury.

Clinical Presentation of CTE

Through family interviews and medical record review of the deceased subjects, McKee et al. provided an initial characterization of clinical symptoms of CTE (McKee et al., 2013). Difficulties in memory, attention and concentration, and executive functions were common throughout the four neuropathological stages, as were disturbances in behavior and mood, particularly depression and related symptoms, aggression, and explosivity. Stern and colleagues conducted a comprehensive investigation on the clinical course and presentation of CTE through retrospective family telephone interviews and medical record reviews of 36 contact sport male athletes (29 American football players, three professional hockey players, one professional wrestler, and three former boxers) who donated their brains to the VA-BU-CLF and were neuropathologically diagnosed with *only* CTE (Stern et al., 2013). Consistent with previous case reports of former boxers, two distinct clinical presentations emerged from this sample:

1. *Behavioral/mood subgroup*: 22 subjects who exhibited initial changes in behavior (e.g., explosivity, impulsivity, physical and verbal violence) or mood (depression, hopelessness, suicidal ideations) at a mean age of 35; and
2. *Cognitive subgroup*: 11 subjects who exhibited initial changes in cognition (e.g., episodic memory and executive dysfunction) at a mean age of approximately 60; this subgroup tended to have more advanced CTE neuropathology.

There was a delay (years to decades) between the end of RHI exposure and symptom onset. Ten of the subjects were diagnosed with dementia, and the initial symptom for seven of these subjects was cognitive impairment. A majority of the individuals classified into the behavioral/mood subgroup later developed cognitive impairment. Three of the subjects from the sample were asymptomatic, including one 17-year-old with Stage I CTE, and the other two had advanced graduate degrees and were professionally very successful, suggesting high cognitive reserve as a possible protective factor in CTE. Cognitive reserve and its effect on age of symptom onset was specifically examined in a sample of 25 former professional American football players with autopsy-confirmed Stage III and Stage IV CTE (Alosco, Mez, et al., 2017). Subjects who achieved a high occupational attainment experienced a delay in cognitive and behavioral/mood symptom onset, compared with those classified as achieving a low occupational attainment.

Motor features (e.g., parkinsonism) were overall infrequent in the sample of 36 former contact sport athletes with CTE examined by Stern et al. (2013), who were predominately former professional football players. This is inconsistent with remote descriptions of CTE in former boxers, in which parkinsonism was a prominent clinical feature (Corsellis et al., 1973). The biomechanical head trauma forces that occur during boxing (e.g., angular acceleration and torsional injury) may place focal stress on brainstem structures to increase vulnerability to parkinsonism.

Traumatic Encephalopathy Syndrome

Clinical research diagnostic criteria for CTE have been proposed by several different author groups (Jordan, 2013; Montenigro et al., 2014; Victoroff, 2013). A detailed comparison of these clinical research diagnostic criteria is provided elsewhere (Baugh, Robbins, Stern, & McKee, 2014). The Jordan and Victoroff criteria are not entirely representative of the current literature on the clinical manifestation of CTE. Montenigro and colleagues published provisional clinical research diagnostic criteria to describe the syndrome of clinical features associated with exposure to RHI, known as traumatic encephalopathy syndrome (TES; Montenigro et al., 2014). TES is based upon a comprehensive literature review of the clinical features of neuropathologically confirmed cases of CTE. To receive a TES diagnosis, an individual must have had a history of multiple impacts to the head (e.g., concussion, moderate or severe TBI, subconcussive head trauma) due to involvement in contact sports, military service, or in other settings of RHI exposure (e.g., domestic violence, head banging). There must be the presence of at least one of the core clinical features, which are based on signs or symptoms found in at least 70% of cases with *only* neuropathologically confirmed CTE (Stern et al., 2013) and include (a) decline in cognitive function, particularly episodic memory, attention, and executive function, that is corroborated by standardized testing; (b) behavioral dysfunction characterized by emotionally explosive and physical and/or verbal aggression; and (c) impairments in mood, namely depression and related symptoms (e.g., hopelessness). At least two of the following supportive features must be present: impulsivity, anxiety, apathy, paranoia, suicidality, headache, motor signs, documented decline, and delayed onset. No other neurological disorder can fully account for the clinical features, and the clinical features must be present for a minimum of 12 months. There are four TES diagnostic subtypes: (a) TES behavioral/mood variant (TES-BMv), (b) TES cognitive variant (TES-COGv), (c) TES mixed variant (TES-MIXv), and (d) TES dementia (TES-D); TES-D requires progressive cognitive worsening and impaired functioning. Modifiers that indicate motor disturbances and clinical course ("stable," "progressive," or "unknown/inconsistent") should be designated. Clinical research involving former NFL players is beginning to provide support for the clinical pheno-type described by the TES criteria. A case-series study of 14 symptomatic former NFL players from an academic memory clinic at the University of California, San Francisco, found three clinical phenotypes (Gardner et al., 2015): (a) delayed-onset (that is, since the end of RHI exposure) behavioral/mood symptoms (e.g., anxiety, depression, irritability, impulsivity); (b) delayed-onset progressive memory and executive dysfunction, with one subject having initial motor signs prior to the cognitive difficulties; and (c) football players who exhibited chronic postconcussive symptoms (e.g., headache, forgetfulness, concentration difficulties, depression). Neuropsychological testing showed impairments in visual and verbal memory, and executive function impairments were most prominent in the cognitive group. All subjects in the behavioral/mood group had clinically elevated scores on the Geriatric Depression Scale (GDS). Elevated depression (Casson, Viano, Haacke, Kou, & LeStrange, 2014; Didehbani et al., 2013; Guskiewicz et al., 2007; Hart et al., 2013; Kerr et al., 2012), and cognitive impairments (Casson et al., 2014; Hart et al., 2013; Randolph, Karantzoulis, & Guskiewicz, 2013; Strain et al., 2015) have been reported in many other samples of former NFL players.

Work by our group and others (Reams et al., 2016) is continuing to refine the Montenigro et al. (2014) TES criteria. However, TES should be considered a provisional clinical research diagnosis and is not meant to indicate underlying CTE neuropathology. The etiology of TES could be from neurodegenerative diseases other than CTE or possibly from chronic or progressive white matter degeneration from recurrent head trauma. However, within the TES classification approach, there are separate diagnostic criteria for Possible CTE, Probable CTE, or Unlikely CTE. A Probable CTE diagnosis requires in vivo biomarker evidence suggestive of the presence of underlying CTE neuropathology, as well as meeting diagnostic criteria for TES. The use of biomarkers is the gold standard for the in vivo diagnosis of AD (Jack et al., 2011; McKhann et al., 2011). Validated available in vivo biomarkers of CTE do not yet exist, but potential targets have been identified.

Possible Biomarkers of CTE

In this subsection, we review studies that have examined potential biomarkers for CTE through the use of various neuroimaging technologies, as well as cerebrospinal fluid and blood protein analysis in former contact sport athletes with a focus on former professional tackle football players

Magnetic Resonance Imaging

MRI assessments of cortical and subcortical gray matter volume (high resolution T1 MRI), white matter microstructure (e.g., DTI), cerebral blood flow (e.g., arterial spin labeling [ASL], single photon emission computed tomography [SPECT]), and neurochemistry (e.g., MRS) can identify potential biomarkers of CTE. Biomarker support for these structural and functional brain alterations is found in the neuropathology of CTE, as described above. However, there is also in vivo research that shows long-term structural, functional, and molecular brain alterations in former professional American football players at high risk for CTE, as reviewed next.

Cavum Septum Pellucidum

A cavum septum pellucidum (CSP) is a separation of the two leaflets of the septum pellucidum and is a common neuropathological finding in autopsy-confirmed cases of CTE (McKee et al., 2013). A CSP can be observed on conventional MRI. Former NFL players exhibit greater rates of CSP (Gardner, Hess, et al., 2016; Gardner, Possin, et al., 2015; Koerte et al., 2016; Kuhn, Zuckerman, Solomon, & Casson, 2016), greater CSP length, and greater ratio of CSP length to septum length (Koerte et al., 2016). Greater CSP length has been identified as a correlate of poorer verbal learning and word reading in former NFL players (Koerte et al., 2016).

Cortical Atrophy and Thinning

In a case series study of former NFL players, seven out of nine had cortical atrophy on MRI (Gardner et al., 2015). Former NFL players have been shown to exhibit smaller hippocampal volumes when compared with age-matched controls (Coughlin et al., 2015). Anterior temporal lobe thinning was reported in former professional football players with a concussion history, with an inverse relationship between orbitofrontal cortical thickness and aggression and errors on a go/no-go task (Goswami et al., 2016). Lower frontal and temporal cortical thickness has also been observed in a sample of 11 former football players, when compared with noncontact sport athlete controls, and greater number of reported concussions was found to predict decreased cortical thickness (Adler et al., 2018). Recent findings from the

DETECT study have further shown smaller amygdala, hippocampus, and cingulate gyrus volumes in symptomatic former NFL players, when compared with controls, and reduced cingulate gyrus and right hippocampal volume correlated with worse psychomotor speed/executive function and visual memory, respectively, in the former NFL players (Lepage et al., 2017).

White Matter Alterations

DTI is an MRI technique that can measure microstructural axonal integrity and is used to investigate the diffuse axonal injuries associated with acute concussion (Giza & Hovda, 2014). Although limited, research has begun to use DTI to examine white matter tract integrity in former professional American football players. Frontal lobe white matter integrity has been correlated with severity of depressive symptoms in a sample of 26 former NFL players (Strain et al., 2013). Lower FA predicted worse scores on a confrontation naming task in former NFL players with specific effects for the forceps minor and major (Strain et al., 2017). Diffusion imaging of the uncinate fasciculus has been found to differentiate former professional football players from healthy controls, and axial diffusivity of the uncinate fasciculus negatively correlated with error rates on a go/no-go task, as well as with aggression (Goswami et al., 2016).

Cerebral Hypoperfusion and Functional Hypoactivity

Cerebral blood flow (CBF) and metabolism has been examined in former NFL players using functional MRI (fMRI), SPECT, and ASL. Among 34 former NFL players and 26 controls who completed ASL MRI, the former NFL players exhibited CBF alterations in multiple regions, including reduced temporal and occipital CBF (Hart et al., 2013). Reduced CBF (as measured by SPECT) was found in another sample of 36 former NFL players (Amen et al., 2016), and hyperactivity and hypoconnectivity of the dorsolateral frontal and frontopolar cortices have also been reported in former NFL players (Hampshire, MacDonald, & Owen, 2013).

Neurochemical Alterations

MRS measures physiological metabolism in vivo. Using a standard MR scanner, it quantifies concentrations of neurometabolic markers that reflect distinct pathology, including neuronal loss (N-acetyl aspartate; NAA), excitotoxicity (glutamate; Glu), axonal injury (Cho), reduced cellular energetics (creatine; Cr), neuroinflammation (glutathione; GSH), and astrocytosis and microglial activation (myo-inositol; mI; Lin et al., 2012). A recent study examined the MRS in former NFL players from the DETECT study. Findings included lower NAA in the parietal white matter among the former NFL players, compared with controls, and robust correlations between anterior cingulate gyrus neurochemistry and clinical function in the former NFL players (Alosco, Tripodis, Rowland, et al., 2017). As previously mentioned, greater RHI exposure also correlated with lower parietal white matter Cr concentrations, suggesting RHI may lead to long-term declines in cellular energy metabolism. Localized Correlated Spectroscopy (L-COSY) is a two-dimensional MRS method that provides a more robust and specific assessment of neurometabolites; it has been examined in five former professional male athletes with a history of RHI exposure (three football players, one professional wrestler, and one baseball player; Lin et al., 2015). Relative to controls, former athletes had >30% Glx (glutamate/glutamine) increases, and 65% higher levels of Cho in the PCG. Spectral regions that contain threonine, fucosylated molecules, lactate, and phenylalanine—metabolites not measured by one-dimensional MRS—were higher in the former athletes. Tremblay and colleagues examined 30 former male college athletes (70% former ice hockey players, 30% former American football players) between the ages of 51 and 75 who were clinically intact and underwent clinical (e.g., neuropsychological testing) and neuroimaging evaluations, including MRS (Tremblay et al., 2013). Among the formerly concussed athletes, there were elevated levels of mI/H_2O in the left medial temporal lobe (MTL) that negatively correlated with episodic memory test performance. There were reductions in Cho in the MTL, and the right prefrontal cortex had increased Cho/H_2O. While MRS is safe and noninvasive, PET radiotracers may offer insight into RHI exposure and neuroinflammation. Former NFL players have been shown to exhibit an increase in binding of [^{11}C]DPA-713 to the translocator protein, suggestive of brain injury and repair, compared with age-match healthy controls (Coughlin, Wang, Minn, et al., 2017; Coughlin, Wang, Munro, et al., 2015).

PET Amyloid and Tau Imaging

MRI does not measure the underlying pathology of CTE, that is, p-tau burden. PET is a nuclear medicine functional imaging method that detects gamma rays emitted from radiolabeled tracers injected into the body. The Food and Drug Administration (FDA) approved PET ligands that bind to beta-amyloid (e.g., [(18)F]-Florbetapir), which are used for the detection of AD. Florbetapir PET may facilitate differential diagnosis of CTE from AD, and other tauopathies. Beta-amyloid is required for the neuropathological diagnosis of AD, but is not a consistent feature of CTE. A negative amyloid PET in an individual who meets the TES diagnostic criteria would be suggestive of CTE, particularly when all other neurological or neuropsychiatric disorders have been ruled out. PET p-tau ligands will optimize clinical diagnostic certainty of CTE, when used in conjunction with amyloid PET. FDDNP is a PET ligand that targets p-tau, and uptake of this radioligand has been shown to be higher among small samples of symptomatic former professional football players (Barrio et al., 2015; Small et al., 2013); the pattern of FDDNP uptake in the Barrio et al. study was inconsistent with the neuropathological descriptions of CTE (McKee et al., 2013). FDDNP lacks diagnostic accuracy and specificity to p-tau, as it binds to beta-amyloid and other proteins. The PET ligand [(18)F]-T807 (also known as AV1451) has improved specificity to p-tau, and a recent case study of a former NFL player supports the diagnostic utility of T807 in CTE (Mitsis et al., 2014). Studies examining T807 PET in former NFL players are currently being completed.

Fluid Biomarkers

PET and other neuroimaging modalities are expensive and time-consuming and can be invasive. Fluid biomarkers derived from blood or cerebrospinal fluid (CSF) are more practical biomarker alternatives that may provide initial screening for underlying CTE neuropathology. Plasma and CSF concentrations of beta-amyloid, total tau, and p-tau (plasma p-tau assays are being refined) are established biomarkers of AD (Olsson et al., 2016). Limited research has examined diagnostic capabilities of fluid biomarkers to detect long-term neurological conditions associated with RHI exposure, including CTE. Stern and colleagues (2016) examined plasma exosomal tau in 78 former NFL players and 16 same-age controls from the DETECT study. Exosomes are nanovesicles released into the periphery and carry the cargo contents of their parent cells. Exosomes can cross the blood–brain barrier. If tau was present in the parent cell, it would be contained in the exosome, and can be isolated by sophisticated analyses of blood assays. The former NFL players from DETECT exhibited higher concentrations of plasma exosomal tau, when compared with the controls, and discriminated the former NFL players from controls with 82% sensitivity and 100% specificity. Greater exosomal tau levels predicted worse memory and psychomotor speed test performance in the former NFL players. These findings require validation using more refined procedures for exosome isolation and p-tau antibodies.

The plasma exosomal tau finding(s) were complemented by a subsequent study in DETECT examining plasma total tau as a potential biomarker for CTE, using new single molecule array technology. There were no differences in plasma total tau levels between former symptomatic NFL players and the controls in DETECT, but the former NFL players exhibited more extreme plasma total tau values. Of the 96 former NFL players in the DETECT sample, 12 had a plasma t-tau concentration greater than or equal to 3.56 pg/mL, whereas no controls had a plasma total tau at this level. As described above, in the former NFL players, greater RHI exposure (estimated using the previously described CHII) predicted higher levels of plasma total tau (Alosco,

Tripodis, Jarnagin, et al., 2017). At the time of this writing, analyses of CSF concentrations in the DETECT sample were being finalized. A recent study examined CSF proteins in professional Swedish ice hockey players who had repeated concussions and were diagnosed with postconcussion syndrome. Findings included increased neurofilament light in players with PCS for more than 1 year, when compared with controls and players whose PCS resolved within one year. Ice hockey players with PCS had lower beta-amyloid levels (Shahim et al., 2016).

CASE STUDY

The authors of this chapter have combined to conduct clinical family interviews for more than 100 cases with autopsy-confirmed CTE as part of ongoing clinicopathological research studies at the VA-BU-CLF. Based on our clinical research experiences with CTE, we present an illustrative case study of a clinically exemplar presentation of an individual with autopsy-confirmed Stage IV CTE. Isolation of a single case was not conducted, in order to preserve confidentiality. The nature of the highly public subjects studied in CTE (e.g., former NFL players) increases susceptibility to confidentiality breaches due to publicly available access to potentially identifiable information.

The case is Mr. A, a 70-year-old, right-handed, Caucasian deceased male who played 16 years of American tackle football. Mr. A played 2 years of youth football, 4 years in high school, four years at a Division I college, and six years professionally. His primary position was offensive lineman. The family estimated that he experienced hundreds of concussions (after being read a modern definition of concussion [Robbins et al., 2014]) that all occurred during his participation in tackle football. None of the concussions resulted in loss of consciousness, or required hospitalization, and he never experienced persistent postconcussive symptoms. He did not participate in any other contact sports, and there is no military history. Mr. A was described to have a "happy" childhood and adolescence, without a history of physical or sexual abuse, or participation in mental health treatment. His premorbid personality was characterized as "bigger than life," "warm," "kind," and "generous." Medical history is remarkable for weight gain following retirement from football at age 28, which led to onset of hypertension and sleep apnea. These were managed with medications and CPAP, respectively. He had numerous orthopedic injuries from football that required surgical repair throughout his life, and he suffered from chronic pain. There is no history of illicit drug use, or misuse of prescription medications. He has no reported family history of mental health illness or dementia.

Following retirement from football at 28, Mr. A married his girlfriend of 10 years. He initially had difficulties adjusting to a nonfootball lifestyle, particularly financially. He spent 2 years exploring different career avenues. In collaboration with other retired football players, he started his own sports apparel business, which quickly became successful. Mr. A had two children by the time he was 31. His wife did not notice any changes in him in the first 5 years of marriage, besides complaints of regular headaches that he managed with Tylenol. At the age of 35, he became less interested in attending family gatherings or recreational activities for his children. He preferred to stay at home and work. He became irritable and short-tempered. Mr. A complained to his wife of interpersonal difficulties with colleagues at work, which included several verbal altercations. At the age of 40, he began to become verbally aggressive with his wife. He was argumentative and made offensive remarks to her, and his wife described him as having a "short fuse." While he historically consumed alcohol occasionally, his use increased at age 40. His use never became excessive, but when he did consume alcohol, he became physically aggressive with his wife. Mr. A's interpersonal difficulties at work worsened, and many of his business partners began to quit. His company began to fail financially forcing him to terminate his business. Mr. A became depressed, and began to withdraw and isolate himself. He expressed suicidal ideations to his wife. He never attempted suicide. His wife was able to convince him to see a psychiatrist at age 45, who prescribed him Celexa. He continued to be monitored by psychiatry and the Celexa stabilized his depression, though his irritability and anger remained and progressively worsened. Mr. A attempted to start several additional businesses, but none ever came to fruition due to his depression, and interpersonal difficulties. There came a point when his family no longer enjoyed his presence, and his wife considered divorce, but she ultimately remained in the marriage for the sake of their children.

At age 55, he began to exhibit lapses in judgment. There was one instance when a stranger approached him and asked for money, and he proceeded to give this individual $1,000. He would also drive two hours to a fast-food restaurant, despite the same restaurant having a location around the corner from his house. He began to make mistakes while performing his lifelong hobby of wood working, such as taking incorrect measurements. At age 57, he began to have memory difficulties, including forgetting recent conversations, misplacing his personal belongings, and trouble remembering scheduled appointments and/or recreational activities. He had mild word-finding difficulties, which caused him to withdraw from conversations with others for fear of making a mistake. His language comprehension was intact, and he never had difficulties with social comportment. His cognitive difficulties progressively worsened over time. By age 60, his wife had to assume responsibility of the household finances because he was forgetting to pay the bills. At this same time, he was starting to become lost while driving around the town in which he had resided for the past 15 years. Mr. A stopped driving at 61 following a motor vehicle accident. He required the assistance of a pillbox and reminders from his wife to manage his medications. Along with the progression of cognitive impairments, his depression and irritability also worsened.

He went to see a neurologist for his cognitive difficulties at age 62. A brain MRI was remarkable for global cortical atrophy. There was mild hippocampal atrophy. A cavum septum pellucidum was present. He had mild small-vessel ischemic disease. Motor exam was unremarkable. Behavioral observations were notable for circumstantial speech and confabulation, as well as low frustration tolerance. His behaviors were otherwise appropriate for the circumstances. Neuropsychological testing showed severe impairment in executive functions, and learning for unstructured (i.e., word lists) and contextualized (i.e., stories) verbal information. His immediate and delayed recall of the information was borderline impaired; although, on the delay trial, he recalled the words he learned. Recognition was low average. Confrontation naming was mildly impaired, as were his performances on tasks of phonemic and semantic fluency. Visual memory, visuospatial abilities, and language expression and comprehension, were all intact. His scores on self-report measures of depression and anxiety were severely elevated. The neurologist diagnosed him with dementia with an unknown etiology. However, he referred him for a florbetapir PET, which was negative for elevated amyloid. His young age of symptom onset in the absence of family history, combined with lack of rapid forgetting, and negative amyloid imaging argued against AD. FTD was considered, but the duration of his clinical course, intact language, and intact social comportment were not fully consistent with what is typically observed in FTD. The neurologist suspected CTE, however, and was aware of the challenges of being able to diagnose this disease during life.

At age 64, his personal hygiene began to decline, as he refused to take showers or clean his clothes. He had minimal activity level. His sleep became disturbed at night because he stopped using his CPAP, and he subsequently napped frequently during the day. There were no signs of a REM sleep behavior disorder. He became physically combative with his wife one day when he was 65, at which time she feared for her safety and she called the police. He was hospitalized, and eventually transitioned into an assisted living facility. He was forced to leave the assisted living facility when he was 67 due to verbal aggression with other residents, and he became fully dependent for all basic self-care tasks. He was placed into a nursing home. The last two years of his life he rarely left his room and had trouble speaking. He developed bilateral tremors and had a shuffling gait, but these appeared to be related to his mood-stabilizing medication. He died at age 70 due to complications from end stage dementia.

For illustrative purposes, Mr. A meets TES criteria based on his head trauma exposure history (years of subconcussive head impact from America football), a decline in both cognitive and behavioral/mood function, presence of at least two supportive features (e.g., suicidal ideations, delayed onset, headaches), and that his clinical features were present for at least 12 months and did not appear to be fully accounted for by another neurological disorder. He did not have motor features. His clinical course was progressive, and he was functionally impaired. Mr. A would therefore be classified as TES-D, mixed subtype. The negative PET amyloid, in conjunction with global atrophy, hippocampal atrophy, and a CSP provides biomarker support for CTE, and permits the designation of Probable CTE.

CLINICAL TAKE-HOME POINTS

1. *The clinical manifestation of CTE has begun to be characterized* through clinical interviews with family members of individuals with autopsy-confirmed CTE, and includes a combination of early in life onset of behavior and mood impairments and later in life cognitive impairments that often lead to dementia.
2. *CTE cannot currently be diagnosed during life* because the clinical presentation of CTE remains ill-defined and validated in vivo biomarkers that can detect the presence of CTE have not yet been developed.
3. *CTE can present clinically similar to neurodegenerative diseases like AD and FTD.* Clinician's should be aware of the association between exposure to RHI and long-term neurological consequences, including CTE, and incorporate clinical assessment of RHI exposure and consider CTE as a potential differential for complex cases when there is a history of RHI exposure and biomarker results (e.g., florbetapir PET, CSF protein analysis) do not support other neurological diagnoses (e.g., AD).

KEY QUESTIONS TO BE ADDRESSED IN THE NEXT 5 YEARS

A 7-year multicenter study, the Diagnostics, Imaging, and Genetics Network for the Objective Study and Evaluation of Chronic Traumatic Encephalopathy (DIAGNOSE CTE) Research Project (PIs: Robert A. Stern

[Contact PI], Jeffrey Cummings, Eric Reiman, Martha Shenton), was recently funded by NINDS to facilitate clinical research on CTE. DIAGNOSE CTE is examining former NFL players with and without symptoms (high RHI exposure group), former college football players with and without symptoms (medium exposure group), and a control group (asymptomatic same-age men without RHI exposure or TBI). At baseline and a three-year follow-up, subjects for DIAGNOSE CTE undergo detailed clinical exams (neurological, motor, neuropsychological, neuropsychiatric, and daily functioning), neuro-imaging (PET tau and amyloid, MRI, fMRI, DTI, MRS), lumbar puncture for CSF protein analysis, and blood draw for DNA extraction and blood protein, and other biomarker analysis. DIAGNOSE CTE will help to address the following questions over the next 5 years:

1. *Can in vivo biomarkers detect the presence of CTE during life and facilitate a Probable CTE diagnosis?* There is a tremendous need for the development and validation of *in vivo* biomarkers that can predict the presence of underlying CTE neuropathology with a high degree of certainty. In vivo biomarkers will permit the designation of a Probable CTE diagnosis, and differentiate CTE from clinically similar neurodegenerative diseases (e.g., AD, FTD), as well as psychiatric disorders (e.g., posttraumatic stress disorder, depression) and postconcussion syndrome that have symptom overlap with CTE. The ability to clinically diagnose CTE during life will facilitate investigations on risk factors for CTE, in addition to longitudinal examinations that incorporate serial neuroimaging to identify the clinical course of CTE, and provide insight into how the acute neurological effects of RHI exposure transition to neurodegeneration.

2. *What is the validity and reliability of the TES clinical research diagnostic criteria?* Clinical research diagnostic criteria for CTE have been proposed, known as TES. The clinical utility and validity of the TES criteria need to be evaluated through inter-rater reliability studies, and clinicopathological investigations that correlate TES with CTE neuropathology. Such studies will be critical to update and refine the TES diagnostic criteria.

3. *What are the risk factors for CTE?* All neuropathologically confirmed cases of CTE to date have had a history of exposure to RHI, but not all individuals exposed to RHI develop CTE. RHI exposure is therefore a necessary but not a sufficient risk factor. Ongoing research will examine other risk factors for CTE, such as genetic, medical, lifestyle, and RHI exposure factors.

4. *What is the prevalence and incidence of CTE and are there available therapeutic interventions on the horizon?* It is the expectation that results from the DIAGNOSE CTE Research Project will eventually lead to epidemiological studies on CTE, the development of therapeutic interventions, and initiation of clinical trials for the treatment of this disease.

CONCLUSIONS AND FUTURE DIRECTIONS

A rapidly evolving literature in former contact sport athletes provides evidence that exposure to recurrent concussion and subconcussive injuries is associated with long-term neuropsychological and neuropsychiatric disturbances. Ex vivo studies have validated CTE as a distinct neurodegenerative disease caused, in part, by exposure to RHI (McKee et al., 2016). The neuropathological features of CTE are relatively well-defined (McKee, Cairns, et al., 2016; McKee, Stein, et al., 2013). However, there remain many knowledge gaps in the science of CTE, particularly in terms of its clinical presentation. Large-scale investigations that focus on the clinical features of CTE and developing methods for detecting CTE in life are of imminent importance due to the millions of individuals exposed to RHI each year, and the many more living individuals who have a history of exposure to RHI.

REFERENCES

Adams, J., Adler, C. M., Jarvis, K., DelBello, M. P., & Strakowski, S. M. (2007). Evidence of anterior temporal atrophy in college-level soccer players. *Clinical Journal of Sport Medicine, 17,* 304–306. http://dx.doi.org/10.1097/JSM.0b013e31803202c8

Adler, C. M., DelBello, M. P., Weber, W., Williams, M., Duran, L. R., Fleck, D., . . . Divine, J. (2018). MRI evidence of neuropathic changes in former college football players. *Clinical Journal of Sport Medicine, 1,* 100–105. http://dx.doi.org/10.1097/JSM.0000000000000391

Alosco, M. L., Jarnagin, J., Tripodis, Y., Platt, M., Martin, B., Chaisson, C. E., . . . Stern, R. A. (2017). Olfactory function and associated clinical correlates in former National Football League players. *Journal of Neurotrauma, 34,* 772–780. http://dx.doi.org/10.1089/neu.2016.4536

Alosco, M. L., Mez, J., Kowall, N. W., Stein, T. D., Goldstein, L. E., Cantu, R. C., . . . McKee, A. C. (2017). Cognitive reserve as a modifier of clinical expression in chronic traumatic encephalopathy: A preliminary examination. *The Journal of Neuropsychiatry and Clinical Neurosciences, 29,* 6–12. http://dx.doi.org/10.1176/appi.neuropsych.16030043

Alosco, M. L., Tripodis, Y., Jarnagin, J., Baugh, C. M., Martin, B., Chaisson, C. E., . . . Stern, R. A. (2017). Repetitive head impact exposure and later-life plasma total tau in former National Football League players. *Alzheimer's & Dementia: Diagnosis, Assessment & Disease Monitoring, 7*, 33–40. http://dx.doi.org/10.1016/j.dadm.2016.11.003

Alosco, M. L., Tripodis, Y., Rowland, B., Liao, H., Martin, B., Chua, A., . . . Lin, A. (2017). *A magnetic resonance spectroscopy investigation in symptomatic former NFL players.* Manuscript under review.

Amen, D. G., Willeumier, K., Omalu, B., Newberg, A., Raghavendra, C., & Raji, C. A. (2016). Perfusion neuroimaging abnormalities alone distinguish National Football League players from a healthy population. *Journal of Alzheimer's Disease, 53*(1), 237–241. http://dx.doi.org/10.3233/JAD-160207

Armstrong, R. A., McKee, A. C., Stein, T. D., Alvarez, V. E., & Cairns, N. J. (2017). A quantitative study of tau pathology in 11 cases of chronic traumatic encephalopathy. *Neuropathology and Applied Neurobiology, 43*, 154–166. http://dx.doi.org/10.1111/nan.12323

Bahrami, N., Sharma, D., Rosenthal, S., Davenport, E. M., Urban, J. E., Wagner, B., . . . Maldjian, J. A. (2016). Subconcussive head impact exposure and white matter tract changes over a single season of youth football. *Radiology, 281*, 919–926. http://dx.doi.org/10.1148/radiol.2016160564

Barrio, J. R., Small, G. W., Wong, K. P., Huang, S. C., Liu, J., Merrill, D. A., . . . Kepe, V. (2015). In vivo characterization of chronic traumatic encephalopathy using [F-18]FDDNP PET brain imaging. *Proceedings of the National Academy of Sciences of the United States of America, 112*, E2039–E2047. http://dx.doi.org/10.1073/pnas.1409952112

Baugh, C. M., Robbins, C. A., Stern, R. A., & McKee, A. C. (2014). Current understanding of chronic traumatic encephalopathy. *Current Treatment Options in Neurology, 16*, 306. http://dx.doi.org/10.1007/s11940-014-0306-5

Bazarian, J. J., Zhu, T., Zhong, J., Janigro, D., Rozen, E., Roberts, A., . . . Blackman, E. G. (2014). Persistent, long-term cerebral white matter changes after sports-related repetitive head impacts. *PLoS One, 9*, e94734. http://dx.doi.org/10.1371/journal.pone.0094734

Bieniek, K. F., Ross, O. A., Cormier, K. A., Walton, R. L., Soto-Ortolaza, A., Johnston, A. E., . . . Dickson, D. W. (2015). Chronic traumatic encephalopathy pathology in a neurodegenerative disorders brain bank. *Acta Neuropathologica, 130*, 877–889. http://dx.doi.org/10.1007/s00401-015-1502-4

Blaylock, R. L., & Maroon, J. (2011). Immunoexcitotoxicity as a central mechanism in chronic traumatic encephalopathy: A unifying hypothesis. *Surgical Neurology International, 2*, 107.

Blumbergs, P. C., Scott, G., Manavis, J., Wainwright, H., Simpson, D. A., & McLean, A. J. (1994). Staining of amyloid precursor protein to study axonal damage in mild head injury. *The Lancet, 344*, 1055–1056. http://dx.doi.org/10.1016/S0140-6736(94)91712-4

Bowman, K. M., & Blau, A. (1940). Psychotic states following head and brain injury in adults and children. In S. Brock (Ed.), *Injuries of the skull, brain and spinal cord: Neuro-psychiatric, surgical, and medico-legal aspects* (pp. 309–360). Baltimore, MD: Williams & Wilkins.

Brandenburg, W., & Hallervorden, J. (1954). *Dementia pugilistica mit anatomischem Befund* [Dementia pugilistica with anatomical findings]. *Virchows Archiv für pathologische Anatomie und Physiologie und für klinische Medizin, 325,* 680–709. http://dx.doi.org/10.1007/BF00955101

Broglio, S. P., Eckner, J. T., Martini, D., Sosnoff, J. J., Kutcher, J. S., & Randolph, C. (2011). Cumulative head impact burden in high school football. *Journal of Neurotrauma, 28,* 2069–2078. http://dx.doi.org/10.1089/neu.2011.1825

Broglio, S. P., Eckner, J. T., Paulson, H. L., & Kutcher, J. S. (2012). Cognitive decline and aging: The role of concussive and subconcussive impacts. *Exercise and Sport Sciences Reviews, 40,* 138–144.

Casson, I. R., Viano, D. C., Haacke, E. M., Kou, Z., & LeStrange, D. G. (2014). Is there chronic brain damage in retired NFL players? Neuroradiology, neuropsychology, and neurology examinations of 45 retired players. *Sports Health, 6,* 384–395. http://dx.doi.org/10.1177/1941738114540270

Caviness, V. S., Jr., Kennedy, D. N., Richelme, C., Rademacher, J., & Filipek, P. A. (1996). The human brain age 7–11 years: A volumetric analysis based on magnetic resonance images. *Cerebral Cortex, 6,* 726–736. http://dx.doi.org/10.1093/cercor/6.5.726

Cherry, J. D., Tripodis, Y., Alvarez, V. E., Huber, B., Kiernan, P. T., Daneshvar, D. H., . . . Stein, T. D. (2016). Microglial neuroinflammation contributes to tau accumulation in chronic traumatic encephalopathy. *Acta Neuropathologica Communications, 4,* 112. http://dx.doi.org/10.1186/s40478-016-0382-8

Cloots, R. J., Gervaise, H. M., van Dommelen, J. A., & Geers, M. G. (2008). Biomechanics of traumatic brain injury: Influences of the morphologic heterogeneities of the cerebral cortex. *Annals of Biomedical Engineering, 36,* 1203–1215. http://dx.doi.org/10.1007/s10439-008-9510-3

Cloots, R. J., van Dommelen, J. A., Nyberg, T., Kleiven, S., & Geers, M. G. (2011). Micromechanics of diffuse axonal injury: Influence of axonal orientation and anisotropy. *Biomechanics and Modeling in Mechanobiology, 10,* 413–422. http://dx.doi.org/10.1007/s10237-010-0243-5

Corsellis, J. A., Bruton, C. J., & Freeman-Browne, D. (1973). The aftermath of boxing. *Psychological Medicine, 3,* 270–303. http://dx.doi.org/10.1017/S0033291700049588

Coughlin, J. M., Wang, Y., Minn, I., Bienko, N., Ambinder, E. B., Xu, X., . . . Pomper, M. G. (2017). Imaging of glial cell activation and white matter integrity in brains of active and recently retired National Football League players. *JAMA Neurology, 74,* 67–74. http://dx.doi.org/10.1001/jamaneurol.2016.3764

Coughlin, J. M., Wang, Y., Munro, C. A., Ma, S., Yue, C., Chen, S., . . . Pomper, M. G. (2015). Neuroinflammation and brain atrophy in former NFL players:

An in vivo multimodal imaging pilot study. *Neurobiology of Disease, 74*, 58–65. http://dx.doi.org/10.1016/j.nbd.2014.10.019

Crisco, J. J., Fiore, R., Beckwith, J. G., Chu, J. J., Brolinson, P. G., Duma, S., . . . Greenwald, R. M. (2010). Frequency and location of head impact exposures in individual collegiate football players. *Journal of Athletic Training, 45*, 549–559. http://dx.doi.org/10.4085/1062-6050-45.6.549

Didehbani, N., Munro Cullum, C., Mansinghani, S., Conover, H., & Hart, J., Jr. (2013). Depressive symptoms and concussions in aging retired NFL players. *Archives of Clinical Neuropsychology, 28*, 418–424. http://dx.doi.org/10.1093/arclin/act028

Epstein, H. T. (1999). Stages of increased cerebral blood flow accompany stages of rapid brain growth. *Brain & Development, 21*, 535–539. http://dx.doi.org/10.1016/S0387-7604(99)00066-2

Ford, J. H., Giovanello, K. S., & Guskiewicz, K. M. (2013). Episodic memory in former professional football players with a history of concussion: An event-related functional neuroimaging study. *Journal of Neurotrauma, 30*, 1683–1701. http://dx.doi.org/10.1089/neu.2012.2535

Gaetz, M. (2004). The neurophysiology of brain injury. *Clinical Neurophysiology, 115*, 4–18. http://dx.doi.org/10.1016/S1388-2457(03)00258-X

Gardner, R. C., Hess, C. P., Brus-Ramer, M., Possin, K. L., Cohn-Sheehy, B. I., Kramer, J. H., . . . Rabinovici, G. D. (2016). Cavum septum pellucidum in retired American pro-football players. *Journal of Neurotrauma, 33*, 157–161. http://dx.doi.org/10.1089/neu.2014.3805

Gardner, R. C., Possin, K. L., Hess, C. P., Huang, E. J., Grinberg, L. T., Nolan, A. L., . . . Rabinovici, G. D. (2015). Evaluating and treating neurobehavioral symptoms in professional American football players: Lessons from a case series. *Neurology. Clinical Practice, 5*, 285–295. http://dx.doi.org/10.1212/CPJ.0000000000000157

Giedd, J. N. (2008). The teen brain: Insights from neuroimaging. *Journal of Adolescent Health, 42*, 335–343. http://dx.doi.org/10.1016/j.jadohealth.2008.01.007

Giza, C. C., & Hovda, D. A. (2014). The new neurometabolic cascade of concussion. *Neurosurgery, 75*(Suppl. 4), S24–S33. http://dx.doi.org/10.1227/NEU.0000000000000505

Goldstein, L. E., Fisher, A. M., Tagge, C. A., Zhang, X. L., Velisek, L., Sullivan, J. A., . . . McKee, A. C. (2012). Chronic traumatic encephalopathy in blast-exposed military veterans and a blast neurotrauma mouse model. *Science Translational Medicine, 4*, 134ra60. Advance online publication. http://dx.doi.org/10.1126/scitranslmed.3003716

Goswami, R., Dufort, P., Tartaglia, M. C., Green, R. E., Crawley, A., Tator, C. H., . . . Davis, K. D. (2016). Frontotemporal correlates of impulsivity and machine learning in retired professional athletes with a history of multiple concussions. *Brain Structure & Function, 221*, 1911–1925. http://dx.doi.org/10.1007/s00429-015-1012-0

Guskiewicz, K. M., Marshall, S. W., Bailes, J., McCrea, M., Cantu, R. C., Randolph, C., & Jordan, B. D. (2005). Association between recurrent concussion and late-life cognitive impairment in retired professional football players. *Neurosurgery, 57*, 719–726. http://dx.doi.org/10.1093/neurosurgery/57.4.719

Guskiewicz, K. M., Marshall, S. W., Bailes, J., McCrea, M., Harding, H. P., Jr., Matthews, A., . . . Cantu, R. C. (2007). Recurrent concussion and risk of depression in retired professional football players. *Medicine and Science in Sports and Exercise, 39*, 903–909. http://dx.doi.org/10.1249/mss.0b013e3180383da5

Gysland, S. M., Mihalik, J. P., Register-Mihalik, J. K., Trulock, S. C., Shields, E. W., & Guskiewicz, K. M. (2012). The relationship between subconcussive impacts and concussion history on clinical measures of neurologic function in collegiate football players. *Annals of Biomedical Engineering, 40*, 14–22. http://dx.doi.org/10.1007/s10439-011-0421-3

Hampshire, A., MacDonald, A., & Owen, A. M. (2013). Hypoconnectivity and hyperfrontality in retired American football players. *Scientific Reports, 3*, 2972. http://dx.doi.org/10.1038/srep02972

Hart, J., Jr., Kraut, M. A., Womack, K. B., Strain, J., Didehbani, N., Bartz, E., . . . Cullum, C. M. (2013). Neuroimaging of cognitive dysfunction and depression in aging retired National Football League players: A cross-sectional study. *JAMA Neurology, 70*, 326–335. http://dx.doi.org/10.1001/2013.jamaneurol.340

Hyman, B. T., Phelps, C. H., Beach, T. G., Bigio, E. H., Cairns, N. J., Carrillo, M. C., . . . Montine, T. J. (2012). National Institute on Aging–Alzheimer's Association guidelines for the neuropathologic assessment of Alzheimer's disease. *Alzheimer's & Dementia: The Journal of the Alzheimer's Association, 8*, 1–13. http://dx.doi.org/10.1016/j.jalz.2011.10.007

Jack, C. R., Jr., Albert, M. S., Knopman, D. S., McKhann, G. M., Sperling, R. A., Carrillo, M. C., . . . Phelps, C. H. (2011). Introduction to the recommendations from the National Institute on Aging–Alzheimer's Association workgroups on diagnostic guidelines for Alzheimer's disease. *Alzheimer's & Dementia: The Journal of the Alzheimer's Association, 7*, 257–262. http://dx.doi.org/10.1016/j.jalz.2011.03.004

Jordan, B. D. (2013). The clinical spectrum of sport-related traumatic brain injury. *Nature Reviews: Neurology, 9*(4), 222–230. http://dx.doi.org/10.1038/nrneurol.2013.33

Kerr, Z. Y., Marshall, S. W., Harding, H. P., Jr., & Guskiewicz, K. M. (2012). Nine-year risk of depression diagnosis increases with increasing self-reported concussions in retired professional football players. *The American Journal of Sports Medicine, 40*, 2206–2212. http://dx.doi.org/10.1177/0363546512456193

Koerte, I. K., Ertl-Wagner, B., Reiser, M., Zafonte, R., & Shenton, M. E. (2012). White matter integrity in the brains of professional soccer players without a symptomatic concussion. *JAMA, 308*, 1859–1861. http://dx.doi.org/10.1001/jama.2012.13735

Koerte, I. K., Hufschmidt, J., Muehlmann, M., Tripodis, Y., Stamm, J. M., Pasternak, O., . . . Shenton, M. E. (2016). Cavum septi pellucidi in symptomatic former professional football players. *Journal of Neurotrauma, 33*, 346–353. http://dx.doi.org/10.1089/neu.2015.3880

Kuhn, A. W., Zuckerman, S. L., Solomon, G., & Casson, I. (2016). 184 Interrelationships among neuroimaging biomarkers, neuropsychological test data, and symptom reporting in a cohort of retired National Football League players. *Neurosurgery, 63*(Suppl. 1), 173. http://dx.doi.org/10.1227/01.neu.0000489753.67038.ae

Langlois, J. A., Rutland-Brown, W., & Wald, M. M. (2006). The epidemiology and impact of traumatic brain injury: A brief overview. *The Journal of Head Trauma Rehabilitation, 21*, 375–378. http://dx.doi.org/10.1097/00001199-200609000-00001

Lepage, C., Muehlmann, M., Tripodis, Y., Hufschmidt, J., Stamm, J., Green, K., . . . Koerte, I. K. (2017). *Limbic system structure volumes and associated neurocognitive functioning in former NFL players*. Manuscript submitted for publication.

Lin, A. P., Liao, H. J., Merugumala, S. K., Prabhu, S. P., Meehan, W. P., III, & Ross, B. D. (2012). Metabolic imaging of mild traumatic brain injury. *Brain Imaging and Behavior, 6*, 208–223. http://dx.doi.org/10.1007/s11682-012-9181-4

Lin, A. P., Ramadan, S., Stern, R. A., Box, H. C., Nowinski, C. J., Ross, B. D., & Mountford, C. E. (2015). Changes in the neurochemistry of athletes with repetitive brain trauma: Preliminary results using localized correlated spectroscopy. *Alzheimer's Research & Therapy, 7*, 13. http://dx.doi.org/10.1186/s13195-015-0094-5

Ling, H., Morris, H. R., Neal, J. W., Lees, A. J., Hardy, J., Holton, J. L., . . . Williams, D. D. (2017). Mixed pathologies including chronic traumatic encephalopathy account for dementia in retired association football (soccer) players. *Acta Neuropathologica, 133*, 337–352. http://dx.doi.org/10.1007/s00401-017-1680-3

Martland, H. S. (1928). Punch drunk. *JAMA, 91*, 1103–1107. http://dx.doi.org/10.1001/jama.1928.02700150029009

Maxwell, W. L., Povlishock, J. T., & Graham, D. L. (1997). A mechanistic analysis of nondisruptive axonal injury: A review. *Journal of Neurotrauma, 14*, 419–440. http://dx.doi.org/10.1089/neu.1997.14.419

McAllister, T. W., Flashman, L. A., Maerlender, A., Greenwald, R. M., Beckwith, J. G., Tosteson, T. D., . . . Turco, J. H. (2012). Cognitive effects of one season of head impacts in a cohort of collegiate contact sport athletes. *Neurology, 78*, 1777–1784. http://dx.doi.org/10.1212/WNL.0b013e3182582fe7

McCrory, P., Meeuwisse, W., Dvořák, J., Aubry, M., Bailes, J., Broglio, S., . . . Vos, P. E. (2017). Consensus statement on concussion in sport—The 5th international conference on concussion in sport held in Berlin, October 2016. *British Journal of Sports Medicine, 51*, 838–847. http://dx.doi.org/10.1136/bjsports-2017-097699

McKee, A. C., Cairns, N. J., Dickson, D. W., Folkerth, R. D., Keene, C. D., Litvan, I., . . . the TBI/CTE Group. (2016). The first NINDS/NIBIB consensus meeting to define neuropathological criteria for the diagnosis of chronic traumatic encephalopathy. *Acta Neuropathologica, 131,* 75–86. http://dx.doi.org/10.1007/s00401-015-1515-z

McKee, A. C., Daneshvar, D. H., Alvarez, V. E., & Stein, T. D. (2014). The neuropathology of sport. *Acta Neuropathologica, 127,* 29–51. http://dx.doi.org/10.1007/s00401-013-1230-6

McKee, A. C., Stein, T. D., Kiernan, P. T., & Alvarez, V. E. (2015). The neuropathology of chronic traumatic encephalopathy. *Brain Pathology, 25,* 350–364. http://dx.doi.org/10.1111/bpa.12248

McKee, A. C., Stein, T. D., Nowinski, C. J., Stern, R. A., Alvarez, V. E., Daneshvar, D. H., . . . Cantu, R. C. (2013). The spectrum of disease in chronic traumatic encephalopathy. *Brain: A Journal of Neurology, 136,* 43–64. http://dx.doi.org/10.1093/brain/aws307

McKhann, G. M., Knopman, D. S., Chertkow, H., Hyman, B. T., Jack, C. R., Jr., Kawas, C. H., . . . Phelps, C. H. (2011). The diagnosis of dementia due to Alzheimer's disease: Recommendations from the National Institute on Aging–Alzheimer's Association workgroups on diagnostic guidelines for Alzheimer's disease. *Alzheimer's & Dementia: The Journal of the Alzheimer's Association, 7,* 263–269. http://dx.doi.org/10.1016/j.jalz.2011.03.005

Medana, I. M., & Esiri, M. M. (2003). Axonal damage: A key predictor of outcome in human CNS diseases. *Brain: A Journal of Neurology, 126,* 515–530. http://dx.doi.org/10.1093/brain/awg061

Mez, J., Daneshvar, D. H., Kiernan, P. T., Abdolmohammadi, B., Alvarez, V. E., Huber, B. R., . . . McKee, A. C. (2017). Clinicopathological evaluation of chronic traumatic encephalopathy in players of American football. *JAMA, 318,* 360–370.

Mez, J., Solomon, T. M., Daneshvar, D. H., Murphy, L., Kiernan, P. T., Montenigro, P. H., . . . McKee, A. C. (2015). Assessing clinicopathological correlation in chronic traumatic encephalopathy: Rationale and methods for the UNITE study. *Alzheimer's Research & Therapy, 7,* 62. http://dx.doi.org/10.1186/s13195-015-0148-8

Millspaugh, J. A. (1937). Dementia pugilistica. *United States Naval Medical Bulletin, 35,* 297–303.

Mitsis, E. M., Riggio, S., Kostakoglu, L., Dickstein, D. L., Machac, J., Delman, B., . . . Gandy, S. (2014). Tauopathy PET and amyloid PET in the diagnosis of chronic traumatic encephalopathies: Studies of a retired NFL player and of a man with FTD and a severe head injury. *Translational Psychiatry, 4,* e441. http://dx.doi.org/10.1038/tp.2014.91

Montenigro, P. H., Alosco, M. L., Martin, B. M., Daneshvar, D. H., Mez, J., Chaisson, C. E., . . . Tripodis, Y. (2017). Cumulative head impact exposure predicts later-life depression, apathy, executive dysfunction, and cognitive impairment in former high school and college football players. *Journal of Neurotrauma, 34*, 328–340. http://dx.doi.org/10.1089/neu.2016.4413

Montenigro, P. H., Baugh, C. M., Daneshvar, D. H., Mez, J., Budson, A. E., Au, R., . . . Stern, R. A. (2014). Clinical subtypes of chronic traumatic encephalopathy: Literature review and proposed research diagnostic criteria for traumatic encephalopathy syndrome. *Alzheimer's Research & Therapy, 6*, 68. http://dx.doi.org/10.1186/s13195-014-0068-z

Mouzon, B. C., Bachmeier, C., Ferro, A., Ojo, J. O., Crynen, G., Acker, C. M., . . . Crawford, F. (2014). Chronic neuropathological and neurobehavioral changes in a repetitive mild traumatic brain injury model. *Annals of Neurology, 75*, 241–254. http://dx.doi.org/10.1002/ana.24064

Olsson, B., Lautner, R., Andreasson, U., Öhrfelt, A., Portelius, E., Bjerke, M., . . . Zetterberg, H. (2016). CSF and blood biomarkers for the diagnosis of Alzheimer's disease: A systematic review and meta-analysis. *The Lancet Neurology, 15*, 673–684. http://dx.doi.org/10.1016/S1474-4422(16)00070-3

Omalu, B. I., Bailes, J., Hamilton, R. L., Kamboh, M. I., Hammers, J., Case, M., & Fitzsimmons, R. (2011). Emerging histomorphologic phenotypes of chronic traumatic encephalopathy in American athletes. *Neurosurgery, 69*, 173–183. http://dx.doi.org/10.1227/NEU.0b013e318212bc7b

Omalu, B. I., Bailes, J., Hammers, J. L., & Fitzsimmons, R. P. (2010). Chronic traumatic encephalopathy, suicides and parasuicides in professional American athletes: The role of the forensic pathologist. *The American Journal of Forensic Medicine and Pathology, 31*, 130–132. http://dx.doi.org/10.1097/PAF.0b013e3181ca7f35

Omalu, B. I., DeKosky, S. T., Hamilton, R. L., Minster, R. L., Kamboh, M. I., Shakir, A. M., & Wecht, C. H. (2006). Chronic traumatic encephalopathy in a National Football League player: Part II. *Neurosurgery, 59*, 1086–1093. http://dx.doi.org/10.1227/01.NEU.0000245601.69451.27

Omalu, B. I., DeKosky, S. T., Minster, R. L., Kamboh, M. I., Hamilton, R. L., & Wecht, C. H. (2005). Chronic traumatic encephalopathy in a National Football League player. *Neurosurgery, 57*, 128–134. http://dx.doi.org/10.1227/01.NEU.0000163407.92769.ED

Omalu, B. I., Fitzsimmons, R. P., Hammers, J., & Bailes, J. (2010). Chronic traumatic encephalopathy in a professional American wrestler. *Journal of Forensic Nursing, 6*, 130–136. http://dx.doi.org/10.1111/j.1939-3938.2010.01078.x

Omalu, B. I., Hamilton, R. L., Kamboh, M. I., DeKosky, S. T., & Bailes, J. (2010). Chronic traumatic encephalopathy (CTE) in a National Football League player: Case report and emerging medicolegal practice questions. *Journal of Forensic Nursing, 6*, 40–46. http://dx.doi.org/10.1111/j.1939-3938.2009.01064.x

Omalu, B. I., Hammers, J. L., Bailes, J., Hamilton, R. L., Kamboh, M. I., Webster, G., & Fitzsimmons, R. P. (2011). Chronic traumatic encephalopathy in an Iraqi war veteran with posttraumatic stress disorder who committed suicide. *Neurosurgical Focus, 31*, E3. http://dx.doi.org/10.3171/2011.9.FOCUS11178

Oppenheimer, D. R. (1968). Microscopic lesions in the brain following head injury. *Journal of Neurology, Neurosurgery, and Psychiatry, 31*, 299–306. http://dx.doi.org/10.1136/jnnp.31.4.299

Povlishock, J. T. (1993). Pathobiology of traumatically induced axonal injury in animals and man. *Annals of Emergency Medicine, 22*, 980–986. http://dx.doi.org/10.1016/S0196-0644(05)82738-6

Randolph, C., Karantzoulis, S., & Guskiewicz, K. (2013). Prevalence and characterization of mild cognitive impairment in retired National Football League players. *Journal of the International Neuropsychological Society, 19*, 873–880. http://dx.doi.org/10.1017/S1355617713000805

Reams, N., Eckner, J. T., Almeida, A. A., Aagesen, A. L., Giordani, B., Paulson, H., . . . Kutcher, J. S. (2016). A clinical approach to the diagnosis of traumatic encephalopathy syndrome: A review. *JAMA Neurology, 73*, 743–749. http://dx.doi.org/10.1001/jamaneurol.2015.5015

Robbins, C. A., Daneshvar, D. H., Picano, J. D., Gavett, B. E., Baugh, C. M., Riley, D. O., . . . Stern, R. A. (2014). Self-reported concussion history: Impact of providing a definition of concussion. *Open Access Journal of Sports Medicine, 5*, 99–103. http://dx.doi.org/10.2147/OAJSM.S58005

Roiger, T., Weidauer, L., & Kern, B. (2015). A longitudinal pilot study of depressive symptoms in concussed and injured/nonconcussed National Collegiate Athletic Association Division I student–athletes. *Journal of Athletic Training, 50*, 256–261. http://dx.doi.org/10.4085/1062-6050-49.3.83

Seichepine, D. R., Stamm, J. M., Daneshvar, D. H., Riley, D. O., Baugh, C. M., Gavett, B. E., . . . Stern, R. A. (2013). Profile of self-reported problems with executive functioning in college and professional football players. *Journal of Neurotrauma, 30*, 1299–1304. http://dx.doi.org/10.1089/neu.2012.2690

Shahim, P., Tegner, Y., Gustafsson, B., Gren, M., Ärlig, J., Olsson, M., . . . Blennow, K. (2016). Neurochemical aftermath of repetitive mild traumatic brain injury. *JAMA Neurology, 73*, 1308–1315. http://dx.doi.org/10.1001/jamaneurol.2016.2038

Shultz, V., Stern, R. A., Tripodis, Y., Stamm, J., Wrobel, P., Lepage, C., . . . Koerte, I. (2018). Age at first exposure to repetitive head impacts is associated with smaller thalamic volumes in former professional football players. *Journal of Neurotrauma, 35*, 278–285. http://dx.doi.org/10.1089/neu.2017.5145

Small, G. W., Kepe, V., Siddarth, P., Ercoli, L. M., Merrill, D. A., Donoghue, N., . . . Barrio, J. R. (2013). PET scanning of brain tau in retired National Football League players: Preliminary findings. *The American Journal of Geriatric Psychiatry, 21*(2), 138–144. http://dx.doi.org/10.1016/j.jagp.2012.11.019

Smith, D. H., Chen, X. H., Nonaka, M., Trojanowski, J. Q., Lee, V. M., Saatman, K. E., . . . Meaney, D. F. (1999). Accumulation of amyloid β and tau and the formation of neurofilament inclusions following diffuse brain injury in the pig. *Journal of Neuropathology and Experimental Neurology, 58*, 982–992. http://dx.doi.org/10.1097/00005072-199909000-00008

Stamm, J. M., Bourlas, A. P., Baugh, C. M., Fritts, N. G., Daneshvar, D. H., Martin, B. M., . . . Stern, R. A. (2015). Age of first exposure to football and later-life cognitive impairment in former NFL players. *Neurology, 84*, 1114–1120. http://dx.doi.org/10.1212/WNL.0000000000001358

Stamm, J. M., Koerte, I. K., Muehlmann, M., Pasternak, O., Bourlas, A. P., Baugh, C. M., . . . Shenton, M. E. (2015). Age at first exposure to football is associated with altered corpus callosum white matter microstructure in former professional football players. *Journal of Neurotrauma, 32*, 1768–1776. http://dx.doi.org/10.1089/neu.2014.3822

Stein, T. D., Alvarez, V. E., & McKee, A. C. (2015). Concussion in chronic traumatic encephalopathy. *Current Pain and Headache Reports, 19*, 47. http://dx.doi.org/10.1007/s11916-015-0522-z

Stein, T. D., Montenigro, P. H., Alvarez, V. E., Xia, W., Crary, J. F., Tripodis, Y., . . . McKee, A. C. (2015). Beta-amyloid deposition in chronic traumatic encephalopathy. *Acta Neuropathologica, 130*, 21–34. http://dx.doi.org/10.1007/s00401-015-1435-y

Stern, R. A., Daneshvar, D. H., Baugh, C. M., Seichepine, D. R., Montenigro, P. H., Riley, D. O., . . . McKee, A. C. (2013). Clinical presentation of chronic traumatic encephalopathy. *Neurology, 81*, 1122–1129. http://dx.doi.org/10.1212/WNL.0b013e3182a55f7f

Stern, R. A., Tripodis, Y., Baugh, C. M., Fritts, N. G., Martin, B. M., Chaisson, C., . . . Taylor, D. D. (2016). Preliminary study of plasma exosomal tau as a potential biomarker for chronic traumatic encephalopathy. *Journal of Alzheimer's Disease, 51*, 1099–1109. http://dx.doi.org/10.3233/JAD-151028

Strain, J., Didehbani, N., Cullum, C. M., Mansinghani, S., Conover, H., Kraut, M. A., . . . Womack, K. B. (2013). Depressive symptoms and white matter dysfunction in retired NFL players with concussion history. *Neurology, 81*, 25–32. http://dx.doi.org/10.1212/WNL.0b013e318299ccf8

Strain, J. F., Didehbani, N., Spence, J., Conover, H., Bartz, E. K., Mansinghani, S., . . . Womack, K. B. (2017). White matter changes and confrontation naming in retired aging national football league athletes. *Journal of Neurotrauma, 34*, 372–379. http://dx.doi.org/10.1089/neu.2016.4446

Strain, J. F., Womack, K. B., Didehbani, N., Spence, J. S., Conover, H., Hart, J., Jr., . . . Cullum, C. M. (2015). Imaging correlates of memory and concussion history in retired National Football League athletes. *JAMA Neurology, 72*, 773–780. http://dx.doi.org/10.1001/jamaneurol.2015.0206

Tagge, C. A., Fisher, A. M., Minaeva, O. V., Gaudreau-Balderrama, A., Moncaster, J. A., Zhang, X. L., . . . Goldstein, L. E. (2018). Concussion, microvascular injury, and early tauopathy in young athletes after impact head injury and an impact concussion mouse model. *Brain: A Journal of Neurology, 141*, 422–458. http://dx.doi.org/10.1093/brain/awx350

Tremblay, S., De Beaumont, L., Henry, L. C., Boulanger, Y., Evans, A. C., Bourgouin, P., . . . Lassonde, M. (2013). Sports concussions and aging: A neuroimaging investigation. *Cerebral Cortex, 23*, 1159–1166. http://dx.doi.org/10.1093/cercor/bhs102

Victoroff, J. (2013). Traumatic encephalopathy: Review and provisional research diagnostic criteria. *NeuroRehabilitation, 32*, 211–224. http://dx.doi.org/10.3233/NRE-130839

Wright, M. J., Woo, E., Birath, J. B., Siders, C. A., Kelly, D. F., Wang, C., . . . Guskiewicz, K. (2016). An index predictive of cognitive outcome in retired professional American football players with a history of sports concussion. *Journal of Clinical and Experimental Neuropsychology, 38*, 561–571. http://dx.doi.org/10.1080/13803395.2016.1139057

III

FACTORS AFFECTING THE VALIDITY OF NEUROPSYCHOLOGICAL RESULTS

7

SEX DIFFERENCES IN SPORTS-RELATED CONCUSSION

TRACEY COVASSIN, ABIGAIL C. BRETZIN,
AND MEGHAN E. FOX

Participation in female high school and collegiate sports has risen tremendously over the past few decades (National Federation of State High School Association [NFHS], 2016). As a result, female athletes are at risk for potential injuries, including concussion. Recently, there has been a focus on sex differences in sports-related concussion (SRC) outcomes. Therefore, this chapter addresses numerous areas related to sex differences in SRC. First, the most recent prevalence and injury rates between male and female athletes at both the high school and collegiate level are provided. Second, an overview of sex differences and concussion outcomes, particularly pertaining to symptom, vestibular, and neurocognitive function, is given. Third, recovery and treatment of SRC are discussed. A case study involving a female concussed soccer athlete is presented. We end the chapter with key take-home points and questions that need to be addressed over the next 5 years on sex differences in SRC.

http://dx.doi.org/10.1037/0000114-008
Neuropsychology of Sports-Related Concussion, P. A. Arnett (Editor)

SEX DIFFERENCES AND EPIDEMIOLOGY IN SPORT

In collegiate and high school athletics, the participation of female athletes has increased dramatically since the implementation of Title IX as part of the Equality in Education Act of 1972. In 2014–2015 the total number of students participating in high school sports was 7,807,047, the most since the NFHS began tracking participation in sports (NFHS, 2016). Girls' participation recorded the highest number ever reaching 3,287,735 athletes, an increase of 20,071 athletes from the previous year (NFHS, 2016). Boys' participation lost 8,682 athletes in 2015, with a total of 4,519,312 athletes (NFHS, 2016). With regard to collegiate athletes, National Collegiate Athletic Association (NCAA) athletic participation increased slightly to over 460,000 athletes (Irick, 2015). Due to this increase in sport participation, it is expected that the annual incidence of SRC will continue to rise.

Epidemiology of SRC is typically reported as either an incidence/prevalence (i.e., percentage of concussions) or an injury rate. An injury rate is defined as the number of injuries in a particular category divided by the number of athlete exposures (AEs) in that category (Kerr et al., 2014). An AE is defined as one student–athlete participating in a sanctioned practice or competition in which he or she was exposed to the possibility of a concussion (Kerr et al., 2014). For this chapter, all injury rates are expressed as 10,000 AEs in order to be consistent throughout the literature.

Recent research suggests that female high school athletes participating in comparable sports have a higher injury rate than male high school athletes (Gessel, Fields, Collins, Dick, & Comstock, 2007; Lincoln et al., 2011; Marar, McIlvain, Fields, & Comstock, 2012; Rosenthal, Foraker, Collins, & Comstock, 2014). Specifically, female athletes participating in soccer, basketball, and softball had a higher injury rate compared with male athletes. Female soccer and softball athletes have almost twice the risk for a SRC compared with their male counterparts. Lacrosse on the other hand, is the one comparable sport where males have an increased risk for a SRC compared with female lacrosse athletes (Xiang, Collins, Liu, McKenzie, & Comstock, 2014).

SRC incidence or injury rates have been reported for collegiate athletes using the NCAA Injury Surveillance Program (ISP; Kerr et al., 2014; see Table 7.1). Hootman, Dick, and Agel (2007) examined 15 years of NCAA ISP data across 16 sports. Similar to high school data, females participating in collegiate soccer, softball, basketball and ice hockey had a greater risk for an SRC than did male collegiate athletes. This study reported similar rates for SRC among male and female lacrosse athletes. An updated study by Kerr and colleagues indicated similar findings for soccer, softball and basketball. However, female lacrosse athletes were now found to have a greater risk of an SRC compared with male lacrosse athletes. Ice hockey was now found to

TABLE 7.1
Reported Concussion Rates by Sport, Sex, and Competition Level
(High School and College)

Sport	High School		College	
	Lincoln (1997–2008)	Rosenthal (2011–2012)	Hootman (1988–2004)	Kerr (2009–2014)
Football	6.0	9.4	3.7	6.7
Ice hockey (W)	—	—	9.1[a]	7.5
Ice hockey (M)	—	—	4.1	7.9
Lacrosse (W)	2.0	2.0	2.5	5.2
Lacrosse (M)	3.0	3.0	2.6	3.2
Soccer (W)	3.5	7.3	4.1	6.3
Soccer (M)	1.7	4.1	2.8	4.9
Wrestling	1.7	5.7	2.5	10.9
Field hockey	1.0	—	1.8	4.0
Basketball (W)	1.6	3.7	2.2	5.9
Basketball (M)	1.0	2.4	1.6	3.9
Softball	1.1	3.0	1.4	3.3
Baseball	0.6	1.4	0.7	0.9
Volleyball	—	1.7	0.9	3.6

Note. Rates per 10,000 AEs.
[a]Data from Lincoln et al. (2011); Rosenthal et al. (2014); Hootman et al. (2007); Kerr et al. (2016).

be fairly similar between male and female NCAA athletes (Kerr, Register-Mihalik, Kroshus, Baugh, & Marshall, 2016).

Females may have a greater risk for an SRC than male athletes for several reasons. Researchers have shown that males and females differ in anthropometrics (Eckner, Oh, Joshi, Richardson, & Ashton-Miller, 2014; Schmidt et al., 2014; Tierney et al., 2005), strength (C. L. Collins et al., 2014; Eckner et al., 2014; Mansell, Tierney, Sitler, Swanik, & Stearne, 2005; Schmidt et al., 2014; Tierney et al., 2005), and in head impact kinematics (Mansell et al., 2005). *Anthropometrics* is the study of human development in reference to height and weight, and is used to quantify dimensions of the body (Malina, Bouchard, & Bar-Or, 2004). When evaluating anthropometrics, females have an increased head–neck segment length (Mansell et al., 2005), as well as lower neck strength measures than males (C. L. Collins et al., 2014; Eckner et al., 2014; Mansell et al., 2005; Schmidt et al., 2014; Tierney et al., 2005). This, in turn, may influence the ability to contract surrounding musculature and couple the head–neck segment to the torso (Tierney et al., 2005). This may subsequently lead to a higher incidence in injury rate, as females are subject to higher forces of angular acceleration (Tierney, Higgins, et al., 2008; Tierney, Sitler, et al., 2005). There are also sex differences in the mechanism of SRC. Female athletes tend to incur their

SRC with a surface or ball contact, while male athletes tend to sustain their SRC due to contact with a player (Dick, 2009). Finally, males may "play through pain" and hide their symptoms. Research indicated that male collegiate athletes were 3 times more likely to not disclose their SRC than were female collegiate athletes (Kerr et al., 2016).

The published epidemiological data for SRC is most likely a conservative estimate, as many concussions go unreported (McCrea, Hammeke, Olsen, Leo, & Guskiewicz, 2004; Register-Mihalik et al., 2013). Moreover, the wide range of published epidemiological findings can be attributed to methodological differences across studies including study design (retrospective vs. prospective); different sources of data collection (athletic trainers, coaches); differences between sample populations (age groups, leagues, rules); and different definitions of injury. Nevertheless, consensus seems to support the notion that female athletes are at a greater risk for an SRC in comparable sports.

SEX DIFFERENCES AND CONCUSSION OUTCOMES IN SPORT

The management of SRC has seen vast improvement over the past decade. Results from empirical studies and consensus statements have refined evaluation and management strategies, benefitting both the sports-medicine professional and injured athletes. More specifically, this progress has seen the suggested abolishment of historically utilized concussion grading scales, improved diagnostic tools, and individual case management recommendations (McCrory et al., 2017). The current recommendation for the evaluation of an SRC involves a multifaceted approach that may include a symptom scale, vestibular/ocular assessment, postural stability assessment, and neurocognitive function (McCrory et al., 2017). Recent research suggests that there are sex differences in concussion outcomes (Berz et al., 2013; Covassin, Elbin, Harris, Parker, & Kontos, 2012; Zuckerman et al., 2012). In this next section, a summary of sex differences in SRC outcomes is presented.

Sex Differences in Concussion Symptoms

Sex differences in baseline symptoms and cognitive function have been well documented. Research has indicated that significantly more baseline symptoms are reported by female athletes compared with male athletes (Covassin, Elbin, Larson, & Kontos, 2012; Covassin, Swanik, et al., 2006). Moreover, female high school and collegiate athletes self-reported more cognitive, emotional, and sleep symptom clusters than male athletes at baseline (Covassin, Elbin, Larson, et al., 2012). With regard to general cognitive function, females performed better on tasks involving verbal memory and perceptual motor speed, whereas males performed better on tasks of visuospatial ability (Weiss et al., 2003). These sex differences have also been documented on neurocognitive measures commonly used for managing concussion (Barr, 2003; Brown, Guskiewicz, & Bleiberg, 2007; Covassin et al., 2006). Specifically, females performed higher on verbal memory, while males demonstrated higher visual memory scores than females (Covassin et al., 2006). Considering these results, discussing sex differences in symptom reports and concussion outcomes is warranted.

Male and female concussed athletes present with a wide variety of signs and symptoms. Multiple studies suggested that female athletes report more total symptoms and increased severity of symptoms compared to male athletes post-concussion (Berz et al., 2013; Covassin, Elbin, Bleecker, Lipchik, & Kontos, 2013; Covassin, Elbin, Harris, et al., 2012; Ono et al., 2015; Zuckerman et al., 2014). Research on adolescents suggests that females present with twice the total symptom scores compared to males on initial concussion assessment (Ono et al., 2015). When managing an SRC, clinicians should be aware of differing symptoms experienced by male and female concussed athletes. Headache is the most commonly reported symptom between both sexes (Guskiewicz, Weaver, Padua, & Garrett, 2000). Males commonly report amnesia and confusion/disorientation, while females report drowsiness and sensitivity to noise more frequently than males (Frommer et al., 2011). High school females experienced greater severity of symptoms for headache, pressure in the head, feeling slowed down, difficulty concentrating, and feeling more emotional, irritable, and sad compared with males (Baker et al., 2016). As a result, health care providers should be aware and mindful of these sex differences in self-reported concussion symptoms when examining concussed athletes.

Neurocognitive Function

Traditionally neuropsychologists used paper-and-pencil tests to determine whether an athlete had incurred an SRC. However, paper-and-pencil tests are time-consuming, costly and inefficient when testing a large number of athletes. As a result, computerized neurocognitive tests have been developed to assist with the evaluation and management of SRC. Computerized neurocognitive tests include Automated Neuropsychological Assessment Metrics (ANAM; Vista Life Sciences, n.d.), Concussion Vital Signs (CNS Vital Signs, 2004), Concussion Resolution Index (CRI) developed by HeadMinder (Erlanger, Feldman, & Kutner, 1999), Computerized Cognitive Assessment Tool (CCAT; Darby & Maruff (2001) marketed in North America by Axon Sports and developed by CogState, and Immediate Post-Concussion Assessment and Cognitive Test (ImPACT; Lovell & Collins,

2002). ImPACT is one of the most widely used computerized neurocognitive assessments available; it assesses verbal memory, visual memory, motor processing speed, and reaction time. Extensive research has been conducted on computerized neurocognitive assessments including sex differences. (See Chapter 9, this volume, on the validity of neuropsychological tests in SRC for a more complete discussion of issues relating to neurocognitive assessment.)

Sex differences in SRC outcomes have been reported in neurocognitive function. Researchers have reported sex differences in visual memory and reaction times (Colvin et al., 2009; Covassin, Elbin, Bleecker, et al., 2013; Covassin, Elbin, Harris, et al., 2012; Sandel, Schatz, Goldberg, & Lazar, 2017). Overall, female high school and collegiate athletes have decreased visual memory and slower reaction time speed compared with their male counterparts. More specifically, females demonstrated cognitive impairment 1.7 times more often than males in simple and choice reaction time (Broshek et al., 2005). These differences may be due to a greater basal rate of glucose metabolism (Andreason, Zametkin, Guo, Baldwin, & Cohen, 1994) and increased cerebral blood flow (Esposito, Van Horn, Weinberger, & Berman, 1996; Ibaraki et al., 2010). An SRC may exacerbate the neurometabolic cascade following injury, resulting in further decreases in cerebral blood flow and increases in glycemic demands (Broshek et al., 2005; Steenerson & Starling, 2017). Another explanation could be sex hormones which may increase neurocognitive impairments in female athletes (Emerson, Headrick, & Vink, 1993). Researchers have reported that following a concussion, females in the luteal phase of their menstrual cycle have high levels of progesterone, which has resulted in poor outcomes (Wunderle, Hoeger, Wasserman, & Bazarian, 2014). Consequently, due to these aforementioned reasons, concussed female athletes may exhibit prolonged neurocognitive impairments compared with males.

Vestibular/Ocular Motor Screening

With the advancing knowledge on SRCs and their resulting impact on the body, new forms of assessment have been developed. Two of these newly innovated assessment tools are the Vestibular and Ocular Motor Screening (VOMS) and the King–Devick (KD) test. The VOMS measures vestibular and ocular motor impairments through symptom provocation and near point convergence (Mucha et al., 2014). The KD measures vision disturbances in terms of saccadic performance (Galetta et al., 2011). Currently, there is very little research on sex differences and the VOMS or the KD.

In the only study to date to examine sex differences in VOMS at baseline, Kontos and colleagues reported that female collegiate athletes were more likely to have abnormal baseline VOMS scores compared with male collegiate athletes (Kontos, Sufrinko, Elbin, Puskar, & Collins, 2016).

Specifically, females had 3 times the risk of males for having one or more item scored above the clinical cutoff levels. The researchers surmised that females' greater proclivity for motion sickness may have played a role in this finding; however, more research is warranted to determine if sex differences exist in baseline vestibular and ocular motor components.

Although the KD was originally developed as an ocular reading test, recently the KD test has been used to assess SRCs. When examining differences among male and female concussed athletes, several researchers reported that sex had no effect on the KD scores (Benedict et al., 2015; Silverberg, Luoto, Öhman, & Iverson, 2014). Certainly, more research needs to be conducted on these assessments before conclusions can be drawn on whether sex differences exist within these new emerging SRC tools. Only minor differences were found on the VOMS with respect to females being at greater odds of having an item score above the established cutoff levels. Therefore, continued research into these findings is warranted.

Imaging

Currently, imaging has not been found to be a useful diagnostic tool for an SRC. However, diffusion tensor imaging (DTI) may be a gateway for SRC diagnosis through the exploration of white matter composition in the brain. With regard to sex differences and DTI, Fakhran, Yaeger, Collins, and Alhilali (2014) found that males have significantly decreased fractional anisotropy (FA) values bilaterally in the uncinate fasciculus (UF), whereas females demonstrated no significant difference in FA after a mild TBI. The UF is a bidirectional white matter tract that connects the lateral orbitofrontal cortex to the anterior temporal lobe and is thought to be partially responsible for memory performance (Fakhran et al., 2014). This may be one explanation for impairments in memory following an SRC. However, future research is needed to replicate the findings of this study, as well as explore other sex differences to determine if any exist in the white matter tracts. (See Chapter 5 for a more detailed discussion of DTI and other neuroimaging parameters in SRC.)

SEX DIFFERENCES AND RECOVERY FROM A SPORTS-RELATED CONCUSSION

Coaches, parents, and sports medicine professionals have a vested interest in ensuring the safety of athletes upon their return to play following concussion. Researchers suggest that 80% to 85% of all SRCs recover in 7 to 10 days (McCrory et al., 2017). In 10% to 20% of individuals, concussive symptoms and impairments may persist for a number of weeks, months, or even years. It is this group that requires close monitoring to determine clinical trajectories and early treatment options.

With regard to sex differences and recovery from an SRC, researchers have reported differences between male and female athletes. Researchers suggest that females demonstrate a protracted symptom recovery compared to male athletes (Baker et al., 2016; Berz et al., 2013; Kostyun & Hafeez, 2015; Zuckerman et al., 2014). Some investigators have suggested that females have taken as long as 23 days to become asymptomatic compared with males, who took 14 days to become asymptomatic (Baker et al., 2016). The higher prevalence of postconcussive symptoms may be related to females being more apt to report symptoms in general or their perceptions of overall injury (Granito, 2002). In addition, females have been shown to have greater concerns about implications on future health resulting from an injury (Granito, 2002).

Although females are reported to have increased deficits and a prolonged recovery following an SRC (Broshek et al., 2005; Covassin, Elbin, Harris, et al., 2012; Covassin, Elbin, Larson, et al., 2012), it has also been reported that recovery time, despite the larger symptom score in females, were the same in both sexes at adolescence (Ono et al., 2015). These contradictory findings on recovery time between sexes suggest that more research is needed to determine if female athletes take longer to recover on other aspects of concussion management besides self-reported symptoms. However, by acknowledging these differences in reporting behaviors, common symptoms reported by sexes, and recovery times between sexes, clinicians can effectively manage concussion as well as educate athletes. Further research is needed to determine best practices for treatment, especially if males and females should be treated differently, which is discussed in the next section.

SEX DIFFERENCES IN TREATMENT
FOR SPORTS-RELATED CONCUSSION

Generally, athletes recover from an SRC within 14 days after injury (McCrea et al., 2004; McCrory et al., 2013, 2017). However, it is the 10% to 20% who require treatment for their concussion symptoms and impairments that are of greatest concern. Moreover, it is suggested that females may report more signs and symptoms (Baker et al., 2016; Covassin, Elbin, Harris, et al., 2012; Kostyun & Hafeez, 2015), and therefore require more treatment strategies (Kostyun & Hafeez, 2015). Researchers have suggested that females are prescribed nearly twice the treatment interventions (2.2 treatment interventions) compared with males (1.3 treatment interventions; Kostyun & Hafeez, 2015). Interventions used to treat these athletes include rest, academic accommodations, vestibular therapy, and medications (Kostyun & Hafeez, 2015).

Rest or Exercise

The initial assessment of an SRC can determine clinical trajectories and treatment options for the concussed athlete. Initially clinicians prescribe physical and cognitive rest until asymptomatic. Immediately after injury the brain undergoes a neurometabolic crisis for which an increase in energy demand may hinder recovery (Silverberg & Iverson, 2013). This crisis leads to the idea that an athlete needs to completely rest following an SRC. A rest intervention that does not depend on the time postconcussion (i.e., 7 days or 30 days) was reported to be beneficial in decreasing symptoms and improving cognitive function (Moser, Glatts, & Schatz, 2012). Sex differences have been reported in the number of individuals who are prescribed rest as an intervention for their SRC. Females have been found to be prescribed rest seven times more often than males following their concussion (Kostyun & Hafeez, 2015). However, recently it has been suggested that rest may not be the best treatment for an SRC. Moderate levels of both physical and cognitive activity were reported to have significantly better performance on cognitive function than athletes participating in low or high levels of activity. This suggests that being under- or overactive may negatively influence concussion recovery (Majerske et al., 2008; Schneider et al., 2013). While considering exercise as a treatment option is a new approach to SRC management, more research is warranted to determine if exercise is beneficial to both male and female concussed athletes. (See Chapter 2 for some additional discussion of the benefits of exercise postinjury in SRC).

Academic Accommodations

In addition to rest and exercise, academic accommodations have also been prescribed to concussed athletes, especially high school and collegiate athletes. Academic accommodations frequently prescribed include extensions for assignments, quizzes or tests; a tutor when absent from the classroom; and modifying the environment such as reduced light and noise (Kostyun & Hafeez, 2015). When examining sex differences and academic accommodations, female concussed athletes were prescribed academic accommodations three times more often than males (Kostyun & Hafeez, 2015). Healthy adolescent girls have been shown to have sleep troubles, report feeling more stressed out, and have increased anxiety compared with adolescent boys (Dumont & Olson, 2012; Grills-Taquechel, Norton, & Ollendick, 2010). It has been suggested that females may need more academic accommodations to ease anxiety concerns over missed assignments or upcoming exams (Kostyun & Hafeez, 2015). In addition, female athletes have been found to take up to 28 days to recover from their SRC; therefore, they may need more academic accommodations compared with males due to an increase in symptom severity and length (Neidecker, Gealt, Luksch, & Weaver, 2017).

Pharmacology

Another common treatment intervention for an SRC is pharmacotherapy. The National Athletic Trainers' Association (NATA) position statement asserts that there is no evidence for medications to speed healing after an SRC (Broglio et al., 2014). In addition, aspirin and nonsteroidal anti-inflammatory drugs should be avoided because they mask symptoms, which could lead to a subsequent impact during competition (Broglio et al., 2014; McCrory et al., 2017). McCrory and colleagues (2017) also warned that medications for neurocognitive impairments (i.e., antidepressants) after an SRC may also mask symptoms when returning to competition, and should therefore be administered with caution. However, in more severe cases of SRC, pharmacotherapy can aid in decreasing symptoms in concussed athletes. For example, concussed athletes who are suffering from migraine symptoms could be prescribed Sumatriptan to decrease their headaches or Xanax for their anxiety symptoms.

With regard to sex differences, female concussed athletes were prescribed medications 4 times more often than male concussed athletes in one study (Kostyun & Hafeez, 2015). These sex differences in medications could be due to females in general having an increase in migraine symptoms (Lipton, Stewart, Diamond, Diamond, & Reed, 2001) and anxiety, therefore, medications could alleviate these symptoms following a concussion. (See Chapter 2 for additional discussion of the pros and cons of medications to treat headache in SRC.)

Vestibular Therapy

A common treatment intervention is vestibular therapy, especially in females (Kostyun & Hafeez, 2015). Females were 8 times more likely to be prescribed vestibular therapy than were males who had a concussion (Kostyun & Hafeez, 2015). Similarly, females were also referred for physical therapies significantly more often than males following their concussion (Vargo et al., 2015). Currently, the most commonly prescribed vestibular rehabilitation exercises following concussion included eye–hand coordination, standing static balance, and ambulation (Alsalaheen et al., 2013). These treatments may be beneficial for females—specifically in collegiate athletes—as they have been reported to score significantly higher (worse) than males using the Balance Error Scoring System following an SRC (Covassin, Elbin, Harris, et al., 2012). Ultimately, treatment of vestibular impairments requires a professionally trained person in neurorehabilitation who can design an individualized plan that targets the current symptoms (M. W. Collins, Kontos, Reynolds, Murawski, & Fu, 2014).

CASE STUDY

As previously mentioned, concussed athletes typically recover within 14 days (McCrory et al., 2017). However, the 10% to 20% of athletes who do not recover within 14 days present unique signs and symptoms to the clinician. The following is an example of a 15-year-old female athlete who incurred an SRC playing soccer. (Identifying information has been changed for the purpose of confidentiality.) The athlete presented on the field with no loss of consciousness and no amnesia; however, she appeared confused and dazed. After it was determined that the athlete did not have a spinal injury, she was moved off the playing field for further examination. The athlete was administered a clinical exam including cranial nerve testing, symptom checklist, standardized assessment of concussion (SAC), and short balance assessment. She scored 44 on the symptom severity scale, scored 23 out of 30 on her SAC test, and presented with mild balance problems. She was immediately removed from participation until cleared from a physician.

This was the athlete's second concussion in 2 years, both occurring in soccer. During the first week following her diagnosed concussion, she completed a postconcussion ImPACT test, which revealed cognitive impairments. Her balance improved the first week of her concussion; however, she still self-reported a high symptom severity score. She was told to avoid physical activity and was held out of school the first 2 days, which took her to the weekend; therefore, she was not in school for 4 days (2 weekdays, 2 weekend days). When the athlete returned to school, she was placed on a modified schedule. This modified schedule included no tests or quizzes, half-day participation, and no homework until her symptoms decreased, and no computer usage. By Day 14 she was still cognitively impaired as indicated by ImPACT and had migraine symptoms (i.e., headache, dizziness, nausea). She had returned to school full time within 2 weeks of her concussion, although she was still on a reduced homework, test, and quiz schedule in order to decrease any cognitive load on her brain. By 1 month postconcussion, she was still cognitively impaired and suffering from postmigraine symptoms. She was prescribed Topamax for her migraine symptoms and placed on a 504 plan for academic accommodations.

By Week 7, she finally presented with no cognitive impairments and no postconcussion symptoms. She was asked to stop taking Topamax to determine if she was truly asymptomatic or if the medication resulted in her being asymptomatic. Two months postconcussion, she was officially cleared by a physician to commence a stepwise return to play progression and was no longer on academic accommodations. Due to the length of her recovery, she was instructed to perform light aerobic (e.g., bike, jogging) activity for the first 14 days to increase her conditioning level. After this period, she returned to sport specific drills with no contact and no heading for another 14-day period. Three months postconcussion she was cleared for contact practice and eventually returned to participating in soccer games. As a result of the timing of her clearance (i.e., winter), she did not return to participate in a game situation until 6 months postconcussion. This is one illustration of a female athlete taking months to return to normal school activities and sport participation in the context of careful postconcussion management.

CLINICAL TAKE-HOME POINTS

It is very important for clinicians to be aware of sex differences in the risk and recovery of concussed athletes. What follows are a few clinical take-home points in relation to this.

1. *Clinicians should be aware that females in comparable sports will report more concussions than male athletes.* Therefore, clinicians should expect to see more female athletes in their practice, and expect them to report more symptoms and possibly take longer to recover than concussed male athletes.
2. *Clinicians should perform a thorough examination that incorporates a multifaceted approach, including a clinical interview, balance, vestibular and ocular motor, paper-and-pencil or computerized cognitive tests.* These results should be interpreted on an individual basis regardless of sex.
3. *Clinicians should prescribe treatment early in the recovery of a concussed athlete.* These treatments can include academic accommodations, medication, or vestibular therapy.

KEY QUESTIONS TO BE ADDRESSED IN THE NEXT 5 YEARS

Over the next 5 years, more research needs to be conducted on sex differences in SRC. Specifically, researchers should investigate three key areas.

1. *More research is warranted on sex differences and recovery from a sports-related concussion.* While the majority of research is conclusive on symptom severity and female athletes, more research

is needed on recovery of other measures such as vestibular, ocular and motor, and cognitive tasks.

2. *Researchers need to examine whether females are at greater risk than males for multiple concussions.* Researchers have suggested that male football athletes have a dose response to SRCs (Guskiewicz et al., 2003); however, no research to date has examined whether female athletes are at a greater risk for subsequent SRCs.

3. *While research is inconclusive on chronic traumatic encephalopathy (CTE), most research has focused on CTE in the brains of male athletes.* Researchers should focus more on the female brain and determine whether subconcussive impacts to the head or multiple sports-related concussions lead to CTE. (See Chapter 6 for a more extensive discussion on CTE.)

REFERENCES

Alsalaheen, B. A., Whitney, S. L., Mucha, A., Morris, L. O., Furman, J. M., & Sparto, P. J. (2013). Exercise prescription patterns in patients treated with vestibular rehabilitation after concussion. *Physiotherapy Research International, 18,* 100–108. http://dx.doi.org/10.1002/pri.1532

Andreason, P. J., Zametkin, A. J., Guo, A. C., Baldwin, P., & Cohen, R. M. (1994). Gender-related differences in regional cerebral glucose metabolism in normal volunteers. *Psychiatry Research, 51,* 175–183. http://dx.doi.org/10.1016/0165-1781(94)90037-X

Baker, J. G., Leddy, J. J., Darling, S. R., Shucard, J., Makdissi, M., & Willer, B. S. (2016). Gender differences in recovery from sports-related concussion in adolescents. *Clinical Pediatrics, 55,* 771–775. http://dx.doi.org/10.1177/0009922815606417

Barr, W. B. (2003). Neuropsychological testing of high school athletes. Preliminary norms and test–retest indices. *Archives of Clinical Neuropsychology, 18,* 91–101. http://dx.doi.org/10.1016/S0887-6177(01)00185-8

Benedict, P. A., Baner, N. V., Harrold, G. K., Moehringer, N., Hasanaj, L., Serrano, L. P., . . . Balcer, L. J. (2015). Gender and age predict outcomes of cognitive, balance and vision testing in a multidisciplinary concussion center. *Journal of the Neurological Sciences, 353,* 111–115. http://dx.doi.org/10.1016/j.jns.2015.04.029

Berz, K., Divine, J., Foss, K. B., Heyl, R., Ford, K. R., & Myer, G. D. (2013). Sex-specific differences in the severity of symptoms and recovery rate following sports-related concussion in young athletes. *The Physician and Sportsmedicine, 41,* 58–63. http://dx.doi.org/10.3810/psm.2013.05.2015

Broglio, S. P., Cantu, R. C., Gioia, G. A., Guskiewicz, K. M., Kutcher, J., Palm, M., & Valovich McLeod, T. C. (2014). National Athletic Trainers' Association position statement: Management of sport concussion. *Journal of Athletic Training, 49,* 245–265. http://dx.doi.org/10.4085/1062-6050-49.1.07

Broshek, D. K., Kaushik, T., Freeman, J. R., Erlanger, D., Webbe, F., & Barth, J. T. (2005). Sex differences in outcome following sports-related concussion. *Journal of Neurosurgery, 102,* 856–863. http://dx.doi.org/10.3171/jns.2005.102.5.0856

Brown, C. N., Guskiewicz, K. M., & Bleiberg, J. (2007). Athlete characteristics and outcome scores for computerized neuropsychological assessment: A preliminary analysis. *Journal of Athletic Training, 42,* 515–523. Retrieved from https://www.ncbi.nlm.nih.gov/pmc/articles/PMC2140078/

CNS Vital Signs, Inc. (2004). *Concussion Vital Signs* [Test]. Morrisville, NC: Author. Retrieved from http://www.concussionvitalsigns.com

Collins, C. L., Fletcher, E. N., Fields, S. K., Kluchurosky, L., Rohrkemper, M. K., Comstock, R. D., & Cantu, R. C. (2014). Neck strength: A protective factor reducing risk for concussion in high school sports. *The Journal of Primary Prevention, 35,* 309–319. http://dx.doi.org/10.1007/s10935-014-0355-2

Collins, M. W., Kontos, A. P., Reynolds, E., Murawski, C. D., & Fu, F. H. (2014). A comprehensive, targeted approach to the clinical care of athletes following sport-related concussion. *Knee Surgery, Sports Traumatology, Arthroscopy, 22,* 235–246. http://dx.doi.org/10.1007/s00167-013-2791-6

Colvin, A. C., Mullen, J., Lovell, M. R., West, R. V., Collins, M. W., & Groh, M. (2009). The role of concussion history and gender in recovery from soccer-related concussion. *The American Journal of Sports Medicine, 37,* 1699–1704. http://dx.doi.org/10.1177/0363546509332497

Covassin, T., Elbin, R. J., Bleecker, A., Lipchik, A., & Kontos, A. P. (2013). Are there differences in neurocognitive function and symptoms between male and female soccer players after concussions? *The American Journal of Sports Medicine, 41,* 2890–2895. http://dx.doi.org/10.1177/0363546513509962

Covassin, T., Elbin, R. J., Harris, W., Parker, T., & Kontos, A. (2012). The role of age and sex in symptoms, neurocognitive performance, and postural stability in athletes after concussion. *The American Journal of Sports Medicine, 40,* 1303–1312. http://dx.doi.org/10.1177/0363546512444554

Covassin, T., Elbin, R. J., III, Larson, E., & Kontos, A. P. (2012). Sex and age differences in depression and baseline sport-related concussion neurocognitive performance and symptoms. *Clinical Journal of Sport Medicine, 22,* 98–104. http://dx.doi.org/10.1097/JSM.0b013e31823403d2

Covassin, T., Swanik, C. B., Sachs, M., Kendrick, Z., Schatz, P., Zillmer, E., & Kaminaris, C. (2006). Sex differences in baseline neuropsychological function and concussion symptoms of collegiate athletes. *British Journal of Sports Medicine, 40,* 923–927. http://dx.doi.org/10.1136/bjsm.2006.029496

Darby, D., & Maruff, P. (2001). *Computerized Cognitive Assessment Tool (CCAT).* Wausau, WI: Axon Sports.

Dick, R. W. (2009). Is there a gender difference in concussion incidence and outcomes? *British Journal of Sports Medicine, 43,* i46–i50. http://dx.doi.org/10.1136/bjsm.2009.058172

Dumont, I. P., & Olson, A. L. (2012). Primary care, depression, and anxiety: Exploring somatic and emotional predictors of mental health status in adolescents. *Journal of the American Board of Family Medicine, 25,* 291–299. http://dx.doi.org/10.3122/jabfm.2012.03.110056

Eckner, J. T., Oh, Y. K., Joshi, M. S., Richardson, J. K., & Ashton-Miller, J. A. (2014). Effect of neck muscle strength and anticipatory cervical muscle activation on the kinematic response of the head to impulsive loads. *The American Journal of Sports Medicine, 42,* 566–576. http://dx.doi.org/10.1177/0363546513517869

Emerson, C. S., Headrick, J. P., & Vink, R. (1993). Estrogen improves biochemical and neurologic outcome following traumatic brain injury in male rats, but not in females. *Brain Research, 608,* 95–100. http://dx.doi.org/10.1016/0006-8993(93)90778-L

Erlanger, D. M., Feldman, D. J., & Kutner, K. (1999). *Concussion Resolution Index* [Assessment tool]. New York, NY: HeadMinder.

Esposito, G., Van Horn, J. D., Weinberger, D. R., & Berman, K. F. (1996). Gender differences in cerebral blood flow as a function of cognitive state with PET. *Journal of Nuclear Medicine, 37,* 559–564.

Fakhran, S., Yaeger, K., Collins, M., & Alhilali, L. (2014). Sex differences in white matter abnormalities after mild traumatic brain injury: Localization and correlation with outcome. *Radiology, 272,* 815–823. http://dx.doi.org/10.1148/radiol.14132512

Frommer, L. J., Gurka, K. K., Cross, K. M., Ingersoll, C. D., Comstock, R. D., & Saliba, S. A. (2011). Sex differences in concussion symptoms of high school athletes. *Journal of Athletic Training, 46,* 76–84. http://dx.doi.org/10.4085/1062-6050-46.1.76

Galetta, K. M., Brandes, L. E., Maki, K., Dziemianowicz, M. S., Laudano, E., Allen, M., . . . Balcer, L. J. (2011). The King–Devick test and sports-related concussion: Study of a rapid visual screening tool in a collegiate cohort. *Journal of the Neurological Sciences, 309,* 34–39. http://dx.doi.org/10.1016/j.jns.2011.07.039

Gessel, L. M., Fields, S. K., Collins, C. L., Dick, R. W., & Comstock, R. D. (2007). Concussions among United States high school and collegiate athletes. *Journal of Athletic Training, 42,* 495–503.

Granito, V. J., Jr. (2002). Psychological response to athletic injury: Gender differences. *Journal of Sport Behavior, 25,* 243. Retrieved from http://www.biomedsearch.com/article/Psychological-response-to-athletic-injury/90527923.html

Grills-Taquechel, A. E., Norton, P., & Ollendick, T. H. (2010). A longitudinal examination of factors predicting anxiety during the transition to middle school. *Anxiety, Stress, and Coping: An International Journal, 23,* 493–513. http://dx.doi.org/10.1080/10615800903494127

Guskiewicz, K. M., McCrea, M., Marshall, S. W., Cantu, R. C., Randolph, C., Barr, W., . . . Kelly, J. P. (2003). Cumulative effects associated with recurrent concussion in collegiate football players: The NCAA Concussion Study. *Journal of* the *American Medical Association, 290,* 2549–2555. http://dx.doi.org/10.1001/jama.290.19.2549

Guskiewicz, K. M., Weaver, N. L., Padua, D. A., & Garrett, W. E., Jr. (2000). Epidemiology of concussion in collegiate and high school football players. *The American Journal of Sports Medicine, 28,* 643–650. http://dx.doi.org/10.1177/03635465000280050401

Hootman, J. M., Dick, R., & Agel, J. (2007). Epidemiology of collegiate injuries for 15 sports: Summary and recommendations for injury prevention initiatives. *Journal of Athletic Training, 42,* 311–319. Retrieved from https://www.ncbi.nlm.nih.gov/pmc/articles/PMC1941297/

Ibaraki, M., Shinohara, Y., Nakamura, K., Miura, S., Kinoshita, F., & Kinoshita, T. (2010). Interindividual variations of cerebral blood flow, oxygen delivery, and metabolism in relation to hemoglobin concentration measured by positron emission tomography in humans. *Journal of Cerebral Blood Flow and Metabolism, 30,* 1296–1305. http://dx.doi.org/10.1038/jcbfm.2010.13

Irick, E. (Ed.). (2015). *Student–athlete participation 1981–82—2014–15: NCAA sports sponsorship and participation rates report.* Retrieved from https://www.ncaa.org/sites/default/files/Participation%20Rates%20Final.pdf

Kerr, Z. Y., Dompier, T. P., Snook, E. M., Marshall, S. W., Klossner, D., Hainline, B., & Corlette, J. (2014). National Collegiate Athletic Association injury surveillance system: Review of methods for 2004–2005 through 2013–2014 data collection. *Journal of Athletic Training, 49,* 552–560. http://dx.doi.org/10.4085/1062-6050-49.3.58

Kerr, Z. Y., Register-Mihalik, J. K., Kroshus, E., Baugh, C. M., & Marshall, S. W. (2016). Motivations associated with nondisclosure of self-reported concussions in former collegiate athletes. *The American Journal of Sports Medicine, 44,* 220–225. http://dx.doi.org/10.1177/0363546515612082

Kontos, A. P., Sufrinko, A., Elbin, R. J., Puskar, A., & Collins, M. W. (2016). Reliability and associated risk factors for performance on the vestibular/ocular motor screening (VOMS) tool in healthy collegiate athletes. *The American Journal of Sports Medicine, 44,* 1400–1406. http://dx.doi.org/10.1177/0363546516632754

Kostyun, R., & Hafeez, I. (2015). Protracted recovery from a concussion: A focus on gender and treatment interventions in an adolescent population. *Sports Health: A Multidisciplinary Approach, 7,* 52–57. http://dx.doi.org/10.1177/1941738114555075

Lincoln, A. E., Caswell, S. V., Almquist, J. L., Dunn, R. E., Norris, J. B., & Hinton, R. Y. (2011). Trends in concussion incidence in high school sports: A prospective 11-year study. *The American Journal of Sports Medicine, 39,* 958–963. http://dx.doi.org/10.1177/0363546510392326

Lipton, R. B., Stewart, W. F., Diamond, S., Diamond, M. L., & Reed, M. (2001). Prevalence and burden of migraine in the United States: Data from the American Migraine Study II. *Headache: The Journal of Head and Face Pain, 41,* 646–657. http://dx.doi.org/10.1046/j.1526-4610.2001.041007646.x

Lovell, M., & Collins, M. (2002). *Immediate Post-Concussion Assessment and Cognitive Test (ImPACT)*. Pittsburgh, PA: ImPact Applications, Inc. Retrieved from https://impacttest.com

Majerske, C. W., Mihalik, J. P., Ren, D., Collins, M. W., Reddy, C. C., Lovell, M. R., & Wagner, A. K. (2008). Concussion in sports: Postconcussive activity levels, symptoms, and neurocognitive performance. *Journal of Athletic Training, 43,* 265–274. http://dx.doi.org/10.4085/1062-6050-43.3.265

Malina, R. M., Bouchard, C., & Bar-Or, O. (2004). *Growth, maturation, and physical activity.* Champaign, IL: Human Kinetics.

Mansell, J., Tierney, R. T., Sitler, M. R., Swanik, K. A., & Stearne, D. (2005). Resistance training and head–neck segment dynamic stabilization in male and female collegiate soccer players. *Journal of Athletic Training, 4,* 310–319. Retrieved from https://www.ncbi.nlm.nih.gov/pmc/articles/PMC1323293/

Marar, M., McIlvain, N. M., Fields, S. K., & Comstock, R. D. (2012). Epidemiology of concussions among United States high school athletes in 20 sports. *The American Journal of Sports Medicine, 40,* 747–755. http://dx.doi.org/10.1177/0363546511435626

McCrea, M., Hammeke, T., Olsen, G., Leo, P., & Guskiewicz, K. (2004). Unreported concussion in high school football players: Implications for prevention. *Clinical Journal of Sport Medicine, 14,* 13–17. http://dx.doi.org/10.1097/00042752-200401000-00003

McCrory, P., Meeuwisse, W. H., Aubry, M., Cantu, B., Dvořák, J., Echemendia, R. J., . . . Turner, M. (2013). Consensus statement on concussion in sport: The 4th International Conference on Concussion in Sport held in Zurich, November 2012. *British Journal of Sports Medicine, 47,* 250–258. http://dx.doi.org/10.1136/bjsports-2013-092313

McCrory, P., Meeuwisse, W. H., Dvořák, J., Aubry, M., Bailes, J., Echemendia, R. J., . . . Vos, P. E. (2017). Consensus statement on concussion in sport—The 5th International Conference on Concussion in sport held in Berlin, October 2016. *British Journal of Sports Medicine, 51,* 838–847. http://dx.doi.org/10.1136/bjsports-2017-097699

Moser, R. S., Glatts, C., & Schatz, P. (2012). Efficacy of immediate and delayed cognitive and physical rest for treatment of sports-related concussion. *The Journal of Pediatrics, 161,* 922–926. http://dx.doi.org/10.1016/j.jpeds.2012.04.012

Mucha, A., Collins, M. W., Elbin, R. J., Furman, J. M., Troutman-Enseki, C., DeWolf, R. M., . . . Kontos, A. P. (2014). A brief vestibular/ocular motor screening (VOMS) assessment to evaluate concussions: Preliminary findings. *The American Journal of Sports Medicine, 42,* 2479–2486. http://dx.doi.org/10.1177/0363546514543775

Neidecker, J. M., Gealt, D. B., Luksch, J. R., & Weaver, M. D. (2017). First-time sports-related concussion recovery: The role of sex, age, and sport. *The Journal of the American Osteopathic Association, 117,* 635–642. http://dx.doi.org/10.7556/jaoa.2017.120

National Federation of State High School Associations. (2016). *Participation in high school sports increases again; confirms the NFHS commitment to stronger leadership.* Retrieved from https://www.nfhs.org/articles/high-school-sports-participation-increases-for-28th-straight-year-nears-8-million-mark/

Ono, K. E., Burns, T. G., Bearden, D. J., McManus, S. M., King, H., & Reisner, A. (2015). Sex-based differences as a predictor of recovery trajectories in young athletes after a sports-related concussion. *The American Journal of Sports Medicine, 44*, 748–752. http://dx.doi.org/10.1177/0363546515617746

Register-Mihalik, J. K., Guskiewicz, K. M., Valovich McLeod, T. C., Linnan, L. A., Mueller, F. O., & Marshall, S. W. (2013). Knowledge, attitude, and concussion—Reporting behaviors among high school athletes: A preliminary study. *Journal of Athletic Training, 48*, 645–653. http://dx.doi.org/10.4085/1062-6050-48.3.20

Rosenthal, J. A., Foraker, R. E., Collins, C. L., & Comstock, R. D. (2014). National high school athlete concussion rates from 2005–2006 to 2011–2012. *The American Journal of Sports Medicine, 42*, 1710–1715. http://dx.doi.org/10.1177/0363546514530091

Sandel, N. K., Schatz, P., Goldberg, K. B., & Lazar, M. (2017). Sex-based differences in cognitive deficits and symptom reporting among acutely concussed adolescent lacrosse and soccer players. *The American Journal of Sports Medicine, 45*, 937–944. http://dx.doi.org/10.1177/0363546516677246

Schmidt, J. D., Guskiewicz, K. M., Blackburn, J. T., Mihalik, J. P., Siegmund, G. P., & Marshall, S. W. (2014). The influence of cervical muscle characteristics on head impact biomechanics in football. *The American Journal of Sports Medicine, 42*, 2056–2066. http://dx.doi.org/10.1177/0363546514536685

Schneider, K. J., Iverson, G. L., Emery, C. A., McCrory, P., Herring, S. A., & Meeuwisse, W. H. (2013). The effects of rest and treatment following sport-related concussion: A systematic review of the literature. *British Journal of Sports Medicine, 47*, 304–307. http://dx.doi.org/10.1136/bjsports-2013-092190

Silverberg, N. D., & Iverson, G. L. (2013). Is rest after concussion "the best medicine?": Recommendations for activity resumption following concussion in athletes, civilians, and military service members. *The Journal of Head Trauma Rehabilitation, 28*, 250–259. http://dx.doi.org/10.1097/HTR.0b013e31825ad658

Silverberg, N. D., Luoto, T. M., Öhman, J., & Iverson, G. L. (2014). Assessment of mild traumatic brain injury with the King–Devick Test in an emergency department sample. *Brain Injury, 28*, 1590–1593. http://dx.doi.org/10.3109/02699052.2014.943287

Steenerson, K., & Starling, A. J. (2017). Pathophysiology of sports-related concussion. *Neurologic Clinics, 35*, 403–408. http://dx.doi.org/10.1016/j.ncl.2017.03.011

Tierney, R. T., Higgins, M., Caswell, S. V., Brady, J., McHardy, K., Driban, J. B., & Darvish, K. (2008). Sex differences in head acceleration during heading while wearing soccer headgear. *Journal of Athletic Training, 43*, 578–584. http://dx.doi.org/10.4085/1062-6050-43.6.578

Tierney, R. T., Sitler, M. R., Swanik, C. B., Swanik, K. A., Higgins, M., & Torg, J. (2005). Gender differences in head–neck segment dynamic stabilization during head acceleration. *Medicine and Science in Sports and Exercise, 37*, 272–279. http://dx.doi.org/10.1249/01.MSS.0000152734.47516.AA

Vargo, M. M., Vargo, K. G., Gunzler, D. D., & Fox, K. W. (2015). Rehabilitation therapies in a concussion clinic cohort: Range, rate, reasons and risk factors. *PM&R, 7*(9, Suppl.), S84. http://dx.doi.org/10.1016/j.pmrj.2015.06.017

Vista Life Sciences. (n.d.). *ANAM Automated Neuropsychological Assessment Metrics* [Library of computer-based assessments of cognitive domains]. Retrieved from https://vistalifesciences.com/anam-intro

Weiss, E. M., Kemmler, G., Deisenhammer, E. A., Fleischhacker, W. W., & Delazer, M. (2003). Sex differences in cognitive functions. *Personality and Individual Differences, 35*, 863–875. http://dx.doi.org/10.1016/S0191-8869(02)00288-X

Wunderle, K., Hoeger, K. M., Wasserman, E., & Bazarian, J. J. (2014). Menstrual phase as predictor of outcome after mild traumatic brain injury in women. *The Journal of Head Trauma Rehabilitation, 29*, E1–E8. http://dx.doi.org/10.1097/HTR.0000000000000006

Xiang, J., Collins, C. L., Liu, D., McKenzie, L. B., & Comstock, R. D. (2014). Lacrosse injuries among high school boys and girls in the United States: Academic years 2008–2009 through 2011–2012. *The American Journal of Sports Medicine, 42*, 2082–2088. http://dx.doi.org/10.1177/0363546514539914

Zuckerman, S. L., Apple, R. P., Odom, M. J., Lee, Y. M., Solomon, G. S., & Sills, A. K. (2014). Effect of sex on symptoms and return to baseline in sport-related concussion: Clinical article. *Journal of Neurosurgery. Pediatrics, 13*, 72–81. http://dx.doi.org/10.3171/2013.9.PEDS13257

Zuckerman, S. L., Solomon, G. S., Forbes, J. A., Haase, R. F., Sills, A. K., & Lovell, M. R. (2012). Response to acute concussive injury in soccer players: Is gender a modifying factor? Clinical article. *Journal of Neurosurgery: Pediatrics, 10*, 504–510. http://dx.doi.org/10.3171/2012.8.PEDS12139

8

ASSESSMENT OF EFFORT IN SPORTS CONCUSSION EVALUATIONS

AMANDA R. RABINOWITZ

Many incidents of sports-related concussion go unreported. Results of one study suggest that athletes disclose only about half of all head injuries (McCrea, Hammeke, Olsen, Leo, & Guskiewicz, 2004). That proportion of unreported injuries may be on the decline, in light of increased concussion awareness among athletes, coaches, athletic trainers, and parents. Nonetheless, diagnosis of concussion often relies heavily on the athlete's self-report of symptoms, which can be subject to biases. In order to offset these biases, objective indicators of injury are considered an important adjunct to athletes' self-reported symptoms. Slowed processing speed, difficulty concentrating, and trouble with memory are hallmark symptoms of concussion. Hence, cognitive tests—standard neuropsychological measures or specially developed computerized testing protocols—have become a cornerstone of the sports-concussion evaluation. However, interpreting cognitive test results is not straightforward. The cognitive effects of concussion can be relatively

http://dx.doi.org/10.1037/0000114-009
Neuropsychology of Sports-Related Concussion, P. A. Arnett (Editor)

subtle (Belanger & Vanderploeg, 2005) and, therefore, difficult to detect. For example, it is a challenge to determine whether memory performance in the low average range (a) is consistent with preinjury expectations or (b) represents a considerable decline from a higher preinjury ability level. For this reason, baseline neuropsychological testing—that is, testing an athlete at the beginning of the athletic season, in theory, before a concussive injury has occurred—has gained widespread popularity.

The logic underlying baseline testing is clear—an athlete's postinjury cognitive performance can be compared to preinjury test results, and hence, cognitive change is directly measured rather than simply inferred. Although this rationale is intuitively appealing, consensus statements have cautioned that there is insufficient evidence to support the routine use of baseline testing (McCrory et al., 2017). Others have gone further, arguing that baseline testing does nothing to reduce risk of reinjury, and may increase risk of premature return to play in some cases (Kirkwood, Randolph, & Yeates, 2009; Randolph, 2011). This chapter highlights issues in the assessment of effort in the context of baseline concussion testing. The differing incentives on good performance for baseline versus postconcussion evaluation raise questions regarding the validity of the baseline test as a comparison standard for determining postconcussion deficits. In addition to traditional performance validity measures, an experimental checklist that may be more sensitive to subtler forms of cognitive underperformance is discussed, as are cases in which normative data should be consulted in addition to or in place of baseline performance.

A major pitfall of baseline concussion testing is athletes' effort towards testing. Although athletes are highly motivated to put forth their best effort after a concussion, they have little incentive to perform well when baseline tests are administered. In fact, there is arguably an incentive to *underperform* at baseline, because underestimation of true ability level may facilitate a more rapid return to play after a future head injury. This phenomenon, called sandbagging, refers to a deliberate attempt to misrepresent one's preinjury cognitive status. In fact, research on baseline testing in sports-concussion assessment has uncovered evidence that baseline performance is, at least sometimes, depressed by poor effort towards testing (Bailey, Echemendia, & Arnett, 2006; Hunt, Ferrara, Miller, & Macciocchi, 2007; Rabinowitz, Merritt, & Arnett, 2015; Schatz, 2010; Solomon & Haase, 2008). Furthermore, emerging evidence from the field of positive psychology suggests that individual differences in effort influence cognitive performance in other contexts. Duckworth and colleagues conducted a meta-analysis of randomized experiments testing the effects of material incentives on intelligence-test performance, and found that incentives increased IQ scores by an average of 0.64 standard deviations (Duckworth, Quinn, Lynam, Loeber, & Stouthamer-Loeber, 2011).

Within the field of clinical neuropsychology, effort is usually discussed in the context of malingering, the act of feigning illness or injury for secondary gain. Individuals who are tested for the purpose of litigation or compensation may be incentivized to perform poorly on cognitive tests despite being neurologically intact. However, within the context of sports-related concussion, the incentive structure is quite different. Athletes are often highly motivated to return to play as quickly as possible following an injury, thus they are rewarded for putting forth their best cognitive performance. A highly motivated approach to testing is not inherently problematic; in fact, neuropsychologists typically instruct examinees to put forth their best effort towards testing. However, problems arise when an athlete's high effort postinjury evaluation is compared to baseline data that were obtained under very different circumstances. Clinicians may find themselves wondering whether an athlete's effort towards testing was comparable across baseline and postconcussion assessments; whether changes in effort level could significantly influence cognitive performance; and whether observed differences in cognitive performance across pre- and postinjury assessments are an accurate reflection of the neurocognitive consequences of concussion, or lack thereof.

Many terms have been used to describe an individual's approach to testing—*malingering, symptom validity, response bias, effort,* and *performance validity.* Often these terms are used interchangeably. However, there are distinctions among these phenomena that are clinically relevant. In fact, conflating these constructs could lead to erroneous conclusions about the extent to which an individual's test results represent their true level of cognitive functioning. An examinee's approach to testing arises from a combination of external incentives, their intentions or goals, and the level of effort they exert towards accomplishing these goals. For example, a malingering litigant could put a tremendous amount of effort towards appearing cognitively impaired. In this case the incentive is financial compensation, the goal is to appear impaired, and the effort level is high. Alternatively, an athlete tested at baseline may intend to demonstrate her true cognitive ability, however, she puts forth little effort because she is bored, distracted, or simply, insufficiently motivated to do her very best. In this example, the athlete's goal may be to perform well, but there is no immediate reward for good performance, and hence, the effort level is low.

EFFORT INFLUENCES COGNITIVE PERFORMANCE

It is clear that malingerers demonstrate cognitive performance that underestimates their true cognitive status—this is inherent in the very definition of malingering. Less is known about how poor effort (without the intent to deceive) may influence neuropsychological test results. However, theoretical and empirical work has addressed this topic, and suggests that incentives and effort are important determinants of cognitive performance. When a reward is at stake, humans and animals alike will increase the amount of effort they expend. This effort could manifest in the form of eagerness, increasing the speed of performance (Knutson, Taylor, Kaufman, Peterson, & Glover, 2005; Tremblay & Schultz, 2000), or in the form of focus, increasing accuracy (Kahneman & Peavler, 1969; Sarter, Gehring, & Kozak, 2006; Wieth & Burns, 2006). Dependent on level of motivation, an individual will increase their effort in response to detrimental mechanisms (Sarter et al., 2006). Detrimental mechanisms are likely to be encountered during any neuropsychological evaluation; mechanisms such as distractions, fatigue, and prolonged time on task. Effort is modulated in a top-down manner to overcome these obstacles and optimize cognitive performance, via a supervisory control system, such as the central executive or anterior attention network (Baddeley, 1986; Posner, 1994; Posner & Dehaene, 1994; Sarter et al., 2006).

A distinction can be drawn between effortful and noneffortful cognitive tasks. For example, research on the cognitive deficits associated with depression has shown that depressed mood selectively affects cognitive tasks that involve effort—tasks such as sustained attention, speeded processing, and free recall (Snyder, 2013; Tancer et al., 1990). By contrast, noneffortful cognitive tasks are those that do not require speeded processing and sustained attention, such as recognition memory (Dehaene, Kerszberg, & Changeux, 1998). This framework provides predictions for which types of tasks should be most influenced by changes in effort level across pre- and postinjury assessments—suggesting that tasks that rely the most heavily on speed and focus should be most affected. These are exactly the tasks that predominate a concussion assessment battery, as they are the very cognitive domains that are most sensitive to concussion. Hence, the results of poor effort at the baseline assessment may look very similar to an impaired postconcussion profile. This state of affairs complicates interpretation of sports-concussion assessment results, particularly in the case where an athlete's cognitive scores show no, or little, change relative to baseline.

A handful of studies have directly examined the role of effort in sports-concussion evaluations. Bailey and colleagues (2006) demonstrated that a proportion of athletes showed a marked *improvement* on cognitive tests after sustaining a concussion, strongly suggesting that their baseline test results underestimated their true cognitive ability level. These investigators characterized athletes with abnormally low baseline scores—at least two standard deviations below the mean—as demonstrating suspect effort. A comparison of pre- and postconcussion performance in the suspect motivation group showed markedly improved performance following concussion, particularly on measures of psychomotor processing speed (Bailey et al., 2006). Another study by our group demonstrated that recently concussed athletes were judged by experimenters as putting forth significantly more effort on cognitive tests, as compared to the same athletes tested at baseline. Furthermore, those rated as putting forth poor effort at baseline exhibited the poorest baseline test performance (Rabinowitz et al., 2015). In this study examiners rated their impression of athletes' effort on a single-item Likert scale ranging from *not trying at all* to *optimal effort*. Other research has shown that the setting of baseline evaluation—one-to-one versus group administration—may play a role in athletes' approach to testing. Moser, Schatz, Neidzwski, and Ott (2011) conducted a study in high school athletes, and found that those completing testing in a group setting scored significantly lower on all neurocognitive indices, compared with athletes tested in an individual setting. Furthermore, there was greater incidence of invalid test performances in those who underwent group administration (Moser et al., 2011).

ACCOUNTING FOR EFFORT IN SPORTS-CONCUSSION NEUROPSYCHOLOGICAL ASSESSMENT

Taken together, these findings clearly demonstrate that baseline testing can serve as a misleading benchmark of an athlete's cognitive ability, at least in some cases. Changes in setting, incentives, motivation, and effort may play a role in this phenomenon. For this reason, accounting for these factors in clinical interpretation of neuropsychological findings is critical. However, to date, there is no gold standard for measuring effort in the context of sports-concussion assessment, leaving those who manage athletes without clear guidelines. Sports medicine professionals play a critical and growing role in baseline and acute postinjury testing for high school and college athletes. With the availability of computerized testing protocols, increasingly, cognitive tests are administered and interpreted by certified athletic trainers (ATs), and not neuropsychologists. ATs do not routinely receive specific training in clinical interpretation of cognitive tests and the myriad nonneurologic factors that may influence performance. For example, one survey of ATs showed that nearly half of those surveyed failed to consult validity indicators for a commonly used computerized testing program (Covassin, Elbin, Stiller-Ostrowski, & Kontos, 2009). In light of the influence of effort on cognitive performance and the need for user friendly assessments, it is clear that more attention must be paid to the following issues: (a) developing a gold standard approach for assessing effort in the context of sports-concussion assessment; (b) developing protocols for handling suspect effort at baseline; and (c) disseminating this information so that it is readily applied by the front-line sports medicine professionals who are most likely to manage recently concussed athletes.

Although there are currently no validated guidelines for baseline effort assessment in sports-concussion management, there is a vast literature on detection of malingering in the context of neuropsychological assessment. Research has shown that clinical judgment on its own is insufficient for determining whether an examinee is putting forth adequate effort on cognitive tests (Arkes, Faust, & Guilmette, 1990; Faust & Guilmette, 1990; Faust, Hart, Guilmette, & Arkes, 1988). Rather, formal performance validity testing is recommended (Bush et al., 2005; Iverson, 2003). A number of objective tests have been developed to assess response bias—both stand-alone measures, and others embedded within standard neuropsychological tests. Most performance validity tests rely on forced-choice recognition memory. Performance that falls below chance (i.e., accuracy less than 50%) is considered a clear indicator of invalid performance. However, other empirical thresholds have been developed based on the performance of individuals with confirmed brain injury, as compared to litigants or uninjured examinees who have been instructed to feign cognitive impairment. Typically, accuracy on forced-choice recognition memory is near 100%, even among neurologically impaired individuals with memory difficulties. Hence, accuracy rates that fall below 90% may be indicative of suspect effort (Allen, Iverson, & Green, 2003; Green, Iverson, & Allen, 1999; Tombaugh, 1997). These more liberal cutoffs increase the sensitivity of performance validity measures but, in turn, increase the rates of false positive identification—that is, misclassifying a sincere examinee as a malingerer. Hence, there is debate over which thresholds are optimal for forced-choice recognition memory measures (Greve, Bianchini, & Doane, 2006). The Test of Memory Malingering (TOMM; Tombaugh, 1997) and the Word Memory Test (WMT; Green, Allen, & Astner, 1996) are common performance validity tests that rely on the forced-choice recognition memory model. The TOMM is administered manually, whereas the WMT is a computer-based assessment. These stand-alone effort measures can be included in a baseline concussion evaluation. Computerized tests, like the WMT are amenable to administration in conjunction with computerized cognitive assessments that are commonly used in concussion management.

Other indices of response bias can be derived from the standard administration of common neuropsychological tests (Meyers, Volbrecht, Axelrod, & Reinsch-Boothby, 2011). For example, Reliable Digit Span (RDS; Greiffenstein, Baker, & Gola, 1994) is derived using indices from the Digit Span subtest of the Wechsler Adult Intelligence Scale. RDS is calculated by adding the longest span of Digit Span forward on which both trials are passed to the longest span on Digit Span backwards on which both trials are passed.

Several studies have examined the use of RDS as an effort measure, and suggest a cutoff of 6 or below (Greve, Ord, Bianchini, & Curtis, 2009; Meyers & Volbrecht, 1998; Meyers & Volbrecht, 2003). The recognition trial from the Auditory Verbal Learning Test (AVLT–Rec) is also considered a test of symptom validity (Slick & Strauss, 2006). AVLT-Rec is scored as the number of True Positive responses on the AVLT Recognition, and scores of 9 or below are considered failures (Meyers & Volbrecht, 2003). Other memory tests with forced choice recognition trials, such as the California Verbal Learning Test (CVLT; Delis, Kramer, Kaplan, & Ober, 2000) can be used in the same manner. Embedded measures are handy in the context of a complete neuropsychological evaluation wherein these tests are being administered for their primary purpose of assessing cognitive function. In this case, deriving effort indices takes little additional work on the examiner's part, and adds no additional time or burden to the examinee. However, in the context of mass baseline testing, one-to-one paper-and-pencil testing is rare, so application of these measures is limited by the time and personnel required.

One advantage of the measures discussed to this point is that they are supported by decades of research. However, it should be noted that the vast majority of these studies have examined these tests as indicators of feigned cognitive impairment. As discussed previously, feigned cognitive impairment is just one of a number of factors that could influence approach to testing in the sports-concussion context. For example, let's return to the scenario alluded to earlier, in which a hypothetical athlete has the sincere intention to demonstrate her true cognitive ability on a baseline cognitive assessment. However, because there is no immediate incentive on optimal performance, she succumbs to fatigue, distractors, and boredom during the testing session, and her effort level is insufficient to overcome these detriments. Still, she easily passes traditional symptom validity tests, such as the TOMM, because these tasks require little mental exertion. Her performance on more effortful cognitive tasks, such as tests of psychomotor processing speed and sustained attention, is within the normal range but at the low end of her true capacity.

Now, let's contrast this approach with the scenario in which the same athlete is tested following a concussion. At this testing session, she is well aware that the results of the assessment will be used to inform return-to-play decisions. Athletic participation is a large part of her identity and daily life as a student–athlete, and hence, she is highly motivated to return to her sport as soon as possible. During this testing session, despite her concussion sequelae, she puts forth maximal effort towards the cognitive tasks. The neurocognitive effects of concussion produce mild deficits in psychomotor processing speed and sustained attention, and comparison of pre- and postinjury assessments reveals roughly equivalent scores across the two test administrations. Does the fact that this athlete passed "effort testing" at baseline indicate that her baseline test provides an accurate benchmark by which to judge her post-injury cognitive performance? Perhaps there is a subtler phenomenon at work that should be accounted for when interpreting these cognitive findings.

In this scenario, the concern is not only the athlete's potentially poor motivation at baseline but also her substantially increased level of motivation postconcussion. There is reason to believe that powerful incentives, like return to play, can serve to enhance motivation and modulate performance via sustained activation of cognitive control regions of the brain (Locke & Braver, 2008). Research has demonstrated that financial incentives result in improved performance on cognitively effortful tasks, and individuals vary in the extent to which they are sensitive to these rewards and modulate cognitive effort accordingly (Locke & Braver, 2008). Other work has shown that financial incentives can even attenuate some of the deleterious cognitive effects of sleep deprivation (Hsieh, Li, & Tsai, 2010). Taken together, this research suggests that an athlete experiencing no or minimal cognitive dysfunction following a head injury may show improved performance postinjury, based purely on incentive-related change in motivation. Furthermore, athletes who are particularly sensitive to the return-to-play incentive may be able to overcome significant cognitive deficits and exhibit stable or even improved performance postconcussion. Traditional symptom validity measures, designed to detect feigned cognitive impairment, are probably not sensitive to these subtler aspects of an athlete's motivational state and the associated changes in effort.

Specialized testing protocols have been designed specifically for repeated administration in the context of sports-concussion assessment. The Immediate Post-Concussion Assessment and Cognitive Testing (ImPACT; Covassin et al., 2009) is a computerized test battery that includes alternate forms for testing athletes at baseline and multiple times postconcussion. Reliable change indices have been calculated to aid in comparison of tests results across multiple administrations. The testing protocol takes approximately 20 minutes to administer, and the computerized platform affords administration to multiple athletes simultaneously without one-to-one attention from a specially trained test administrator. Hence, ImPACT has multiple advantages for cognitive assessment in a sports-concussion context, and, not surprisingly, it is widely used to manage sports-related head injuries at the high school and collegiate level. The creators of the ImPACT have recognized that suspect effort, distraction, technical difficulties, and other factors may influence the validity of baseline assessment. In response to this issue, they have established red flags and validity indicators for poor performance, generally based on scores two standard deviations (SDs) below the mean on certain test indices.

Research evaluating ImPACT's validity indicators and red flags as measures of effort has revealed that the base rate of invalid performance among high school and collegiate athletes falls between 4% and 11% (Schatz, Moser,

Solomon, Ott, & Karpf, 2012), with younger athletes (ages 10–12) exhibiting a higher rate of invalid scores (Lichtenstein, Moser, & Schatz, 2014), and desktop administration, as opposed to web-based administration, resulting in a greater proportion of invalid scores (Schatz et al., 2012). Studies examining the sensitivity of these validity indicators have instructed participants to deliberately underperform on ImPACT, and found that red flags and validity indicators correctly identified most intentional underperformers; however, 11% were able to fake lower scores without detection in one study (Erdal, 2012), and 30% to 35% of intentional underperformers evaded detection in another study (Schatz & Glatts, 2013). One of the advantages of computerized neurocognitive testing is the ability to test a large group of athletes at once. However, group administration may be problematic, as research has demonstrated that athletes tested with ImPACT in a large group format exhibit poorer overall performance and a higher rate of invalid scores, as compared with those tested in a one-to-one (Moser et al., 2011) or small group setting (Lichtenstein et al., 2014; see Chapter 9, this volume, for a more detailed discussion of validity issues as they pertain to computerized testing formats in sports concussion).

KNOWLEDGE GAPS IN RESEARCH AND PRACTICE

The ImPACT's performance-based validity indicators are an important tool for clinicians to use in interpreting baseline test results. When baseline testing is invalid, repeated administration has been recommended, and Schatz and colleagues (2014) showed that nearly 90% of athletes with invalid scores produced valid results with a second administration. However, a survey of athletic trainers suggests that nearly half of ATs never examine ImPACT validity indicators (Covassin et al., 2009). This finding demonstrates that there is an urgent need for evidence-based protocols for handling invalid baseline performance. ATs who manage sports concussions should be aware of threats to test validity and the evidence in support of repeating cognitive assessment in the case of invalid baseline scores. Developing and disseminating evidence-based guidelines for using ImPACT's validity indicators and red flags is needed to improve the use of neurocognitive testing in concussion management. However, even with improved testing protocols, at least one study has demonstrated performance-based validity indicators fail to capture all cases of faking cognitive deficits (Erdal, 2012), which, in theory, should have a more pronounced influence on test performance than poor effort without the intent to deceive. Furthermore, it is possible that incremental changes in effort level may have an important influence on neuropsychological test performance in a way that goes unappreciated by categorical approaches to effort testing that flag patients' profiles as "suspect" or "invalid."

Our group has designed an observational checklist to assess effort toward testing called the Motivation Behavior Checklist (MBC; Rabinowitz, Merritt, & Arnett, 2016). Test administrators rate the frequencies of 18 behaviors that may reveal an athlete's effort toward testing. Examples of behaviors rated on the MBC include "Mentions being tired or hungry" and "Moves in more closely when test materials are presented." The intent of this checklist is to provide an objective way of quantifying variation in approach to testing with more granularity than simply classifying test results as "valid" or "invalid." A continuous measure, such as the MBC, may have the sensitivity to detect subtle but impactful changes in approach towards testing across pre- and postinjury test sessions. Our initial investigation has demonstrated that the MBC has good inter-rater reliability and internal consistency. The MBC items represent four latent factors, Complaints, Poor Focus, Psychomotor Agitation, and Impulsivity, and its construct validity is supported by correlation with examiner- and self-ratings of effort and cognitive performance (Rabinowitz et al., 2016). Although more research is needed to further validate this measure, it could be a useful adjunct to sports-related concussion testing protocols. The MBC takes only about two minutes to complete by the test administrator posttesting, hence it is a very practical measure.

The MBC is, to our knowledge, the first measure of its kind designed to assess effort across the full continuum, ranging from poor to exceptional effort. It was developed based on a model positing that incentives and motivation-related incremental changes in effort influence cognitive performance. Hence, fine-grained assessment of effort is relevant for valid interpretation of neuropsychological assessment. It should be noted that this is a broader conceptualization of effort than what is typically considered in clinical neuropsychology and measured by traditional effort tests. This narrow definition of effort has been a limitation for the field of clinical neuropsychological assessment, and this limitation has come to the fore in the context of sports-related concussion where good cognitive performance is rewarded with return to play. The MBC represents one approach for accounting for this phenomenon— an observational checklist that is completed by examiners. Research to develop other measures based on a broad conceptualization of effort, particularly measures that are performance or physiologically based, would be a great asset to the field.

CONCLUSIONS

In summary, as the popularity of baseline testing for sports-concussion has grown, so too has evidence suggesting that poor effort can compromise the validity of baseline assessment results. There are now multiple studies demonstrating that a proportion of athletes exhibit poor effort at baseline, demonstrated by failure of formal effort testing or marked improvements following concussion. These findings are consistent with research showing that incentives serve to increase an individual's motivational state, which, in turn, leads to effort-related modulation of top-down cognitive control mechanisms that improve focus and speed. Younger athletes and those tested in a group format may be particularly susceptible to poor effort at baseline. Traditional approaches to formal effort testing are predominantly designed to detect feigned cognitive impairment. These measures may not be sensitive to subtle changes in effort due to the presence of a powerful return-to-play incentive after injury that is absent at baseline. The development of tools for measuring this latter phenomenon is hampered by the fact that the cognitive domains that are most sensitive to effort also happen to be those that are most sensitive to concussion. Clinical observation on its own has been shown to be insufficient in detecting poor effort, however, augmented with behavioral checklists, such as the recently developed MBC, it may provide information that aids in clinical interpretation of sports-concussion assessment results.

Although it is clear that more research is needed, the issues discussed above have important clinical implications, and recommendations follow from the current state of the research evidence. Given that baseline testing can be problematic, it is reasonable to ask whether it is necessary at all (see Arnett, Meyer, Merritt, & Guty, 2016, for a description of an evidence-based approach without the use of baseline testing). A number of authors have questioned whether evidence supports the routine use of baseline testing. There is a growing consensus that there is insufficient evidence in support of this practice (De Marco & Broshek, 2016; Echemendia et al., 2013; Kontos, Sufrinko, Womble, & Kegel, 2016). However, baseline testing may be particularly useful for subgroups of individuals with preinjury conditions or circumstances that are known to influence cognitive test results, such as premorbid attention-deficit/hyperactivity disorder, learning disability, or differences in primary language background or educational status (Jones et al., 2014; Littleton et al., 2015; Ott, Blake, Villanyi, & Schatz, 2014). Yet, in many cases, baseline test results may offer little advantage over normative data (Echemendia et al., 2013). Despite caution from the scientific community, baseline testing is intuitively appealing. For many scholastic athletic programs, it represents a major pillar of concussion management protocols, and offers reassurance to parents and students. Furthermore, baseline testing is a lucrative business for private test developers and a revenue source for providers who administer tests. Hence, it is likely that baseline testing is here to stay.

The literature suggests certain steps that may optimize the utility of baseline testing to remove distraction and mitigate other threats to test validity. Most importantly, testing in a large group format is ill-advised (Moser et al., 2011). One-to-one baseline testing is preferable, because it eliminates social distractions and most closely mimics the circumstances of postconcussion assessment, but small groups of no more than three athletes are superior to testing in large-group format (Lichtenstein et al., 2014). Baseline assessments should always include formal effort testing. As discussed above, traditional performance validity tests are not ideal measures of subtle changes in effort; however, these measures can detect feigned cognitive impairment, referred to as "sandbagging" in the context of sports-related concussion. When baseline performance is impaired, failure on a traditional performance validity measure is highly suggestive of sandbagging. Computerized performance validity tests, such as the WMT are most amenable to inclusion with popular computerized testing batteries. When tests include embedded validity indicators, these should always be consulted in the short term following test administration, bearing in mind that technical difficulties, failure to read directions, and poor effort can all lead to an invalid result. Evidence supports re-administering baseline testing when the initial test administration is invalid (Schatz et al., 2014). Postconcussion test batteries should include the same effort and performance validity measures that were included at baseline, in order to examine longitudinal changes in approach to testing.

Regarding interpreting change in cognitive performance from baseline, practitioners are cautioned to remember that cognitive test results do not exist in a vacuum. It is critical to consider the examinee's context, psychological state, goals, and personality as factors that interact with cognitive functioning to produce test results. In addition to consulting the results of effort testing, practitioners should use a clinical interview to gather information about academic history, prior conditions, and other factors that are related to cognitive performance. Baseline test results should be regarded as suspect when they deviate substantially from norm-based expectations, or are inconsistent with other data, such as academic records and standardized test scores. When poor effort at baseline is suggested by formal effort testing, clinical observation, or performance falling well below norm- or personal history-based expectations, post-injury performance that suggests no change from baseline should be interpreted with extreme caution. In cases for which baseline testing is suspect or invalid, practitioners should consider consulting an evidence-based model for interpreting performance when baseline testing is unavailable (Arnett et al., 2016).

CASE STUDY[1]

A college freshman joins the women's soccer team with a true premorbid verbal memory ability of 120 standard score points. She comes to the baseline testing session directly after a rigorous workout. The purpose

---

[1]Some of the original details of this case have been changed to protect the confidentiality of the individual tested.

of baseline testing has been explained to her, however, some details have been forgotten amidst the demands of acclimating to her new campus, team, and schedule of courses. She is surprised to learn that the testing session will take an hour, which interferes with her plans to purchase textbooks before meeting teammates for dinner. The examiner encourages her to put forth her best effort. She is friendly and cooperative, although slightly fatigued and distracted. She asks the examiner about the length of testing multiple times. On a test of verbal memory she receives a score of 100 standard score points, underestimating her true premorbid ability of 120 standard score points. Overall, her baseline test performance is well within the normal range, and does not trigger performance invalidity indicators. The test administrator completes the MBC after testing, and notes her distracted behavior. Later that season, she sustains a concussion and experiences problems with memory. Despite her deficit, she is highly motivated to perform well on the postconcussion assessment. She is eager to return to play, and wants to present an accurate impression of her current cognitive functioning so that her team physician can make an informed return-to-play decision. During the postconcussion test session, she is focused and does not engage the test administrator in test-irrelevant conversation. She receives a verbal memory score of 100 standard score points, technically "back to baseline," but still substantially below her true premorbid ability level. The examiner completes the MBC again after testing and finds that her postconcussion MBC score falls 20 points below her baseline MBC score, indicating a more motivated approach to testing after concussion. Although her baseline performance was "valid," according to standard validity indicators, the MBC, a continuous measure that captures incremental changes in approach to testing, did reveal a change in approach to testing as compared with baseline. This hypothetical scenario demonstrates that valid cognitive performance may not be optimal, and continuous measures of approach towards testing may provide information that allows the examiner to distinguish between optimal performance and performance that is merely "valid."

CLINICAL TAKE-HOME POINTS

1. *Poor effort at baseline, and/or exceptional effort postconcussion, influences cognitive performance and complicates interpretation of neuropsychological test results.*
2. *Administering baseline testing in a large group format (more than two or three athletes at once) compounds the influence of poor effort at baseline.* One-to-one baseline test administration is advised.

3. *Formal effort testing should always be included in baseline and postconcussion neuropsychological assessment.* When poor effort at baseline is suggested by formal effort testing, clinical observation, or performance falling well below norm- or personal history-based expectations, postinjury performance that suggests no change from baseline should be interpreted with extreme caution.

KEY QUESTIONS TO BE ADDRESSED IN THE NEXT 5 YEARS

There are pressing questions that should be addressed within the next 5 years.

1. *Are there cognitive domains that are sensitive to concussion, but not sensitive to changes in effort?* This endeavor requires identifying neurocognitive functions that are sensitive to effort but not concussion and vice versa. For example, Heitger and colleagues (2009) have demonstrated that eye movements are not influenced by malingering, depression, or intellectual ability, but are impaired in individuals with postconcussion syndrome (Heitger et al., 2009).

2. *For whom is baseline testing necessary (i.e., superior to norm-based comparisons)?* Ultimately, the primary purpose of pre- and postinjury neuropsychological testing is to inform return-to-play decision making.

REFERENCES

Allen, L. M., III, Iverson, G. L., & Green, P. (2003). Computerized assessment of response bias in forensic neuropsychology. *Journal of Forensic Neuropsychology, 3*, 205–225. http://dx.doi.org/10.1300/J151v03n01_02

Arkes, H. R., Faust, D., & Guilmette, T. J. (1990). Response to Schmidt's (1988) comments on Faust, Hart, Guilmette, and Arkes (1988). *Professional Psychology: Research and Practice, 21*, 3–4. Retrieved from http://psycnet.apa.org/buy/2010-03284-001

Arnett, P., Meyer, J., Merritt, V., & Guty, E. (2016). Neuropsychological testing in mild traumatic brain injury: What to do when baseline testing is not available. *Sports Medicine and Arthroscopy Review, 24*, 116–122. http://dx.doi.org/10.1097/JSA.0000000000000123

Baddeley, A. (1986). *Working memory, 11*. Oxford, England: Clarendon Press.

Bailey, C. M., Echemendia, R. J., & Arnett, P. A. (2006). The impact of motivation on neuropsychological performance in sports-related mild traumatic brain injury. *Journal of the International Neuropsychological Society, 12*, 475–484. http://dx.doi.org/10.1017/S1355617706060619

Belanger, H. G., & Vanderploeg, R. D. (2005). The neuropsychological impact of sports-related concussion: A meta-analysis. *Journal of the International Neuropsychological Society, 11*, 345–357. http://dx.doi.org/10.1017/S1355617705050411

Bush, S. S., Ruff, R. M., Tröster, A. I., Barth, J. T., Koffler, S. P., Pliskin, N. H., . . . Silver, C. H. (2005). Symptom validity assessment: Practice issues and medical necessity NAN policy & planning committee. *Archives of Clinical Neuropsychology, 20*, 419–426. http://dx.doi.org/10.1016/j.acn.2005.02.002

Covassin, T., Elbin, R. J., III, Stiller-Ostrowski, J. L., & Kontos, A. P. (2009). Immediate post-concussion assessment and cognitive testing (ImPACT) practices of sports medicine professionals. *Journal of Athletic Training, 44*, 639–644. http://dx.doi.org/10.4085/1062-6050-44.6.639

De Marco, A. P., & Broshek, D. K. (2016). Computerized cognitive testing in the management of youth sports-related concussion. *Journal of Child Neurology, 31*, 68–75. http://dx.doi.org/10.1177/0883073814559645

Delis, D. C., Kramer, J. H., Kaplan, E., & Ober, B. A. (2000). *CVLT-II: California verbal learning test: Adult version*. San Antonio, TX: The Psychological Corporation/Harcourt.

Dehaene, S., Kerszberg, M., & Changeux, J. P. (1998). A neuronal model of a global workspace in effortful cognitive tasks. *Proceedings of the National Academy of Sciences of the United States, 95*, 14529–14534. http://dx.doi.org/10.1073/pnas.95.24.14529

Duckworth, A. L., Quinn, P. D., Lynam, D. R., Loeber, R., & Stouthamer-Loeber, M. (2011). Role of test motivation in intelligence testing. *Proceedings of the National Academy of Sciences of the United States of America, 108*, 7716–7720. http://dx.doi.org/10.1073/pnas.1018601108

Echemendia, R. J., Iverson, G. L., McCrea, M., Macciocchi, S. N., Gioia, G. A., Putukian, M., & Comper, P. (2013). Advances in neuropsychological assessment of sport-related concussion. *British Journal of Sports Medicine, 47*, 294–298. http://dx.doi.org/10.1136/bjsports-2013-092186

Erdal, K. (2012). Neuropsychological testing for sports-related concussion: How athletes can sandbag their baseline testing without detection. *Archives of Clinical Neuropsychology, 27*, 473–479. http://dx.doi.org/10.1093/arclin/acs050

Faust, D., & Guilmette, T. J. (1990). To say it's not so doesn't prove that it isn't: Research on the detection of malingering: Reply to Bigler. *Journal of Consulting and Clinical Psychology, 58*, 248–250. http://dx.doi.org/10.1037/0022-006X.58.2.248

Faust, D., Hart, K. J., Guilmette, T. J., & Arkes, H. R. (1988). Neuropsychologists' capacity to detect adolescent malingerers. *Professional Psychology: Research and Practice, 19*, 508–515. http://dx.doi.org/10.1037/0735-7028.19.5.508

Green, P., Allen, L. M., & Astner, K. (1996). *The Word Memory Test: A user's guide to the oral and computer-administered forms, US Version 1.1.* Durham, NC: CogniSyst.

Green, P., Iverson, G. L., & Allen, L. (1999). Detecting malingering in head injury litigation with the Word Memory Test. *Brain Injury, 13*, 813–819. http://dx.doi.org/10.1080/026990599121205

Greiffenstein, M. F., Baker, W. J., & Gola, T. (1994). Validation of malingered amnesia measures with a large clinical sample. *Psychological Assessment, 6*, 218–224. http://dx.doi.org/10.1037/1040-3590.6.3.218

Greve, K. W., Bianchini, K. J., & Doane, B. M. (2006). Classification accuracy of the test of memory malingering in traumatic brain injury: Results of a known-groups analysis. *Journal of Clinical and Experimental Neuropsychology, 28*, 1176–1190. http://dx.doi.org/10.1080/13803390500263550

Greve, K. W., Ord, J. S., Bianchini, K. J., & Curtis, K. L. (2009). Prevalence of malingering in patients with chronic pain referred for psychologic evaluation in a medico–legal context. *Archives of Physical Medicine and Rehabilitation, 90*, 1117–1126. http://dx.doi.org/10.1016/j.apmr.2009.01.018

Heitger, M. H., Jones, R. D., Macleod, A. D., Snell, D. L., Frampton, C. M., & Anderson, T. J. (2009). Impaired eye movements in post-concussion syndrome indicate suboptimal brain function beyond the influence of depression, malingering or intellectual ability. *Brain: A Journal of Neurology, 132*, 2850–2870. http://dx.doi.org/10.1093/brain/awp181

Hsieh, S., Li, T.-H., & Tsai, L.-L. (2010). Impact of monetary incentives on cognitive performance and error monitoring following sleep deprivation. *Sleep, 33*, 499–507. http://dx.doi.org/10.1093/sleep/33.4.499

Hunt, T. N., Ferrara, M. S., Miller, L. S., & Macciocchi, S. (2007). The effect of effort on baseline neuropsychological test scores in high school football athletes. *Archives of Clinical Neuropsychology, 22*, 615–621. http://dx.doi.org/10.1016/j.acn.2007.04.005

Iverson, G. L. (2003). Detecting malingering in civil forensic evaluations. In A. M. Horton, Jr. & L. C. Hartlage (Eds.), *Handbook of forensic neuropsychology* (pp. 137–177). New York, NY: Springer.

Jones, N. S., Walter, K. D., Caplinger, R., Wright, D., Raasch, W. G., & Young, C. (2014). Effect of education and language on baseline concussion screening tests in professional baseball players. *Clinical Journal of Sport Medicine, 24*, 284–288. http://dx.doi.org/10.1097/JSM.0000000000000031

Kahneman, D., & Peavler, W. S. (1969). Incentive effects and pupillary changes in association learning. *Journal of Experimental Psychology, 79*, 312–318. http://dx.doi.org/10.1037/h0026912

Kirkwood, M. W., Randolph, C., & Yeates, K. O. (2009). Returning pediatric athletes to play after concussion: The evidence (or lack thereof) behind baseline neuropsychological testing. *Acta Paediatrica*, 98, 1409–1411. http://dx.doi.org/10.1111/j.1651-2227.2009.01448.x

Knutson, B., Taylor, J., Kaufman, M., Peterson, R., & Glover, G. (2005). Distributed neural representation of expected value. *The Journal of Neuroscience*, 25, 4806–4812. http://dx.doi.org/10.1523/JNEUROSCI.0642-05.2005

Kontos, A. P., Sufrinko, A., Womble, M., & Kegel, N. (2016). Neuropsychological assessment following concussion: An evidence-based review of the role of neuropsychological assessment pre- and post-concussion. *Current Pain and Headache Reports*, 20, 38. http://dx.doi.org/10.1007/s11916-016-0571-y

Lichtenstein, J. D., Moser, R. S., & Schatz, P. (2014). Age and test setting affect the prevalence of invalid baseline scores on neurocognitive tests. *The American Journal of Sports Medicine*, 42, 479–484. http://dx.doi.org/10.1177/0363546513509225

Littleton, A. C., Schmidt, J. D., Register-Mihalik, J. K., Gioia, G. A., Waicus, K. M., Mihalik, J. P., & Guskiewicz, K. M. (2015). Effects of attention deficit hyperactivity disorder and stimulant medication on concussion symptom reporting and computerized neurocognitive test performance. *Archives of Clinical Neuropsychology*, 30, 683–693. http://dx.doi.org/10.1093/arclin/acv043

Locke, H. S., & Braver, T. S. (2008). Motivational influences on cognitive control: Behavior, brain activation, and individual differences. *Cognitive, Affective, & Behavioral Neuroscience*, 8, 99–112. http://dx.doi.org/10.3758/CABN.8.1.99

McCrea, M., Hammeke, T., Olsen, G., Leo, P., & Guskiewicz, K. (2004). Unreported concussion in high school football players: Implications for prevention. *Clinical Journal of Sport Medicine*, 14, 13–17. http://dx.doi.org/10.1097/00042752-200401000-00003

McCrory, P., Meeuwisse, W., Dvořák, J., Aubry, M., Bailes, J., Broglio, S., . . . Vos, P. E. (2017). Consensus statement on concussion in sport—The 5th international conference on concussion in sport held in Berlin, October 2016. *British Journal of Sports Medicine*, 51, 838–847. http://dx.doi.org/10.1136/bjsports-2017-097699

Meyers, J. E., & Volbrecht, M. (1998). Validation of reliable digits for detection of malingering. *Assessment*, 5, 303–307. http://dx.doi.org/10.1177/107319119800500309

Meyers, J. E., & Volbrecht, M. E. (2003). A validation of multiple malingering detection methods in a large clinical sample. *Archives of Clinical Neuropsychology*, 18, 261–276. http://dx.doi.org/10.1093/arclin/18.3.261

Meyers, J. E., Volbrecht, M., Axelrod, B. N., & Reinsch-Boothby, L. (2011). Embedded symptom validity tests and overall neuropsychological test performance. *Archives of Clinical Neuropsychology*, 26, 8–15. http://dx.doi.org/10.1093/arclin/acq083

Moser, R. S., Schatz, P., Neidzwski, K., & Ott, S. D. (2011). Group versus individual administration affects baseline neurocognitive test performance. *The*

American Journal of Sports Medicine, 39, 2325–2330. http://dx.doi.org/10.1177/0363546511417114

Ott, S., Blake, M., Villanyi, E., & Schatz, P. (2014). Bilingual Spanish speakers perform significantly better on ImPACT in English than Spanish. Archives of Clinical Neuropsychology, 29, 572. http://dx.doi.org/10.1093/arclin/acu038.182

Posner, M. I. (1994). Attention: The mechanisms of consciousness. Proceedings of the National Academy of Sciences of the United States of America, 91, 7398–7403.

Posner, M. I., & Dehaene, S. (1994). Attentional networks. Trends in Neurosciences, 17, 75–79. http://dx.doi.org/10.1016/0166-2236(94)90078-7

Rabinowitz, A. R., Merritt, V. C., & Arnett, P. A. (2015). The return-to-play incentive and the effect of motivation on neuropsychological test-performance: Implications for baseline concussion testing. Developmental Neuropsychology, 40, 29–33. http://dx.doi.org/10.1080/87565641.2014.1001066

Rabinowitz, A. R., Merritt, V., & Arnett, P. A. (2016). A pilot investigation of the Motivation Behaviors Checklist (MBC): An observational rating scale of effort towards testing for baseline sports-concussion assessment. Journal of Clinical and Experimental Neuropsychology, 38, 599–610. http://dx.doi.org/10.1080/13803395.2015.1123224

Randolph, C. (2011). Baseline neuropsychological testing in managing sport-related concussion: Does it modify risk? Current Sports Medicine Reports, 10, 21–26. http://dx.doi.org/10.1249/JSR.0b013e318207831d

Sarter, M., Gehring, W. J., & Kozak, R. (2006). More attention must be paid: The neurobiology of attentional effort. Brain Research Reviews, 51, 145–160. http://dx.doi.org/10.1016/j.brainresrev.2005.11.002

Schatz, P. (2010). Long-term test–retest reliability of baseline cognitive assessments using ImPACT. The American Journal of Sports Medicine, 38, 47–53. http://dx.doi.org/10.1177/0363546509343805

Schatz, P., & Glatts, C. (2013). "Sandbagging" baseline test performance on ImPACT, without detection, is more difficult than it appears. Archives of Clinical Neuropsychology, 28, 236–244. http://dx.doi.org/10.1093/arclin/act009

Schatz, P., Kelley, T., Ott, S. D., Solomon, G. S., Elbin, R. J., Higgins, K., & Moser, R. S. (2014). Utility of repeated assessment after invalid baseline neurocognitive test performance. Journal of Athletic Training, 49, 659–664. http://dx.doi.org/10.4085/1062-6050-49.3.37

Schatz, P., Moser, R. S., Solomon, G. S., Ott, S. D., & Karpf, R. (2012). Prevalence of invalid computerized baseline neurocognitive test results in high school and collegiate athletes. Journal of Athletic Training, 47, 289–296. http://dx.doi.org/10.4085/1062-6050-47.3.14

Slick, D. J., & Strauss, E. (2006). Measures of suboptimal performance derived from neuropsychological tests. In A. M. Poreh (Ed.), The quantified process approach to neuropsychological assessment (pp. 327–340). New York, NY: Psychology Press/Taylor & Francis.

Snyder, H. R. (2013). Major depressive disorder is associated with broad impairments on neuropsychological measures of executive function: A meta-analysis and review. *Psychological Bulletin, 139,* 81–132. http://dx.doi.org/10.1037/a0028727

Solomon, G. S., & Haase, R. F. (2008). Biopsychosocial characteristics and neuro-cognitive test performance in National Football League players: An initial assessment. *Archives of Clinical Neuropsychology, 23,* 563–577. http://dx.doi.org/10.1016/j.acn.2008.05.008

Tancer, M. E., Brown, T. M., Evans, D. L., Ekstrom, D., Haggerty, J. J., Jr., Pedersen, C., & Golden, R. N. (1990). Impaired effortful cognition in depression. *Psychiatry Research, 31,* 161–168. http://dx.doi.org/10.1016/0165-1781(90)90118-O

Tombaugh, T. N. (1997). The Test of Memory Malingering (TOMM): Normative data from cognitively intact and cognitively impaired individuals. *Psychological Assessment, 9,* 260–268. http://dx.doi.org/10.1037/1040-3590.9.3.260

Tremblay, L., & Schultz, W. (2000). Reward-related neuronal activity during go–nogo task performance in primate orbitofrontal cortex. *Journal of Neurophysiology, 83,* 1864–1876. http://dx.doi.org/10.1152/jn.2000.83.4.1864

Wieth, M., & Burns, B. D. (2006). Incentives improve performance on both incremental and insight problem solving. *Quarterly Journal of Experimental Psychology, 59,* 1378–1394. http://dx.doi.org/10.1080/17470210500234026

9

THE VALIDITY OF NEUROPSYCHOLOGICAL TESTS IN SPORTS-RELATED CONCUSSIONS

ARTHUR MAERLENDER

Studies of neuropsychological testing in the management of sports-related concussion (SRC) have a long history (see e.g., Grindel, Lovell, & Collins, 2001). The author informally searched PubMed and identified over 250 articles with the key words "neuropsychological testing" and "sports-related concussion." With the availability of computerized neuropsychological tests, the acquisition of data has become easier, allowing for empirical analysis of test scores. However, this ease of data collection also raises questions about quality control and the accuracy of data that would reduce the validity of findings. But test validity has always been a focus for neuropsychology, long before computers. The purpose of this chapter is to review the concept of validity in neuropsychological testing as it relates to SRC, including challenges and criticisms. I provide a survey of peer-reviewed research that includes findings of validity of various tests used in the assessment and management of SRC. Note that this does not include the assessment of performance validity that is the subject of Chapter 8 of this volume.

http://dx.doi.org/10.1037/0000114-010
Neuropsychology of Sports-Related Concussion, P. A. Arnett (Editor)

TYPES OF TEST VALIDITY

Neuropsychology is the study of brain–behavior relationships, that is, the ways in which specific neural (brain) structures and activity are reflected in cognitive and physical behavior. The terms *neuropsychological* and *cognitive* are often used interchangeably (as in neuropsychological testing, cognitive testing, and neurocognitive testing). For the purposes of this chapter, these terms can be understood as equivalent.

The concept of test validity appears to have first been formulated by Kelley (1927), who stated that a test is valid if it measures what it claims to measure. According to the Standards for Educational and Psychological Testing (American Educational Research Association [AERA], American Psychological Association, National Council on Measurement in Education, & Joint Committee on Standards for Educational and Psychological Testing, 2014), *validity* refers to the extent to which a test measures the construct of interest. However, validity is not a single state to be measured, but establishing validity is a process. Validation usually starts with an explicit statement about the proposed interpretation of the test scores. The relevance of the interpretation is also important, as is the specification of the construct in question (the concept or characteristic that is to be measured). Different uses of the test require different forms of validity. Establishing validity is necessary before a test can be accepted as clinically useful, while the specific types of validity that are established must be understood and adhered to in clinical use (AERA, 2014). A single interpretation of any test result may require several propositions to be true (or may be questioned by any one of a set of threats to its validity). Evidence for validity comes from multiple sources: the test content, the actual processes used in taking the test, the internal structure of the test, relationships to other variables, and evidence of the consequences of test results.

Internal Validity

There are two broad types on validity: internal and external. *Internal validity* refers to whether the effects observed in a study are due to the manipulation of the independent variable and not some other factor. In other words, there is a causal relationship between the independent (subject state) and dependent (test) variables.

Internal validity can be improved by controlling extraneous variables, using standardized instructions, counter balancing test order, eliminating demand characteristics and investigator effects (to name a few factors). Figure 9.1 depicts the relationship of various types of validity.

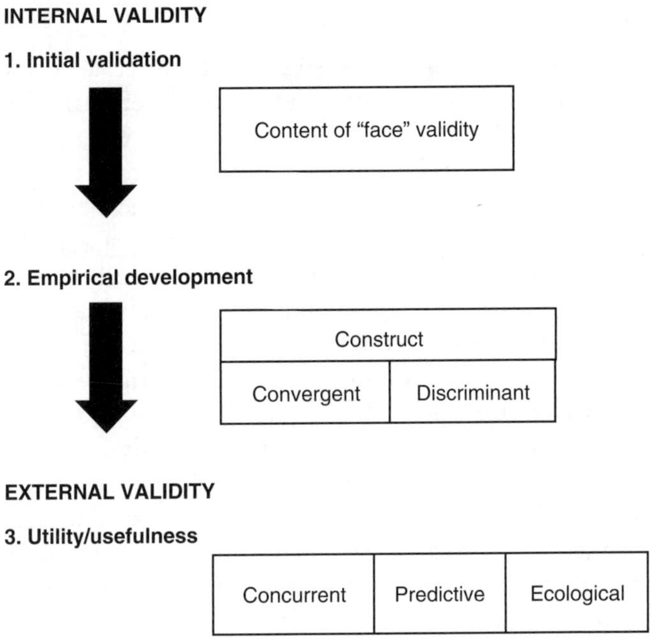

INTERNAL VALIDITY

1. Initial validation

Content of "face" validity

2. Empirical development

Construct	
Convergent	Discriminant

EXTERNAL VALIDITY

3. Utility/usefulness

Concurrent	Predictive	Ecological

Figure 9.1. Process and types of validity. Data from the American Educational Research Association (AERA), American Psychological Association, National Council on Measurement in Education, and Joint Committee on Standards for Educational and Psychological Testing (2014).

Content Validity

A test has *content validity* if it measures knowledge of the content domain of which it was designed to measure knowledge. Another way of saying this is that content validity concerns, primarily, the adequacy with which the test items adequately and representatively sample the content area to be measured. To establish the content validity of a measuring instrument, the researcher must identify the overall content to be represented. Items must then be randomly chosen from this content that will accurately represent the information in all areas. By using this method, the researcher should obtain a group of items that is representative of the content of the trait or property to be measured.

It is not easy to identify a universe of content; therefore, it is typical to have a panel of experts in the field to be studied identify the content area. Content validity may also be established by systematic observations or surveys of competencies, domains of knowledge, activity, etc. In general, content validity is the least empirically derived form of validity.

Construct Validity

"Construct validity must be investigated whenever no criterion or universe of content is accepted as entirely adequate to define the quality to be measured" (Cronbach & Meehl, 1955, p. 282).

A test has *construct validity* if it accurately measures a theoretical, nonobservable construct or trait. Most targets of psychological research are theoretical and nonobservable. The construct validity of a test is established over a period of time on the basis of an accumulation of evidence. The theory underlying the construct to be measured must first be considered. Second, how well the test measures the construct must be evaluated.

There are a number of ways to establish construct validity. The two most frequently employed methods of establishing a test's construct validity are convergent/discriminant validation and factor analysis.

A test has *convergent validity* if it has a high correlation with another test that measures the same construct. By contrast, a test's *discriminant validity* (sometimes called *divergent validity*) is demonstrated through a low correlation with a test that measures a different construct (the two tests measure different traits). This involves demonstrating that the construct can be differentiated from other constructs that may be somewhat similar. It should be shown that the construct being measured is not the same as one that was measured under a different name or some universal construct. The multitrait–multimethod matrix was first proposed by Campbell and Fiske (1959) and is one way to assess a test's convergent and discriminant validity at the same time. In this approach, multiple constructs are measured by multiple methods, with each construct measured by each method.

Campbell and Fiske (1959) went on to articulate the process of the multitrait–multimethod analysis of construct validity, by which constructs of interest (traits) are measured by multiple means (methods). In this way, better construct specification can be obtained while controlling for shared method variance. They also noted that

> for the justification of novel trait measures, for the validation of test interpretation, or for the establishment of construct validity, *discriminant* validation as well as convergent validation is required. Tests can be invalidated by too high correlations with other tests from which they were intended to differ. (p. 100)

Each test used is a trait–method unit, which contains both trait features and measurement features that are not specific to the trait content. "In order to examine discriminant validity, and in order to estimate the relative contributions of trait and method variance, *more than one trait* as well as *more than one method* must be employed in the validation process" (Campbell & Fiske, 1959, p. 100; emphasis in original). Systematic variance among test scores is related to both test-response features and trait content features. By utilizing a multitrait–multimethod matrix, trait and method features can be more clearly isolated. A similar approach is used in structural equation (measurement) modeling (SEM) when multiple trait–method units are obtained (Cole, Howard, & Maxwell, 1981).

Exploratory factor analysis (e.g., principal components analysis) is a complex statistical procedure that assesses the relationship of test scores and tests to each other to establish underlying statistical relationships. The grouping of items and tests from the analysis suggests the underlying constructs. For instance, the most commonly used computerized neuropsychological battery in sports-concussion testing, the Immediate Post-Concussion Assessment and Cognitive Test (ImPACT) test, provides four composite scores: (a) Verbal Memory, (b) Visual Memory, (c) Visual Motor Speed, and (d) Reaction Time. When factor analyzed, the scores from a sample of participants grouped into two factors with both memory composites and speed composites "clumping" together (Schatz & Maerlender, 2013). The interpretation was that the test has two underlying factors: memory and speed. Memory (including working memory) and speed of processing (including reaction time) are often noted as sensitive factors in mild traumatic brain injury (mTBI; e.g., see Allen & Gfeller, 2011). Indeed, working memory has long been identified as sensitive to brain injury (see McDonald, Saykin, & McAllister, 2012).

Confirmatory factor analysis utilizes SEM to determine if data fit a theoretical model of constructs that are hypothesized to exist. This is a more powerful analytic approach and is sometimes used to confirm the structure identified in the exploratory model.

Additionally, tests measuring certain developmental constructs can be shown to have construct validity if the scores on the tests show predictable developmental changes over time. Experimental intervention can also be used to support construct validity if scores should change following an experimental manipulation, in the direction predicted by the theory underlying the construct.

External Validity

External validity is the extent to which the results of a study can be generalized to other situations and to other people.

Concurrent Versus Predictive Validity (Validation)

The term *validation* refers to the procedures used to determine how valid a predictor is. There are two types of validation procedures. In *concurrent validation*, the predictor and criterion data are collected at or about the same time. This kind of validation is appropriate for tests designed to asses a person's current criterion status. It is often used for developing diagnostic tests. In *predictive validation*, the predictor scores are collected first and criterion data are collected at some later point, typically to asses a person's future status on a criterion. A test has *criterion-related validity* if it is useful for predicting a person's behavior in a specified situation, including diagnostic status.

In many cases when using predictor tests, the goal is to predict whether or not a person will meet or exceed a minimum standard of criterion performance—the criterion cutoff point. When a predictor is to be used in this manner, the goal of the validation study is to set an optimal predictor cut-off score: an examinee who scores at or above the predictor cutoff is predicted to score at or above the criterion cutoff.

The number or percentage of *true positives* (or valid acceptance) accurately identified by the predictor as meeting the criterion standard is compared to the number of *false positives* (or false acceptance)—those scores that are incorrectly identified by the predictor as meeting the criterion standard. *True negatives* (valid rejection) are cases accurately identified by the predictor as not meeting the criterion standard and *false negatives* (invalid rejection) are cases that meet the criterion standard, even though the predictor indicated the case would not. The ratios of these conditions determine how *sensitive* the test is (the ratio of true positive identifications—those with the condition of interest that are accurately identified—to the total number of those with the condition in the sample). The test's *specificity* is determined by the ratio of true negatives—those without the condition who are accurately identified—to the total number of those without the condition in the sample.

Ecological Validity

Ecological validity refers to a test's ability to measure some functional or real-world attribute, outside of a tightly controlled laboratory. Studies of ecological validity are difficult and rare. They often require naturalistic designs to capture functioning in daily living. In the sports world, one approach would be to compare test results with game or meet performance before and after mTBI. To our knowledge, no such studies currently exist.

FACTORS AFFECTING THE VALIDITY OF NEUROPSYCHOLOGICAL TESTS

As sensitive tools, neuropsychological tests are used to characterize cognitive functions including (but not limited to) memory, speed, and efficiency of information processing, executive functions and visual–perceptual functions. The validity of a test is crucial for allowing the clinician to rely on the outcomes as part of an assessment process. Thus, not only the development and use of the test, but the process of administration is critical. Further, examinee characteristics can influence the outcome of testing, including the manner in which the test is taken, state effects of the individual (including motivation), and environmental factors. Indeed, intraindividual variation in "normal" subjects is well-established and complicates validity studies (Rabinowitz & Arnett, 2013).

The influence of intrinsic and extrinsic factors on neuropsychological test performance has long been studied; clinicians attempt to minimize effects through standardized procedures and the testing environment.

In the sports-concussion context, McCrory and colleagues listed a number of individual factors (e.g., genetics, general cognitive level of functioning, gender, ethnicity, mood) and methodological factors (e.g., testing environment, practice and learning effects, administrative expertise) that may influence test outcomes (see Table 9.1). Symptom load as a state factor should also be considered as a factor that affects test performance (McCrory, Makdissi, Davis, & Collie, 2005). Score interpretation depends on reliable administration and proper consideration of all of these factors, some of which are reduced with computerized testing (McCrory et al., 2005).

Using trained test administrators and testing in appropriate environments are fairly obvious requirements, although there are no data on the actual

TABLE 9.1
Threats to the Validity of Neuropsychological Tests

Past history	Psychological factors	Genetic factors	Methodological factors	Other factors
Previous concussions	Test anxiety	Age	Testing situation	Cognitive function
Other head injuries	Depression, other emotional states	Intelligence	Practice and learning effects	Symptom load
Education		Sex	Administrator expertise/ competence	Test setting and distractions
Background		Race		Motivation
Previous testing		Handedness	Procedural fidelity	Fatigue
Drug use		Visual acuity		Random variance and chance
Alcohol use		Auditory acuity		

training or test environments currently in use. Group testing, the way in which most baseline assessments are administered, appears to systematically lower scores compared with individualized administration (Erdal, 2012; Moser, Schatz, Neidzwski, & Ott, 2011; Schatz & Sandel, 2013).

Age and sex are well-known contributors to score differences in all educational and psychological tests. Test standardization requires validity studies that determine these differences and thus the presentation of separate norms (see AERA et al., 1999). Most published tests (including ImPACT, CogSport, and Concussion Resolution Index [CRI]), provide age and gender normative standards or references. Unless tests have been shown to be insensitive to gender differences, they are expected to offer separate scoring parameters.

Higher academic achievement has been linked to higher computerized neuropsychological test scores. One study looked at neuropsychological test scores in more than 300 Division I NCAA schools. Athletes with the highest levels of academic achievement based on the Scholastic Aptitude Test (SAT) had higher scores on the Automated Neuropsychological Assessment Metrics (ANAM) test battery than did those athletes with lower SAT scores (Brown, Guskiewicz, & Bleiberg, 2007). Comorbid conditions such as attention-deficit/hyperactivity disorder (ADHD), and learning disabilities (LD; Collins et al., 1999) also may be reflected in test scores. Some medications can also affect scores, including antiepileptic drugs and psychostimulants.

Poor effort is somewhat more difficult to detect and control but is a factor that lowers scores. This has been documented in the general traumatic brain injury (TBI) literature (Green, 2007; Lange, Iverson, Brooks, & Rennison, 2010). A major concern in sports concussion is willful lowering of baseline scores in order to establish an easier threshold for "return to baseline" (Gaudet & Weyandt, 2017). The ImPACT test has embedded validity indicators to help examiners determine atypically low scores on specific subtests, although several authors have identified additional markers of questionable validity (Schatz & Glatts, 2013). However, individuals with neurologic or developmental disorders or those under acute stress may legitimately score low on these indicators; thus, individual analysis is required before declaring a test "invalid." There are also specific tests and profiles within neuropsychological tests that are used to detect poor effort, "malingering," or suboptimal performance (see Chapter 8, this volume, for a detailed discussion of the influence of motivational factors in sports concussion testing).

In the clinical pediatric population, sleep debt does not appear to interfere with neuropsychological testing, although it is strongly implicated in poor school performance (see Beebe, 2012, for review). There have been mixed results of sleep the night before baseline testing and test outcomes. Two research teams (Maerlender & Alt, 2012; Silverberg, Berkner, Atkins,

Zafonte, & Iverson, 2016) found that the duration of sleep the night before testing as recorded on the ImPACT program showed strong relationships with symptom reporting, with females reporting more than males. However, McClure, Zuckerman, Kutscher, Gregory, and Solomon (2014) found a relationship between less than 7 hours of sleep the night before testing and the ImPACT Verbal Memory, Visual Memory and Reaction Time composite scores. Note that the McClure et al. study included college students, while the other two studies were limited to high school students.

Mood and anxiety have long been known to affect neuropsychological test performance in clinical patients. Bailey and colleagues and Maerlender and colleagues have presented data demonstrating that mood and anxiety scores on independent measures were related to specific test score patterns on ImPACT and on a paper-and-pencil neuropsychological battery. The Bailey study administered the Personality Assessment Inventory together with the CRI and found that a significant amount of variance in baseline scores was accounted for by mood and anxiety symptom load (Bailey, Samples, Broshek, Freeman, & Barth, 2010; Maerlender et al., 2010). Using the symptom scale that is part of the ImPACT battery, Covassin and colleagues found that athletes with high levels of depression reported more concussion-like symptoms and had lower ImPACT test scores on baseline tests (Covassin, Elbin, Larson, & Kontos, 2012).[1] The ANAM battery has validated a mood scale and demonstrated its relationship to test scores (Johnson et al., 2008). Given the increased use of neuropsychological testing at baseline and post injury, the effect of these factors is important to understand and highlights the need for interpretation by experienced providers. The relationship between mood and anxiety and neuropsychological performance in concussed athletes could be that both are end results of the same brain injury, that depression and anxiety symptoms are in reaction to difficulties in cognitive performance, or that depression and anxiety have direct negative effects on neurocognitive performance. There is evidence to support each of these three possibilities (Chen et al., 2007; Pardini et al., 2010). Although most studies of athletes have used older samples, there is no reason to believe that the state effects of anxiety, mood, or stress would be any different in a younger population; however, there are no systematic studies in athletes younger than high school age. (See Chapter 3 for a more detailed discussion of the assessment and impact of depression and anxiety in SRC.)

Fazio and colleagues demonstrated that symptoms associated with the injury were related to lower test scores as well (Fazio, Lovell, Pardini, & Collins, 2007). When comparing groups of concussed athletes with and without

---

[1]High school athletes reported more somatic or migraine symptoms than college athletes, whereas college athletes reported more emotional and sleep symptoms than their high school counterparts.

reported symptoms to nonconcussed athletes, they found significant differences among all three groups on each of the four ImPACT composites, with the symptomatic group obtaining the lowest scores, the asymptomatic group having the next lowest scores compared to the control group. This suggested that the presence of symptoms was related to lower test scores (a "feeling bad" effect).

Pain has also been shown to affect cognition in some groups of patients. Gosselin and colleagues (2012) compared groups of adolescents with mTBI ($n = 24$; 50% were sports-related injuries), noninjured controls ($n = 16$), and athletes with orthopedic injuries ($n = 29$). Levels of pain were the dependent measure and fMRI BOLD (blood oxygenation level dependent) activation during a working memory task was the outcome. While results were somewhat complicated, the authors interpreted the results as demonstrating that behavioral performance and cerebral function were related to levels of pain.

Experimenter expectancies can also bias outcomes. This is the logic behind the blinding procedure in randomized trials. While developing new tests requires the "experimenter" to conduct initial trials to assess the test, independent assessments are necessary to fully establish the validity of the test. More and more professional journals are requiring statements about conflicts of interest that include this form of bias. However, it is important to seek independent confirmation of initial findings to avoid this type of bias. As an example, a recent systematic review of the King–Devick Test was published by the King–Devick group, with the majority of articles reviewed from the same group (Galetta et al., 2016). It is difficult to overestimate the likely effect of expectation bias in such situations. Journal editors have a role to play in this regard.

VALIDITY OF COMPUTERIZED TESTS

The presentation format of a computer-based test presents different limitations and strengths compared with paper-and-pencil testing (Bauer et al., 2012). For instance, memory is a complex function, and computerized tests of memory are limited to recognition formats. This format limitation may be one reason for difficulty in isolating specific cognitive functions, as there may be overlap between, for example, processing speed and working memory (Maerlender et al., 2010). However, answering questions about identification and recovery may not require such construct specification.

Collie, Darby, and Maruff (2001) raised concerns with paper-and-pencil testing due to interrater reliability issues, the general lack of alternative forms, and the effect of practice in repeat testing. McCrory and colleagues (2005) noted that computerized testing offered advantages such as standardized and randomized presentation of stimuli, shorter time length, central data storage, and more accurate temporal calculations. Furthermore, standard paper-and-pencil tests do not typically have normative standards specifically for athletes. Additionally, computerized tests allow for easier repeat (serial) testing to track cognitive recovery. Indeed, an entire industry, with its corresponding potential financial conflicts of interest, has developed around providing baseline and serial postinjury testing to thousands of athletes. By 2003, the brief paper-and-pencil test battery was becoming replaced by computerized test batteries such as ImPACT, CogSport, ANAM, and CRI (see, e.g., Cernich, Reeves, Sun, & Bleiberg, 2007; Collie et al., 2003; Collins et al., 2003; Erlanger et al., 2003; Kontos, Braithwaite, Dakan, & Elbin, 2014). Although there are concerns with their use, they continue to represent a large portion of concussion management activity. However, addressing these threats to the validity of the tests is important in both research and clinical activities.

THREATS TO VALIDITY IN SPORTS-CONCUSSION TESTING

Chapter 8 discusses the testing of effort in concussion management assessment. Effort in baseline testing is a significant threat to internal validity. Postinjury effort is seen as less of a concern, as most athletes and students have motivation to be cleared and so put forth good effort. However, this is not always the case, as some individuals see test failure as a means for quitting a sport they no longer want to play or feel pressured to play. Each of the computerized tests utilize some embedded indicators of invalidity for use (primarily) in baseline testing. However, effort is not the only cause for exceeding invalidity measures. Nelson et al. (2016) studied various subject characteristics in relation to "tripping" embedded validity measures. History or presence of ADHD, LD, low grade point average, and low single-word reading score (often used as a proxy for IQ) was found to be a predictor of "failure" on computerized tests. Separate norms for clinical populations should be provided but often are not. Resch, McCrea, and Cullum (2013) published a review of validity studies of computerized neuropsychological tests (CNT) used in concussion management. They summarized their survey noting the variability and limits of the findings:

> In terms of validity, highly variable evidence has been reported for each CNT. In terms of sensitivity and specificity, values ranged from 1% to 94.6% for sensitivity and 86% to 100% for specificity for each CNT, including metrics for the battery, subtest, and summary scores. Limited data on other forms of validity have been reported in the literature. (pp. 345–346)

This summary is consistent with the Institute of Medicine report (IOM & NRC, 2013) and highlights the need for continued work to establish validity of these tests.

An often neglected aspect of the validity of computerized tests involves the technology itself. Rahman-Filipiak and Woodard (2013) noted that most studies utilizing computer-based tests provide poor descriptions of administration methods and testing conditions. In their review, no studies described the assessment protocol sufficiently to deduce whether guidelines for computer-based testing had been followed. While the presence of a proctor was often noted, many researchers did not clarify the identity or training level of the proctor. They provide a table of other guidelines related to administration that tend not to be described. They noted that the absence of this information would not necessarily invalidate the results, but did make it difficult to draw firm conclusions regarding the internal validity of studies' conclusions.

With the move to tablet-based testing, entirely new issues have evolved. Schatz, Ybarra, and Leitner (2015) analyzed the timing mechanisms of several tablets. There were significant differences documented between tablet devices and timing intervals. The actual variation in timing accuracy was quite consistent, suggesting that while specific tablet devices have greater inherent error, this error is standardized and consistent. They opined that software developers should be aware of the platform differences and should either provide parameters for interpretation of reaction time data or conduct internal calibration or normalization of data prior to clinical output.

Burke et al. (2017) compared the two reaction-time tasks of C3Logix to a standard continuous performance test. Sixty healthy young adults completed simple reaction time (SRT) and complex reaction time (CRT) tasks using a traditional test platform and mobile platforms on two occasions. The SRT was similar across test modality: 300, 287, and 280 milliseconds (ms) for the traditional, iPad, and iTouch, respectively. The CRT was similar within mobile devices, though slightly faster on the traditional: 359, 408, and 384 ms for traditional, iPad, and iTouch, respectively (independent tests of validity of other C3Logix tests have not yet been published).

ESTABLISHING INTERNAL VALIDITY

As the previous discussion of types of validity suggests, the question of a test's validity is not always a simple matter. Construct validity helps clarify the usefulness of a test in specific contexts. For instance, if the construct of interest is specifically memory, the clinician must understand what aspect of memory the test is assessing. While there is some variability, particularly in assessment methodologies, most or all of the tests used in SRC have demonstrated some level of construct validity (see Table 9.2).

TABLE 9.2
Validity Studies by Test and Validation Type

Test	Study author(s)	Age range	Subjects (n)	Type of validity	Comparisons	Findings
ANAM	Bleiberg, Kane, Reeves, Garmoe, & Halpern, 2000	High school and college	122	Concurrent	Trail Making Test Part B, ACT total score, PASAT, HVLT, Stroop Color–Word test	PASAT r MTH = .66; PASAT r with Sternberg Memory = .45; PASAT r with SPD = .33; Trails B r Matching to Sample = –.50//PASAT & Trails B correlated with MTH, Sternberg Memory, SPD & Matching to Sample
ANAM	Bleiberg et al., 2004	College	68 concussed of 729; 18 controls tested at same interval	Predictive	Test intervals: 0 to 23 hours, 1–2 days, 3–7 days, and 8–14 days	< 24 hr: SPD $p < .01$; MTH < .05; 1–2 change in SPD < .05; no other findings
ANAM	Mihalik et al., 2013	College	132 concussed	Predictive	Percentage exceeding RCI; RCI values based on separate healthy sample.	Sensitivity at 80%, 90%, and 95% all < 15%; specificity > 90%
ANAM	Woodard et al., 2002	High school	20 nonconcussed	Concurrent	Healthy athletes ANAM and paper-and-pencil tests	Significant correlations between individual ANAM scores and HVLT, COWAT, Digit Symbol, Symbol Search
CogSport	Collie et al., 2003	Mean age 22	240 elite Australian rules football players, 160 healthy volunteers	Concurrent	Trails, DSMT; ICCs calculated from z scores	ICCs stronger for DSMT than Trails; speed scores better than accuracy.

(continues)

TABLE 9.2

Validity Studies by Test and Validation Type (*Continued*)

Test	Study author(s)	Age range	Subjects (*n*)	Type of validity	Comparisons	Findings
CogSport/ Axon	Makdissi et al., 2010	16–35	88 concussed Australian rules football players	Predictive	Trails B, Digit Symbol and CogSport; symptomatic vs. asymptomatic at time of testing	Both CogSport and paper-and-pencil showed more RCI changes for symptomatic than asymptomatic; significantly more athletes showed RCI changes on CogSport than paper-and-pencil for both.
CogSport/ Axon	Moriarity et al., 2012		96 amateur boxers	Predictive	Baseline to postbout	2 of 96 had low scores but no concussion; conclusion was unclear. Note: some took baseline tests in dorm room
CogSport	Schatz & Putz, 2006	18–23 college students	30	Concurrent	SRT: CogSport, Head-minder, Trails A, Digit Symbol; CRT: ImPACT, CogSport, Head-minder, Trails A, Trails B, Digit Symbol; Memory: CogSport visual and learning, ImPACT verbal and visual; Pro-cessing Speed: ImPACT, CogSport, Trails B, Digit Symbol,	SRT no significant *r*; CRT to Impact RT *r* = .649; to Trails A *r* = .544; to Trails B *r* = .535; Memory to CogSport Learning *r* = .723

Test	Reference	Age	Sample	Validity	Method	Results
CogSport	Louey et al., 2014	16–26	29 rugby and Australian rules football players	Predictive	Baseline-adjusted change scores comparing concussed to normative sample on 4 indices	Significant differences on all 4 indices; all $p < .001$
ImPACT	Iverson, Brooks, Lovell, & Collins, 2006	Mean age 17	72 amateur	Concurrent	Tested within 21 days of concussion; correlated with Symbol Digit	All composites and symptom total significantly correlated with SDMT
ImPACT	Iverson, Lovell, & Collins, 2005 (abstract)	None given	72 amateur	Concurrent–construct	Tested within 20 days of injury; BVMT–R, Trail Making, Symbol Digit Modalities	SDMT and BVMT–R delayed significantly correlated with all 4 Impact composites. Both Trails correlated with processing speed
ImPACT	Schatz, Pardini, Lovell, Collins, & Podell, 2006	High school	72 concussed athletes	Predictive	Concussed compared to controls within 72 hrs of injury	Significant differences between groups on all Impact composites and symptoms; 1 discriminant function included Visual memory, Processing Speed, Impulse Control and symptom total: sensitivity = 82%, specificity = 89%
ImPACT	Schatz & Putz, 2006	18–23	30 College students	Concurrent	Indices from CogSport, Headminder, ImPACT, and Trails A & B, SDMT.	Complex RT to Headminder $r = .407$; to CogSport $r = .649$; to Trails A $r = .641$; to Trails B $r = .442$; to DigSymbol $r = -.455$; Memory no significant r; Processing Speed to Headminder $r = -.373$

(continues)

TABLE 9.2
Validity Studies by Test and Validation Type (Continued)

Test	Study author(s)	Age range	Subjects (n)	Type of validity	Comparisons	Findings
ImPACT	Schatz & Sandel, 2013	High school and college, 13–21	Concussed symptomatic athletes (81); concussed asymptomatic athletes (37)	Predictive	Concussed evaluated within hrs of injury compared to controls' baseline testing; also compared scores of symptomatic athletes to asymptomatic athletes to matched controls	Symptomatic athletes: sensitivity = .75; specificity = .89; PPP = .91, NPP = .69; Asymptomatic: sensitivity, specificity, PPP, NPP = .97 (only 2 cases were misclassified)
ImPACT	Tsushima, Shirakawa, & Geling, 2013	High school	26 concussed vs. 25 controls	Criterion	Score comparisons at 6 days	No difference in test scores at 6 days, significant difference in sx; authors felt it replicated previous findings of no test score difference at 7 days.
ImPACT	Maerlender et al., 2010	College	54 nonconcussed	Convergent, concurrent, construct	ImPACT to paper-and-pencil and to in-scanner behavioral tests	High correlations between similar measures for all 4 composites
ImPACT	Maerlender et al., 2013	College	54 nonconcussed (same sample as 2010 study)	Discriminant, concurrent construct	ImPACT to paper-and-pencil and to in-scanner behavioral tests	Poor discriminant validity for 3 or 4 composites—high correlations with dissimilar paper-and-pencil measures, except for reaction time.
ImPACT	Allen & Gfeller, 2011	College	100 nonconcussed	Construct	Factor analysis of Impact and paper-and-pencil battery	Five Impact factors accounted for 69% of variance; Significant correlations between Impact composites and paper-and-pencil tests (except Impulse Control)

Test	Author	Age	Sample	Validity	Description	Findings
Pediatric ImPACT	Newman et al., 2013	5–12	164 concussed	Concurrent–construct	Tested an average of 12 days from injury; correlations with paper-and-pencil and fluency tests	Response Speed Composite r: Digit Span, forward & backward, ACT, Symbol Digit memory; Response Speed Composite was more strongly associated with traditional speed measures than it was with the Learning & Memory Composite, indicating relative independence of the Response Speed and Learning & Memory Accuracy
Pediatric ImPACT	Gioia et al., 2013 (abstract)	22 age 5–7, 67 age 8–12	< 7 days post-concussion	Criterion–predictive	Response speed and symptoms by age	Response speed and symptoms together correctly classified by age.
CRI/ HeadMinder	Erlanger et al., 2003	13–35	414	Concurrent	CRI factors correlated with paper-and-pencil tests (Processing Speed, SRT, CRT)	SDMT & Grooved pegs (bilateral) correlated with all 3 factors; Trails A correlated with SRT and CRT; Trails B and Stroop interference correlated with Processing Speed; Digit Symbol (WAIS-III) correlated with simple RT.
CRI/ HeadMinder	Erlanger et al., 2003	18–87	66 out of a larger sample	Concurrent	4 factors identified (Response Speed, Processing Speed, Memory, Attention) and correlated with paper-and-pencil tests	SDMT correlated with all 4 factors; Symbol Search & Digit Span correlated with Response Speed, Processing Speed, Reaction Time; Bushke Selective Reminding correlated with Response Speed, Memory, Attention; Trails A & B correlated with Response Speed.

(continues)

TABLE 9.2
Validity Studies by Test and Validation Type   (Continued)

Test	Study author(s)	Age range	Subjects (n)	Type of validity	Comparisons	Findings
CRI/ HeadMinder	Schatz & Putz, 2006	18–23 College	30	Concurrent	SRT: CogSport, Head-minder, Trails A, Digit Symbol; CRT: ImPACT, CogSport, Head-minder, Trails A, Trails B, Digit Symbol; Memory: Cog-Sport visual and learning, ImPACT verbal and visual; Processing Speed: ImPACT, CogSport, Trails B, DSMT	SRT to Trails A = .428; to Digit Symbol r = -.526; CRT no significant r; Processing Speed to Trails B r = .601; to Digit Symbol r = -.610; to Impact r = -.373
Affective Word List	Meyer & Arnett, 2015	18–23 college	420 divided across 4 forms of test	Concurrent	RBMT Story Memory, BVMT–R, Trials 1–3, HVLT–R Trials 1–3, CARB), SDMT, Trail Making Test A and B, RBMT Story Memory Delayed Recall, HVLT–R Delayed Recall, BVMT–R Delayed Recall, AWL Trials 1–3, Vigil Continuous Perfor-mance Test, Digit Span, Stroop Color Word Test, PSU	Strong correlations with learning trials of memory tests and strong correla-tions with Beck Depres-sion; good discriminant validity with processing speed and reaction time scores

Test	Author	Population	N	Validity	Method	Results
RTclin	Eckner et al., 2010	College	64	Concurrent	Compared RTclin to CogState SRT	r = .445, p < .001
RTclin	Eckner et al., 2014	College and high school	28 concussed, equal comparisons	Predictive	Compared RTclin after RCI adjustment	Specificity better than sensitivity at each CI except 60% CI; 95 CI sensitivity = 39%, specificity = 93%
CNSVS	Gualtieri & Johnson, 2006	Adults	145 normal, 15 mTBI, 13 PCS, 113 sTBI	Predictive	11 CNSVS domain and 15 test scores by 5 groups (MANOVA)	No significant differences between mTBI and controls; significant ROC found between PCS and more severe TBI on composite NCI and in the domains of psychomotor speed and cognitive flexibility.
CNSVS	Barker-Collo et al., 2015	> 16	427 acute to 227 at 12 mo	Predictive	Pearson's or Spearman's correlations 2 weeks, 1 month, 6 months, 12 months postinjury	At 2 weeks > 20% had very low scores on executive ability, complex attention and cognitive flexibility. At 1 and 6 month > 20% were very low on complex attention, with 16.3% remaining so at 12 months. Executive abilities and speed were related to postconcussion symptoms, mood, and self-reported cognition at 12 months.

(continues)

TABLE 9.2
Validity Studies by Test and Validation Type (Continued)

Test	Study author(s)	Age range	Subjects (n)	Type of validity	Comparisons	Findings
CNSVS	Hume et al., 2017	Former athletes	Former elite contact 103, recreational contact 193, noncontact 65	Predictive	Effect sizes of differences among groups and between groups with and without concussion histories	Elite worse than noncontact on complex attention, processing speed, executive functioning, and cognitive flexibility; recreational worse than noncontact on executive functioning and cognitive flexibility; elite and recreational worse than norms on processing speed, cognitive flexibility and executive functioning; recreational worse than norms on memory; all 3 groups worse than norms on verbal memory and reaction time. Former players with 1 or more concussions had worse scores on cognitive flexibility, executive functioning, and complex attention.

Note. Portions of the data from Institute of Medicine and National Research Council (2013). ACT = Auditory Consonant Trigrams; AWL = Affective Word List; ANAM = Automated Neuropsychological Assessment Metrics; BVMT–R = Brief Visual Memory Test—Revised; CARB = Computerized Assessment of Response Bias; r = correlation coefficient; COWAT = Controlled Oral Word Fluency; CNSVS = CNS Vital Signs; HVLT = Hopkins Verbal Learning Test; ICC = Intraclass correlation; PSU = Penn State University Cancellation Test; MTH = ANAM Mathematical Processing; PASAT = Paced Auditory Serial Addition test; PCS = Post-Concussion Syndrome; CRT = Reaction Time complex; SRT = Reaction Time simple; RCI = Reliable change index; ROC = Receiver Operating Characteristics; RBMT = Rivermead Behavioral Memory Test; SPD = ANAM Spatial Processing; SDMT = Symbol Digit Modalities Test; sx = symptoms; WAIS-III = Wechsler Adult Intelligence Scale, Third Edition.

Paper-and-pencil tests such as Trail Making, the Paced Auditory Serial Attention Test (PASAT), Symbol Digit Modalities Test (SDMT), and Digit Span have long been used in documenting cognitive deficits in TBI. The earlier neuropsychological literature on TBI has documented several specific areas of typical deficit, with processing speed, attention, and memory typically showing the most significant deficits. Sports concussions may have the following effects: (a) reduced planning and ability to switch mental set (Barth, Alves, et al., 1989; Barth, Freeman, et al., 2000; Barth, Macciocchi, et al., 1983; Rimel, Giordani, Barth, & Jane, 1982), (b) impaired memory and learning (Gronwall & Wrightson, 1981; Guskiewicz, 2001; Lovell et al., 2003), (c) reduced attention and ability to process information (Maddocks, Dicker, & Saling, 1995), and (d) slowed reaction times and increased variability in response (Collins et al., 2003; Makdissi et al., 2001).

These tests have become something of a standard in TBI assessment, although variability based on clinician preference certainly exists. The National Hockey League (NHL) neuropsychological test protocol under the direction of Ruben Echemendia, PhD, chair of the NHL and NHL Players' Association Working Concussion Group, includes most of these measures in addition to ImPACT. Similarly, the National Football League (NFL) battery includes most of these as well. However, group differences between baseline and postinjury performance on this battery failed to identify significant cognitive declines approximately 1 day after injury, and all scores were within normal limits (Pellman, Lovell, Viano, Casson, & Tucker, 2004).

Several studies have looked at the concurrent and convergent validity of computerized tests with paper-and-pencil tests. Bleiberg, Kane, Reeves, Garmoe, and Halpern (2000) administered a battery of paper-and-pencil tests together with the ANAM computerized battery. The intercorrelation matrix of significant correlations between ANAM scores (Math Processing Throughput, Accuracy and Reaction Time, Sternberg Memory Throughput and Reaction Time, Matching to Sample Throughput and Reaction Time, Spatial Processing Throughput and Reaction Time) and paper-and-pencil test scores (Trails B, Auditory Consonant Trigrams, PASAT, Hopkins Verbal Learning Test—Revised [HVLT–R], and Stroop) demonstrated a wide range of convergence among tests. Although correlations were labeled as significant, no adjustment for multiple comparisons was made and p-values were not presented. A principal components analysis of the ANAM reaction time and response accuracy scores obtained a three-factor solution with the first two factors representing response speed and response accuracy as predicted; the third factor was made up of only Matching to Sample Accuracy and was difficult to interpret due to its solitary nature. When both batteries were included, a four-factor solution was obtained: Factors 1 and 2 were interpreted as representing different aspects of reaction time, resistance to interference, and working memory. Factor 3 reflected a shared motor-speed component, and Factor 4 appeared to be a memory component (Bleiberg et al., 2000).

Schatz and Putz (2006) had 40 undergraduates take different combinations of computerized and paper-and-pencil tests over 3 days. While there were multiple intercorrelations between CNT indices, the relationships among paper-and-pencil tests and these three CNTs were somewhat more illuminating. For SRT, HeadMinder correlated highly with Trails A and Digit Symbol, but not Trails B. CogSport did not correlate with any paper-and-pencil SRT tests, and ImPACT does not have an SRT index. ImPACT and CogSport CRT indices correlated highly with Trails A and B, and ImPACT also correlated highly with Digit Symbol. HeadMinder did not correlate with any, suggesting poor CRT convergence. HeadMinder and ImPACT processing speed indices correlated highly with Digit Symbol and Trails B. Thus, CogSport did not demonstrate construct validity for processing speed or simple reaction time but did for CRT. ImPACT demonstrated good construct validity in the processing speed and CRT domains, and HeadMinder demonstrated good construct validity for SRT and processing speed but not CRT. As there was no paper-and-pencil memory test, no valid construct validity support could be inferred. Note that test-takers were not athletes, and the actual sample sizes were quite small with no consistency of participants across all tests.

Allen and Gfeller (2011) compared the NFL paper-and-pencil battery with the ImPACT computerized battery in a series of factor analytic studies. A four-factor solution explaining 70% of variance was found with the NFL battery. The factors were labeled as (a) general memory, (b) mental processing speed, (c) verbal memory and processing speed, and (d) auditory and verbal working memory. A five-factor solution explaining 69% of the variance was found with the ImPACT battery, with components assessing (a) forced choice efficiency, (b) verbal and visual memory, (c) inhibitory cognitive abilities, (d) visual processing abilities with a memory component, and (e) a factor with a single loading from Color Match Total Commissions. Correlations between the two batteries were mixed. When data were constrained to two factors, both batteries clearly assessed memory and cognitive efficiency (speed).

Only three studies mention the discriminating ability of the tests: that is, whether a particular test shows low correlations with other tests that it should not be highly correlated with. For example, while the ImPACT test has high correlations between the composite scores and similar paper-and-pencil tests (convergent construct validity), the same sample showed high correlations with dissimilar paper-and-pencil measures (Maerlender et al., 2010). On the other hand, Newman and colleagues showed good discrimination of the new Pediatric ImPACT test between speed of processing and memory tests (Newman, Reesman, Vaughan, & Gioia, 2013). Using a factor-analytic approach, Allen and Gfeller (2011) also demonstrated construct validity for ImPACT. Maerlender et al. (2010) demonstrated adequate convergent validity of ImPACT with both paper-and-pencil and experimental tasks, but weak discriminant validity (2012). ANAM (Bleiberg, Cernich, et al., 2004; Bleiberg, Garmoe, et al., 1997; Bleiberg, Kane, et al., 2000; Prichep, McCrea, Barr, Powell, & Chabot, 2013), CogSport, (Collie et al., 2003; Makdissi et al., 2010; Moriarity et al., 2012), and CRI (Erlanger et al., 2003) have been shown to possess various types of validity.

Mihalik et al. (2013) used a healthy sample of college football players to establish reliable change confidence intervals (CIs) for common clinical concussion measures and applied the reliable change parameters to a sample of concussed players examined before and after injury. Outcome measures included symptom severity scores, ANAM computerized neuropsychological battery throughput scores, and Sensory Organization Test (SOT) composite scores. Concussed athletes were assessed within 5 days of injury ($n = 132$). Based on the percentage of athletes with reliable change scores below or above various CI cutoffs (80%, 90%, and 95%), they calculated sensitivity and specificity based on the percentage of cases that declined by more than the reliable change metric. At all three CIs, individual tests and total battery scores exceeded 90% specificity, indicating that no change or improvement was predictive of not having a concussion. However, score declines were not predictive of having a concussion. Although having at least one score decline across the entire battery improved sensitivity, it was still at 50%. The authors cite the importance of a total battery in the assessment of concussion. In this battery, score declines did not predict concussion better than chance (Mihalik et al., 2013).

The CNS Vital Signs (CNSVS) is a computerized battery of tests with reported psychometrics (Gualtieri & Johnson, 2008) obtained from a variety of clinical samples. A small sample of adults with postconcussion syndrome (PCS) and severe TBI were included. Concurrent and convergent validity with comparable paper-and-pencil tests were obtained for a large normative group. Means and standard deviations for the normative group for ages 7 through 90 are available in multiple languages. However, Gualtieri and Johnson (2008) have developed a concussion battery that includes a general Neurocognitive Index, Verbal and Visual Memory, Psychomotor Speed, Executive Function, Cognitive Flexibility and Reaction Time.

While computerized and tablet neuropsychological tests have become more frequently used, development of nondigital tests continues. A simple reaction-time test (RTclin) has been developed that uses a long stick with a weight on the end that the athlete must grasp as it is dropped through the fingers. After eight trials, the mean measurements on the stick are calculated to reflect speed of reaction (Eckner, Kutcher, & Richardson, 2010). Following standardized procedures, 64 Division I NCAA athletes completed both the

RTclin and the CogState reaction-time tests. Good concurrent validity was established and the authors noted less variability in the RTclin scores than in the CogState tests.

Meyer and Arnett (2015) developed a promising new measure, the Affective Word List (AWL), to assess affective bias in the context of a verbal learning and memory test. Because it is designed as a traditional list-learning task, the cognitive indices of the AWL have the added potential to be used as measures of verbal learning and memory. The AWL was administered as part of a standard battery that included the HVLT–R, ImPACT, Rivermead Story Memory test, Vigil Continuous Performance Test (CPT), Computerized Assessment of Response Bias (CARB), and the Penn State Cancellation test. Factor analysis confirmed a three-factor model (memory, processing speed, reaction time), while the intercorrelations reflected positive correlations among memory tests and weak correlations with the nonmemory tests. Thus, construct validity was demonstrated for both convergent and discriminant functions.

Other newer tests are coming into the market and have yet to show independent peer-reviewed validity. The older, more established tests have demonstrated adequate to excellent internal validity relative to their typical functions. Reaction times and processing speed are clearly important constructs to measure, while working memory and memory encoding (which relies on working memory) are also important functions impacted by mTBI. While strong convergent validity is often demonstrated, the specificity of functions as demonstrated by discriminant validity is often not reported. Clinicians need to be aware of the strengths and limitations of various tests and use them accordingly. Computerized tests appear to be less specific than paper-and-pencil neuropsychological tests. The use of computers also adds a layer of complexity that can affect the validity of findings. As Schatz et al. (2015) noted, timing mechanisms for speeded tasks may vary by platform.

ESTABLISHING EXTERNAL VALIDITY

Predictive and Criterion-Related Validity of Injury and Diagnosis

Identifying specific brain injury or lesion is not always possible with neuropsychological tests, and, as SRC has typically been defined as a transient alteration of brain function, the search for a biological signature of concussion has been a challenge. While several studies have identified physiologic changes apparently due to concussion, only one study has linked those changes to neuropsychological testing and thus contributed to the validity of these tests. McAllister et al. (2014) assessed a large number of collegiate athletes at preseason, a postinjury subgroup, and postseason. Both contact (football and hockey) and noncontact athletes were compared. A subgroup of athletes and noncontact comparison subjects who performed worse than predicted on the CVLT-II total words recalled measure (defined by scores 1.5 SDs below the predicted score) were compared at the postseason assessment. The contact group showed more change in diffusion tensor imaging metrics (DTI) of mean diffusivity (MD) in the corpus callosum ($p = .017$) relative to the normally performing group of athletes. Further, in the larger sample, there was a significant association between head impact metrics and postseason white matter measures in a number of regions, including the corpus callosum, amygdala, cerebellum, and hippocampus. Thus, in those who scored below expectation on the CVLT-II, the contact athletes had more white matter change than normally performing athletes. DTI metrics and biomechanical force exposure were related across samples, lending inferential support to the validity of CVLT-II to white matter changes and levels of biomechanical force.

The usefulness of tests to diagnose a disease entity (i.e., their ability to detect a person with disease or exclude a person without disease), is often described by the test's sensitivity, specificity, positive predictive value, and negative predictive value. These functions specify the proportions of cases that are known to have the disease (or not) compared with those who should have the disease (or not) based on test scores. Although sensitivity and specificity are the characteristics most reported for a diagnostic test, the users of the test are likely to be more interested in the predictive values (the chance that a person identified by the test as concussed actually had a concussion—positive predictive value—and the chance that a person identified as not having a concussion was actually free of a recent concussion—negative predictive value). The predictive value changes depending on what fraction of the athletes tested truly had a concussion.

Studies of the ability of neuropsychological tests to provide accurate diagnoses of concussion typically have tests administered within 72 hours of the injury. They include studies comparing groups of concussed individuals to nonconcussed individuals by comparing group-level score changes. Group studies include cross-sectional designs and within-subjects designs that use baseline or multiple test points for comparisons. Another approach is to compare the number of accurately identified to misidentified cases (diagnostic accuracy). However, it should be noted that neuropsychological tests are traditionally not used to make diagnoses, but to characterize function. So it is of interest to determine if neuropsychological tests contribute to diagnosis.

As the term *criterion-related validity* indicates, a test is compared with a criterion. When using diagnosis as the criterion, several threats immediately stand out. First, there is no clear biomarker of the injury, making it necessary to rely on less-objective criteria. The diagnostic criterion of a "temporary alteration in consciousness" is operationalized to distinguish mild from moderate injury along with the presence of any of 22 symptoms that are present in temporal proximity to a presumed mechanism of injury. The presence of false positives is a concern, particularly when symptom reporting is largely a subjective activity. In one study, 50% of diagnosed concussions were identified more than 24 hours after the incident, while 30% of these had no identifiable biomechanical impacts on the day of the reported injury, based on accelerometer readings in the helmets (Duhaime et al., 2012). Determining diagnostic efficiency of a test will be impacted by the validity of actual diagnoses. Thus, variability in this process can produce conflicting or limited results when studying the predictive ability of any tool.

Given the relatively rapid time course of the injury, the temporal aspects of the injury are also significant factors in studying the phenomena. Broglio and Puetz (2008) noted that comparing athletes who are assessed at different time points from injury likely invalidates the findings. Controlling for diagnosis and time of testing, baseline exposure to the tests, and other factors all add to the complexity of studying concussions at the group and individual levels, particularly in the immediate aftermath of the injury when symptoms are typically high.

As noted by McCrory and colleagues (2005), the presence of symptoms may preclude accurate (valid) test results. Symptoms may interfere in test performance through any or all attention mechanisms, reducing arousal, orienting, focus, sustaining focus, etc. Or symptoms may make the individual feel too bad to participate (a type of motivational effect). Unfortunately, the actual evidence is limited, as few studies directly test the hypothesis that symptoms (either in total or individually) account for significant variance in test scores.

As a practical matter, the test scores may reflect the overall status of the individual, but the inclusion of symptom-related error into the test scores may interfere in the psychometric accuracy of the test. Studies indirectly point to the correlation of symptoms and test scores (Collins et al., 2003; Fazio et al., 2007), particularly immediately after injury when symptoms tend to be highest. Thus, the mediating effect of symptoms on test scores in the immediate aftermath of the injury likely reduces the predictive power of tests alone. Two studies have looked at the sensitivity of CNTs in asymptomatic athletes. Schatz and Sandel (2013) and Nelson et al. (2016) utilized asymptomatic (or at least concussed athletes reporting no symptoms) for determining sensitivity and specificity of CNTs. Schatz and Sandel noted a finding of higher sensitivity of ImPACT scores for the asymptomatic athletes at 3 days postinjury than for symptomatic athletes. However, the asymptomatic athletes were presumed to be underreporting symptoms and were selected because at least one test score was below baseline validity values.

Nelson et al. (2016) rigorously compared three CNTs (ImPACT, Axon, and ANAM), using reliable change indices to determine sensitivity and specificity at several time points postconcussion. They compared concussed athletes with matched nonconcussed controls. The predictive validity approach was to establish the rates of false-positive findings based on a criterion of symptom presentation. Overall, they found that ANAM, Axon, and ImPACT showed moderate group-level sensitivity within 24 hours of injury, but that further out than 8 days, effect sizes were generally small. These tests added some value within a narrow window when the outcome was to make a diagnosis. In terms of sensitivity, this is consistent with the previous meta-analyses (Belanger & Vanderploeg, 2005; Broglio & Puetz, 2008).

The group studies through 2007 have been described in two meta-analytic studies (Belanger & Vanderploeg, 2005; Broglio & Puetz, 2008). Although there was considerable overlap in the studies reviewed, Broglio and Puetz (2008) were interested in the effect of using multimodal assessments, whereas Belanger and Vanderploeg (2005) were focused on neuropsychological assessments only.

Group studies have generally shown that a significant proportion of concussed athletes have neurocognitive decrements compared with controls (or compared with baseline performances) in the initial days following the injury, but scores returning to normal or baseline by 7 days postinjury. Belanger and Vanderploeg (2005) analyzed 21 studies from 1994 to 2004. All had multiple assessment points using control groups tested at the same interval. They found significant acute effects (changes in scores reflecting worsening in the first 24 hours after injury) for most cognitive domains (delayed memory: $d = 1.00$; memory acquisition: $d = 1.03$; and global cognitive functioning: $d = 1.42$). However, across all studies no group residual neuropsychological reductions were found when testing was completed beyond 7 days postinjury.

Broglio and Puetz (2008) conducted a meta-analysis that included 39 studies from 1970 to 2006 that met their inclusion criteria: studies of concussed athletes who were evaluated using symptom assessment, balance assessment, and/or neuropsychological/cognitive assessment. One postinjury assessment had to have been completed within 14 days of injury and compared with a baseline measure or control group. Three types of cognitive assessments were included: the SAC, paper-and-pencil batteries, and computerized batteries. They found significant effects of concussion on all three assessment modalities immediately after injury. The type of cognitive assessment was determined to be a moderator effect, as was the time from injury to assessment. The largest effect was for the SAC immediately after injury.

Further, both of these meta-analyses documented neuropsychological test score changes through the recovery period. Belanger and Vanderploeg (2005) found significant improvement between Days 7 and 10 for verbal memory retention scores only. Broglio and Puetz (2008) found significant effects of concussion with all three assessment modalities immediately after injury, and reduced but large effects for the cognitive assessment at the 14-day postinjury interval. Both the type of cognitive assessment and time from injury to assessment were identified as moderators. The paper-and-pencil batteries had significantly greater effects than the SAC or computer batteries at 14 days postinjury.

Van Kampen, Lovell, Pardini, Collins, and Fu (2006) tested the added benefit of neuropsychological testing to symptom load in diagnosis. One hundred twenty-two athletes diagnosed with concussion were compared on baseline to postinjury symptoms and test scores. Change in symptom total provided 93% positive predictive power, but only 59% negative predictive power. When ImPACT was used in the absence of symptom data, the predictive value of having at least one abnormal[2] neurocognitive test score was 83%, and the predictive value of a negative test result was 70%. However, when criteria for concussion classification were changed to require at least one abnormal ImPACT test and an abnormal symptom total score (significant increase from baseline), the predictive value was 81%, and the predictive value of having a negative score was 83%.

Several other studies have demonstrated strong diagnostic efficiency of neuropsychological tests. Schatz and colleagues (2006) also obtained 82% sensitivity and 89% specificity comparing ImPACT tests scores ($n = 72$) within 72 hours of injury to scores of nonconcussed athletes ($n = 66$).

Broglio, Macciocchi, and Ferrara (2007) compared the sensitivity of concussion-assessment tests in three distinct cohorts. Athletes with diagnosed concussions were evaluated using self-reported symptoms, postural control assessment, and one of three cognitive assessment methodologies: (a) ImPACT, (b) HeadMinder, or (c) paper-and-pencil tests. At Day 1 postinjury, ImPACT had the highest sensitivity (79.2%) and HeadMinder CRI was next (78.6%). These were followed in sensitivity by concussion-related symptoms (68.0%), the postural control evaluation (61.9%), and the paper-and-pencil assessment (43.5%). When the assessments were combined, the sensitivity ranged from 89% to 96%. However, no control for practice effects or regression to the mean was provided, raising questions about the actual score changes.

Gualtieri and Johnson (2008) included 15 mTBI adults in a sample of postconcussive subjects and two severe TBI groups, and compared with a normative sample. The goal was to "evaluate the discriminant validity of the CNSVS battery in patients with a spectrum of TBIs" (mild, severe, and a postconcussive group compared with a noninjured group). It seems this study would more properly be considered a between-groups predictive validity study.

---

[2]*Abnormal* here means a change from baseline to postinjury score outside the 80% confidence interval for reliable change. This does not necessarily imply clinical abnormality.

Overall, the mTBI patients performed as well as normal controls on all tests. Sensitivity was established between those with PCS and more severe TBI.

Hume et al. (2017) established predictive validity by comparing differences in CNSVS scores between retired elite and recreational rugby players and noncontact athletes to the CNSVS normative data. They also compared test scores between those with reported histories of concussion to normative values. Past participation in rugby or a history of concussion were associated with small to moderate neurocognitive deficits (as indicated by worse CNSVS scores) in athletes postretirement from competitive sport. Thus, there have been mixed findings of predictive validity in CNSVS in sports concussion and/or mTBI. Concurrent validity appears strong across a variety of disorders, but sports-concussion findings are limited.

The RTclin reaction-time test was shown be specific to noninjury with weak sensitivity after adjustments for practice effects (Eckner, Kutcher, Broglio, & Richardson, 2014). The authors compared 28 concussed athletes with 28 same-team controls, all tested within 48 hours of injury. The control test results were used to establish reliable change parameters. Across five CIs, sensitivity was lower than specificity except at the 60% CI.

Monitoring (Tracking) Recovery

Neuropsychological testing has been used extensively in the rehabilitation setting to document and track cognitive recovery. In sports concussion, the standard as promulgated by Zurich and other consensus statements (McCrory et al., 2017) has been that recovery takes place when symptoms, cognition, and balance have returned to the athlete's baseline (or typical) performance (Halstead, Walter, & The Council on Sports Medicine and Fitness, 2010; Harmon et al., 2013). Using that as the benchmark, studies have generally found neuropsychological testing to be useful for aiding in the determination of an athlete's recovery for return to competition. Although the variability of methodological rigor in studies has been noted (Comper, Hutchison, Magrys, Mainwaring, & Richards, 2010), the ability of neuropsychological tests to detect subtle changes in cognitive function is well established. The two meta-analyses described above provide evidence for the use of neuropsychological tests to track cognitive recovery. A more recent study using ANAM found that several subtest scores differentiated mild from moderate concussions on the day of injury, but not at 8 days from injury (Prichep et al., 2013).

Prediction of the Length of Time to Recovery

Research evidence has consistently demonstrated that most individuals recover within a short time span. While most studies point to a 2-week window, some studies have noted longer durations. Any outcome linked to recovery is hampered by the lack of a biomarker to understand when the injury is no longer present. Further, the outcome presumes the individual wants to return to play as soon as possible. While there are no empirical studies, clinical experience with middle and high school students suggests that this not a universal goal. Many younger student athletes participate in sports for social reasons and when injured simply disappear. When finally tracked down by an athletic trainer, months may have passed. When these individuals are included in outcome studies of time to recovery, the length of time is skewed by poor motivation to return.

With that being said, it is of clinical importance to be able to predict those who may take longer to recover. In its simplest form, the question of a dose–response relationship is valuable and adds to the clinical validity of tests. Prediction of recovery status is obviously important.

In a retrospective sample of 114 high school football players, Iverson (2007) found that athletes with a complex concussion performed significantly more poorly on neuropsychological tests (ImPACT) and reported more sub-jective symptoms than those athletes with simple concussions at 72 hours postinjury. While all concussed athletes showed some cognitive declines after injury, those with persistent symptoms (more than 10 days) were 18 times more likely to have clinically and statistically significant neurocognitive impairments at 3 days postconcussion. A more recent study of the predictive ability of computerized neurocognitive testing (Lau et al., 2011) determined that visual memory and processing speed were significantly worse in athletes suffering a complex concussion, as were subjective reports of migraine, sleep disturbances, and cognitive problems.

McCrea and colleagues (2013) analyzed data from 570 high school and college athletes with concussions taken at several time points after injury. The study stratified concussions based on symptom resolution at less than 7 days (typical) and more than 7 days (prolonged recovery). Neuropsychological test scores at less than 2 days postinjury were not predictive of recovery group. This finding was similar to findings in the two meta-analytic studies reported on previously (Belanger & Vanderploeg, 2005; Broglio & Puetz, 2008). It should be noted that, since 90% of cases are recovered by the end of 2 weeks (typically), group analyses may obscure the effect of the 10% of scores that continues to suggest injury.

Prediction of Outcomes: What Is the Criterion?

An ongoing challenge to establishing predictive or criterion-related validity is the lack of an unambiguous criterion for concussion. Neurophysio-logical differences in concussed athletes weeks and months after injury (and "recovery") are being reported with some regularity. The functional implication of these findings is not clear. While predicting "recovery" on the basis of test scores appears to be valid, developing research suggests continuing impact on white matter microstructures, and electrophysiological changes long after "recovery" (Broglio, Pontifex, O'Connor, & Hillman, 2009; Dettwiler et al., 2013; Prichep et al., 2013; Zhu et al., 2015). The functional implications of these findings are yet unclear, but need consideration. (See Chapter 5 for a more detailed discussion of neuroimaging parameters underlying concussion.)

One line of evidence of the ability to track and determine recovery is provided by the specificity statistics cited in the diagnostic studies. Specificity is the ability to detect when someone does not have a disease, disorder, or injury when the test results indicate that they should not. As Table 9.1 demonstrates, the specificity of the computerized tests is typically higher than the sensitivity—generally above the 80% level. This indicates that these tests are very good at determining when someone should not be, or should no longer be, diagnosed with the injury

Judged in this light, CNTs appear to do a better job identifying noninjury (or a point of cognitive recovery) than they do for predicting injury itself. From a clinical management point of view, this may be more salient since the goal is to minimize risk of return to play (I do not dismiss the possibility that the residual physiologic abnormalities noted in several studies may be indications of incomplete recovery; however, this has not yet been established).

Based on a theory of secondary prevention, the reduction of risk of second injury is important. Thus, another predictive validity perspective may be the number of repeat injuries athletes receive. Using tests to determine when the condition is no longer present is actually how most CNTs are used in practice (as opposed to diagnosing the injury).

While sensitivity to injury is quite weak, specificity and negative predictive power have rarely been considered important validation indices. While sensitivity is the rate at which an instrument correctly classifies a disorder or condition, specificity is the degree to which the test accurately identifies those without the disorder, disease, injury. From the secondary prevention perspective, specificity is more useful than sensitivity, since secondary prevention assumes the injury has already occurred. Concussion management is a postinjury endeavor. Specificity (and negative predictive power) are typically higher in studies than are sensitivity and positive predictive power. As Table 9.1 demonstrates, ImPACT has shown specificity rates between 89% and 97%, while ANAM has shown specificity over 85%.

Van Kampen and colleagues (2006) demonstrated that neuropsychological testing provides improvement in diagnostic accuracy, particularly in ruling out concussion if test results are normal or typical relative to an appropriate individual or group norm (baseline).

Inspection of Nelson and colleagues' (2016) data shows that, across the three batteries, the negative predictive power (the ability to identify no concussion) was better than sensitivity at 8 and 45 days, and > 70% for most comparisons, indicating that high scores on neuropsychological tests likely reflects resolution of cognitive problems associated with acute concussion.

SUMMARY

Establishing the validity of a test or test battery is a process that includes attention to both internal aspects of the test (how it is validated and the conditions or purposes under which it is used, including the concordance with the desired construct), as well as external features (the utility or usefulness). Thus, both the test's development and its use impact the validity of the results it provides. Not all uses of neuropsychological tests have been shown to be consistently valid in the field of SRCs. Independent studies continue to be needed, as developer-initiated studies—while important—necessarily contain bias.

The promise of easy data through large-scale use of computerized testing has provided a large amount of data whose validity in individual studies must be questioned. Most commercially available computerized test batteries have demonstrated some evidence of concurrent validity with traditional paper-and-pencil tests. But the ease of data acquisition from computerized tests belies the threats to internal validity. Easy data is often not good data, and clinicians and researchers must attend to the threats to validity in both development and administration.

Direct and indirect studies of the validity of both paper-and-pencil and computerized neuropsychological tests demonstrate that appropriate administration is important for obtaining external validity. While most studies of diagnostic utility indicate weak validity of neuropsychological tests to diagnose, there is a long history of neuropsychological test usage to track recovery from brain injury; neuropsychological tests are currently accepted as reflecting functional cognitive recovery. Group studies of sports concussion show that the combination of test scores and symptoms appears to identify neuropsychological changes at least up to 7 to 14 days, although roughly 10% of individuals continue to demonstrate score and symptom differences beyond that point. As symptoms resolve, some studies demonstrate continued cognitive declines, while two meta-analyses indicated no effect of neuropsychological test scores after 7 to 14 days. Of note is the consistent finding of better specificity than sensitivity of neuropsychological tests. This means that identifying the disorder is less certain than identifying when the disorder is not present, thus supporting their use in determining recovery.

Lesion identification is only partially validated, in part due to the lack of lesion identification associated with SRC. Identifying an end stage also appears quite valid, at least as best we understand recovery at this point in time. The lack of a biomarker criterion of the injury is an ongoing problem for validating any instrument or tool. Specificity and negative predictive power have not typically been considered relevant metrics; however, given the use of tests for determining when the injury is no longer present, clinicians would be advised to consider these test psychometrics more carefully.

In the world of SRC, the most consistently identified constructs of interest are memory (primarily working memory) and speed (including efficient, rapid output). Accurate assessment of these constructs provides the best utility. The eventual identification of a single biomarker or set of biomarkers will provide a gold standard criterion against which to measure tests. Tracking repeat concussions appears to be a useful metric for establishing predictive validity of outcomes. From a clinical perspective, the accurate interpretation of neuropsychological test results is understudied, as the multiple factors impinging on test performance and outcome requires advanced clinical knowledge and skill for individual results to be valid. Tests are but tools and misuse and misinterpretation limit a test's validity and individual clinical usefulness.

REFERENCES

Allen, B. J., & Gfeller, J. D. (2011). The Immediate Post-Concussion Assessment and Cognitive Testing battery and traditional neuropsychological measures: A construct and concurrent validity study. *Brain Injury*, 25, 179–191. http://dx.doi.org/10.3109/02699052.2010.541897

American Educational Research Association (AERA), American Psychological Association, National Council on Measurement in Education, & Joint Committee on Standards for Educational and Psychological Testing. (1999). *Standards for educational and psychological testing.* Washington, DC: American Educational Research Association.

American Educational Research Association (AERA), American Psychological Association, National Council on Measurement in Education, & Joint Committee on Standards for Educational and Psychological Testing. (2014). *Standards for educational and psychological testing.* Washington, DC: American Educational Research Association.

Bailey, C. M., Samples, H. L., Broshek, D. K., Freeman, J. R., & Barth, J. T. (2010). The relationship between psychological distress and baseline sports-related concussion testing. *Clinical Journal of Sport Medicine*, 20, 272–277. http://dx.doi.org/10.1097/JSM.0b013e3181e8f8d8

Barker-Collo, S., Jones, K., Theadom, A., Starkey, N., Dowell, A., McPherson, K., . . . Feigin, V. (2015). Neuropsychological outcome and its correlates in the first year after adult mild traumatic brain injury: A population-based New Zealand study. *Brain Injury, 29*(13–14), 1604–1616. http://dx.doi.org/10.3109/02699052.2015.1075143

Barth, J. T., Alves, W. M., Ryan, T. V., Macciocci, S. N., Rimel, R. W., Jane, J. A., & Nelson, W. E. (1989). Mild head injury in sports: Neuropsychological sequelae and recovery of function. In H. S. Levin, H. M. Eisenberg, & A. L. Benton (Eds.), *Mild head injury* (pp. 257–275). New York, NY: Oxford University Press.

Barth, J. T., Freeman, J. R., & Winters, J. E. (2000). Management of sports-related concussions. *Dental Clinics of North America, 44*, 67–83. Retrieved from https://www.ncbi.nlm.nih.gov/pubmed/10635469

Barth, J. T., Macciocchi, S. N., Giordani, B., Rimel, R., Jane, J. A., & Boll, T. J. (1983). Neuropsychological sequelae of minor head injury. *Neurosurgery, 13*, 529–533. http://dx.doi.org/10.1227/00006123-198311000-00008

Bauer, R. M., Iverson, G. L., Cernich, A. N., Binder, L. M., Ruff, R. M., & Naugle, R. I. (2012). Computerized neuropsychological assessment devices: Joint position paper of the American Academy of Clinical Neuropsychology and the National Academy of Neuropsychology. *Archives of Clinical Neuropsychology, 27*, 362–373. http://dx.doi.org/10.1093/arclin/acs027

Beebe, D. W. (2012). A brief primer on sleep for pediatric and child clinical neuropsychologists. *Child Neuropsychology, 18*, 313–338. http://dx.doi.org/10.1080/09297049.2011.602014

Belanger, H. G., & Vanderploeg, R. D. (2005). The neuropsychological impact of sports-related concussion: A meta-analysis. *Journal of the International Neuropsychological Society, 11*, 345–357. http://dx.doi.org/10.1017/S1355617705050411

Bleiberg, J., Cernich, A. N., Cameron, K., Sun, W., Peck, K., Ecklund, P. J., . . . Warden, D. L. (2004). Duration of cognitive impairment after sports concussion. *Neurosurgery, 54*, 1073–1080. http://dx.doi.org/10.1227/01.NEU.0000118820.33396.6A

Bleiberg, J., Garmoe, W. S., Halpern, E. L., Reeves, D. L., & Nadler, J. D. (1997). Consistency of within-day and across-day performance after mild brain injury. *Neuropsychiatry, Neuropsychology, and Behavioral Neurology, 10*, 247–253.

Bleiberg, J., Kane, R. L., Reeves, D. L., Garmoe, W. S., & Halpern, E. (2000). Factor analysis of computerized and traditional tests used in mild brain injury research. *The Clinical Neuropsychologist, 14*, 287–294. http://dx.doi.org/10.1076/1385-4046(200008)14:3;1-P;FT287

Broglio, S. P., Macciocchi, S. N., & Ferrara, M. S. (2007). Neurocognitive performance of concussed athletes when symptom free. *Journal of Athletic Training, 42*, 504–508. Retrieved from https://www.ncbi.nlm.nih.gov/pmc/articles/PMC2140076/

Broglio, S. P., Pontifex, M. B., O'Connor, P., & Hillman, C. H. (2009). The persistent effects of concussion on neuroelectric indices of attention. *Journal of Neurotrauma, 26*, 1463–1470. http://dx.doi.org/10.1089/neu.2008.0766

Broglio, S. P., & Puetz, T. W. (2008). The effect of sport concussion on neurocognitive function, self-report symptoms and postural control: A meta-analysis. *Sports Medicine, 38*, 53–67. http://dx.doi.org/10.2165/00007256-200838010-00005

Brown, C. N., Guskiewicz, K. M., & Bleiberg, J. (2007). Athlete characteristics and outcome scores for computerized neuropsychological assessment: A preliminary analysis. *Journal of Athletic Training, 42*, 515–523. Retrieved from https://www.ncbi.nlm.nih.gov/pmc/articles/PMC2140078/

Burke, D., Linder, S., Hirsch, J., Dey, T., Kana, D., Ringenbach, S., . . . Alberts, J. (2017). Characterizing information processing with a mobile device: Measurement of simple and choice reaction time. *Assessment, 24*, 885–895. http://dx.doi.org/10.1177/1073191116633752

Campbell, D. T., & Fiske, D. W. (1959). Convergent and discriminant validation by the multitrait–multimethod matrix. *Psychological Bulletin, 56*, 81–105. http://dx.doi.org/10.1037/h0046016

Cernich, A., Reeves, D., Sun, W., & Bleiberg, J. (2007). Automated Neuropsychological Assessment Metrics sports medicine battery. *Archives of Clinical Neuropsychology, 22*, S101–S114. http://dx.doi.org/10.1016/j.acn.2006.10.008

Chen, H., Richard, M., Sandler, D. P., Umbach, D. M., & Kamel, F. (2007). Head injury and amyotrophic lateral sclerosis. *American Journal of Epidemiology, 166*, 810–816. http://dx.doi.org/10.1093/aje/kwm153

Cole, D., Howard, G. S., & Maxwell, S. E. (1981). Effects of mono- versus multiple-operationalization in construct validation efforts. *Journal of Consulting and Clinical Psychology, 49*, 395–405. http://dx.doi.org/10.1037/0022-006X.49.3.395

Collie, A., Darby, D., & Maruff, P. (2001). Computerised cognitive assessment of athletes with sports related head injury. *British Journal of Sports Medicine, 35*, 297–302. http://dx.doi.org/10.1136/bjsm.35.5.297

Collie, A., Maruff, P., Makdissi, M., McCrory, P., McStephen, M., & Darby, D. (2003). CogSport: Reliability and correlation with conventional cognitive tests used in postconcussion medical evaluations. *Clinical Journal of Sport Medicine, 13*, 28–32. http://dx.doi.org/10.1097/00042752-200301000-00006

Collins, M. W., Grindel, S. H., Lovell, M. R., Dede, D. E., Moser, D. J., Phalin, B. R., . . . McKeag, D. B. (1999). Relationship between concussion and neuropsychological performance in college football players. *JAMA, 282*, 964–970. http://dx.doi.org/10.1001/jama.282.10.964

Collins, M. W., Iverson, G. L., Lovell, M. R., McKeag, D. B., Norwig, J., & Maroon, J. (2003). On-field predictors of neuropsychological and symptom deficit following sports-related concussion. *Clinical Journal of Sport Medicine, 13*, 222–229. http://dx.doi.org/10.1097/00042752-200307000-00005

Comper, P., Hutchison, M., Magrys, S., Mainwaring, L., & Richards, D. (2010). Evaluating the methodological quality of sports neuropsychology concussion research: A systematic review. *Brain Injury, 24*, 1257–1271. http://dx.doi.org/10.3109/02699052.2010.506854

Covassin, T., Elbin, R. J., III, Larson, E., & Kontos, A. P. (2012). Sex and age differences in depression and baseline sport-related concussion neurocognitive performance and symptoms. *Clinical Journal of Sport Medicine, 22*, 98–104. http://dx.doi.org/10.1097/JSM.0b013e31823403d2

Cronbach, L. J., & Meehl, P. E. (1955). Construct validity in psychological tests. *Psychological Bulletin, 52*, 281–302. http://dx.doi.org/10.1037/h0040957

Dettwiler, A., Murugavel, M., Putukian, M., Echemendia, R., Cubon, V., Furtado, J., & Osherson, D. (2013). Persistent differences in patterns of brain activation after sports-related concussion: A longitudinal fMRI study. *British Journal of Sports Medicine, 47*, e1.21. http://dx.doi.org/10.1136/bjsports-2012-092101.28

Duhaime, A.-C., Beckwith, J. G., Maerlender, A. C., McAllister, T. W., Crisco, J. J., Duma, S. M., . . . Greenwald, R. M. (2012). Spectrum of acute clinical characteristics of diagnosed concussions in college athletes wearing instrumented helmets. *Journal of Neurosurgery, 117*, 1092–1099. http://dx.doi.org/10.3171/2012.8.JNS112298

Eckner, J. T., Kutcher, J. S., Broglio, S. P., & Richardson, J. K. (2014). Effect of sport-related concussion on clinically measured simple reaction time. *British Journal of Sports Medicine, 48*, 112–118. http://dx.doi.org/10.1136/bjsports-2012-091579

Eckner, J. T., Kutcher, J. S., & Richardson, J. K. (2010). Pilot evaluation of a novel clinical test of reaction time in National Collegiate Athletic Association Division I football players. *Journal of Athletic Training, 45*, 327–332. http://dx.doi.org/10.4085/1062-6050-45.4.327

Erdal, K. (2012). Neuropsychological testing for sports-related concussion: How athletes can sandbag their baseline testing without detection. *Archives of Clinical Neuropsychology, 27*, 473–479. http://dx.doi.org/10.1093/arclin/acs050

Erlanger, D., Feldman, D., Kutner, K., Kaushik, T., Kroger, H., Festa, J., . . . Broshek, D. (2003). Development and validation of a web-based neuropsychological test protocol for sports-related return-to-play decision-making. *Archives of Clinical Neuropsychology, 18*, 293–316. http://dx.doi.org/10.1093/arclin/18.3.293

Fazio, V. C., Lovell, M. R., Pardini, J. E., & Collins, M. W. (2007). The relation between post concussion symptoms and neurocognitive performance in concussed athletes. *NeuroRehabilitation, 22*, 207–216. Retrieved from https://content.iospress.com/articles/neurorehabilitation/nre00369

Galetta, K., Liu, M., Leong, D. F., Ventura, R. E., Galetta, S. L., & Balcer, L. J. (2016). The King–Devick test of rapid number naming for concussion detection: Meta-analysis and systematic review of the literature. *Concussion, 1*, 1–15. http://dx.doi.org/10.2217/cnc.15.8

Gaudet, C. E., & Weyandt, L. L. (2017). Immediate Post-Concussion and Cognitive Testing (ImPACT): A systematic review of the prevalence and assessment of invalid performance. *Clinical Neuropsychologist, 31*, 43–58. http://dx.doi.org/10.1080/13854046.2016.1220622

Gioia, G., Isquith, P., & Vaughan, C. (2013). Classification analyses of pediatric concussion assessment battery. *British Journal of Sports Medicine, 47*, e1. Retrieved from http://bjsm.bmj.com/content/47/5/e1.39

Gosselin, N., Chen, J. K., Bottari, C., Petrides, M., Jubault, T., Tinawi, S., . . . Ptito, A. (2012). The influence of pain on cerebral functioning after mild traumatic brain injury. *Journal of Neurotrauma, 29*, 2625–2634. http://dx.doi.org/10.1089/neu.2012.2312

Green, P. (2007). The pervasive influence of effort on neuropsychological tests. *Physical Medicine and Rehabilitation Clinics of North America, 18*, 43–68. http://dx.doi.org/10.1016/j.pmr.2006.11.002

Grindel, S. H., Lovell, M. R., & Collins, M. W. (2001). The assessment of sport-related concussion: The evidence behind neuropsychological testing and management. *Clinical Journal of Sport Medicine, 11*, 134–143. http://dx.doi.org/10.1097/00042752-200107000-00003

Gronwall, D., & Wrightson, P. (1981). Memory and information processing capacity after closed head injury. *Journal of Neurology, Neurosurgery & Psychiatry, 44*, 889–895. http://dx.doi.org/10.1136/jnnp.44.10.889

Gualtieri, C. T., & Johnson, L. G. (2006). Reliability and validity of a computerized neurocognitive test battery, CNS Vital Signs. *Archives of Clinical Neuropsychology, 21*, 623–643. http://dx.doi.org/10.1016/j.acn.2006.05.007

Gualtieri, C. T., & Johnson, L. G. (2008). A computerized test battery sensitive to mild and severe brain injury. *Medscape Journal of Medicine, 10*, 90. Retrieved from https://www.ncbi.nlm.nih.gov/pmc/articles/PMC2390690/

Guskiewicz, K. M. (2001). Postural stability assessment following concussion: One piece of the puzzle. *Clinical Journal of Sport Medicine, 11*, 182–189. http://dx.doi.org/10.1097/00042752-200107000-00009

Halstead, M. E., Walter, K. D., & The Council on Sports Medicine and Fitness. (2010). Sport-related concussion in children and adolescents. *Pediatrics, 126*, 597–615. http://dx.doi.org/10.1542/peds.2010-2005

Harmon, K. G., Drezner, J. A., Gammons, M., Guskiewicz, K. M., Halstead, M., Herring, S. A., . . . Roberts, W. O. (2013). American Medical Society for Sports Medicine position statement: Concussion in sport. *British Journal of Sports Medicine, 47*, 15–26. http://dx.doi.org/10.1136/bjsports-2012-091941

Hume, P. A., Theadom, A., Lewis, G. N., Quarrie, K. L., Brown, S. R., Hill, R., & Marshall, S. W. A. (2017). A comparison of cognitive function in former rugby union players compared with former non-contact-sport players and the impact of concussion history. *Sports Medicine, 47*, 1209–1220. Retrieved from https://www.ncbi.nlm.nih.gov/pubmed/27558141

Institute of Medicine (IOM) and National Research Council (NRC). (2013). *Sports-related concussions in youth: Improving the science, changing the culture*. Washington, DC: The National Academies Press. Retrieved from https://www.nap.edu/resource/18377/concussions-RB.pdf

Iverson, G. (2007). Predicting slow recovery from sport-related concussion: The new simple-complex distinction. *Clinical Journal of Sport Medicine, 17*, 31–37.

Iverson, G. L., Brooks, B. L., Lovell, M. R., & Collins, M. W. (2006). No cumulative effects for one or two previous concussions. *British Journal of Sports Medicine, 40*(1), 72–75.

Iverson, G., Lovell, M., & Collins, M. (2005). Validity of ImPACT for measuring processing speed following sports-related concussion. *Clinical and Experimental Neuropsychology, 27*, 683–689. http://dx.doi.org/10.1081/13803390490918435

Johnson, D. R., Vincent, A. S., Johnson, A. E., Gilliland, K., & Schlegel, R. E. (2008). Reliability and construct validity of the Automated Neuropsychological Assessment Metrics (ANAM) mood scale. *Archives of Clinical Neuropsychology, 23*, 73–85. http://dx.doi.org/10.1016/j.acn.2007.10.001

Kelley, T. L. (1927). *Interpretation of educational measurements.* Yonkers-on-Hudson, NY: World Book.

Kontos, A. P., Braithwaite, R., Dakan, S., & Elbin, R. J. (2014). Computerized neuro-cognitive testing within 1 week of sport-related concussion: Meta-analytic review and analysis of moderating factors. *Journal of the International Neuropsychological Society, 20*, 324–332. http://dx.doi.org/10.1017/S1355617713001471

Lange, R. T., Iverson, G. L., Brooks, B. L., & Rennison, V. L. A. (2010). Influence of poor effort on self-reported symptoms and neurocognitive test performance following mild traumatic brain injury. *Journal of Clinical and Experimental Neuropsychology, 32*, 961–972. http://dx.doi.org/10.1080/13803391003645657

Lau, B. C., Kontos, A. P., Collins, M. W., Mucha, A., & Lovell, M. R. (2011). Which on-field signs/symptoms predict protracted recovery from sport-related concussion among high school football players? *American Journal of Sports Medicine, 39*, 2311–2318. http://dx.doi.org/10.1177/0363546511410655

Louey, A. G., Cromer, J. A., Schembri, A. J., Darby, D. G., Maruff, P., Makdissi, M., & Mccrory, P. (2014). Detecting cognitive impairment after concussion: Sensitivity of change from baseline and normative data methods using the CogSport/Axon Cognitive Test Battery. *Archives of Clinical Neuropsychology 29*, 432–441. http://dx.doi.org/10.1093/arclin/acu020

Lovell, M. R., Collins, M. W., Iverson, G. L., Field, M., Maroon, J. C., Cantu, R., . . . Fu, F. H. (2003). Recovery from mild concussion in high school athletes. *Journal of Neurosurgery, 98*, 296–301. http://dx.doi.org/10.3171/jns.2003.98.2.0296

Maddocks, D. L., Dicker, G. D., & Saling, M. M. (1995). The assessment of orientation following concussion in athletes. *Clinical Journal of Sport Medicine, 5*, 32–35. http://dx.doi.org/10.1097/00042752-199501000-00006

Maerlender, A., & Alt, A. (2012). The effect of sleep the night before on baseline neuropsychological screening and symptom reporting [Abstract]. *Journal of the International Neuropsychological Society, 18*, 165.

Maerlender, A., Flashman, L., Kessler, A., Kumbhani, S., Greenwald, R., Tosteson, T., & McAllister, T. (2010). Examination of the construct validity of ImPACT computerized test, traditional, and experimental neuropsychological measures.

The Clinical Neuropsychologist, 24, 1309–1325. http://dx.doi.org/10.1080/13854046.2010.516072

Maerlender, A., Flashman, L., Kessler, A., Kumbhani, S., Greenwald, R., Tosteson, T., & McAllister, T. (2013). Discriminant construct validity of ImPACT™: A companion study. *The Clinical Neuropsychologist, 27,* 290–299. http://dx.doi.org/10.1080/13854046.2012.744098

Makdissi, M., Collie, A., Maruff, P., Darby, D. G., Bush, A., McCrory, P., & Bennell, K. (2001). Computerised cognitive assessment of concussed Australian Rules footballers. *British Journal of Sports Medicine, 35,* 354–360. http://dx.doi.org/10.1136/bjsm.35.5.354

Makdissi, M., Darby, D., Maruff, P., Ugoni, A., Brukner, P., & McCrory, P. R. (2010). Natural history of concussion in sport: Markers of severity and implications for management. *The American Journal of Sports Medicine, 38,* 464–471. http://dx.doi.org/10.1177/0363546509349491

McAllister, T. W., Ford, J. C., Flashman, L. A., Maerlender, A., Greenwald, R. M., Beckwith, J. G., . . . Jain, S. (2014). Effect of head impacts on diffusivity measures in a cohort of collegiate contact sport athletes. *Neurology, 82,* 63–69. http://dx.doi.org/10.1212/01.wnl.0000438220.16190.42

McClure, D. J., Zuckerman, S. L., Kutscher, S. J., Gregory, A. J., & Solomon, G. S. (2014). Baseline neurocognitive testing in sports-related concussions: The importance of a prior night's sleep. *The American Journal of Sports Medicine, 42,* 472–478. http://dx.doi.org/10.1177/0363546513510389

McCrea, M., Guskiewicz, K., Randolph, C., Barr, W. B., Hammeke, T. A., Marshall, S. W., . . . Kelly, J. P. (2013). Incidence, clinical course, and predictors of prolonged recovery time following sport-related concussion in high school and college athletes. *Journal of the International Neuropsychological Society, 19,* 22–33. http://dx.doi.org/10.1017/S1355617712000872

McCrory, P., Makdissi, M., Davis, G., & Collie, A. (2005). Value of neuropsychological testing after head injuries in football. *British Journal of Sports Medicine, 39,* i58–i63. http://dx.doi.org/10.1136/bjsm.2005.020776

McCrory, P., Meeuwisse, W., Dvorák, J., Aubry, M., Bailes, J., Broglio, S., . . . Vos, P. E. (2017). Consensus statement on concussion in sport–The 5th international conference on concussion in sport held in Berlin, October 2016. *British Journal of Sports Medicine, 51,* 838–847. http://dx.doi.org/10.1136/bjsports-2017-097699

McDonald, B. C., Saykin, A. J., & McAllister, T. W. (2012). Functional MRI of mild traumatic brain injury (mTBI): Progress and perspectives from the first decade of studies. *Brain Imaging and Behavior, 6,* 193–207. http://dx.doi.org/10.1007/s11682-012-9173-4

Meyer, J. E., & Arnett, P. A. (2015). Validation of the Affective Word List as a measure of verbal learning and memory. *Journal of Clinical and Experimental Neuropsychology, 37,* 316–324. http://dx.doi.org/10.1080/13803395.2015.1012486

Mihalik, J. P., Lengas, E., Register-Mihalik, J. K., Oyama, S., Begalle, R. L., & Guskiewicz, K. M. (2013). The effects of sleep quality and sleep quantity on concussion baseline assessment. *Clinical Journal of Sport Medicine, 23,* 343–348. http://dx.doi.org/10.1097/JSM.0b013e318295a834

Moriarity, J. M., Pietrzak, R. H., Kutcher, J. S., Clausen, M. H., McAward, K., & Darby, D. G. (2012). Unrecognised ringside concussive injury in amateur boxers. *British Journal of Sports Medicine, 46,* 1011–1015. http://dx.doi.org/10.1136/bjsports-2011-090893

Moser, R. S., Schatz, P., Neidzwski, K., & Ott, S. D. (2011). Group versus individual administration affects baseline neurocognitive test performance. *The American Journal of Sports Medicine, 39,* 2325–2330. http://dx.doi.org/10.1177/0363546511417114

Nelson, L. D., LaRoche, A. A., Pfaller, A. Y., Lerner, E. B., Hammeke, T. A., Randolph, C., . . . McCrea, M. A. (2016). Prospective, head-to-head study of three computerized neurocognitive assessment tools (CNTs): Reliability and validity for the assessment of sport-related concussion. *Journal of the International Neuropsychological Society, 22,* 24–37. http://dx.doi.org/10.1017/S1355617715001101

Newman, J. B., Reesman, J. H., Vaughan, C. G., & Gioia, G. A. (2013). Assessment of processing speed in children with mild TBI: A "first look" at the validity of pediatric ImPACT. *The Clinical Neuropsychologist, 27,* 779–793. http://dx.doi.org/10.1080/13854046.2013.789552

Pardini, J. E., Pardini, D. A., Becker, J. T., Dunfee, K. L., Eddy, W. F., Lovell, M. R., & Welling, J. S. (2010). Postconcussive symptoms are associated with compensatory cortical recruitment during a working memory task. *Neurosurgery, 67,* 1020–1028. http://dx.doi.org/10.1227/NEU.0b013e3181ee33e2

Pellman, E. J., Lovell, M. R., Viano, D. C., Casson, I. R., & Tucker, A. M. (2004). Concussion in professional football: Neuropsychological testing—Part 6. *Neurosurgery, 55,* 1290–1305. http://dx.doi.org/10.1227/01.NEU.0000149244.97560.91

Prichep, L. S., McCrea, M., Barr, W., Powell, M., & Chabot, R. J. (2013). Time course of clinical and electrophysiological recovery after sport-related concussion. *The Journal of Head Trauma Rehabilitation, 28,* 266–273. http://dx.doi.org/10.1097/HTR.0b013e318247b54e

Rabinowitz, A. R., & Arnett, P. A. (2013). Intraindividual cognitive variability before and after sports-related concussion. *Neuropsychology, 27,* 481–490. http://dx.doi.org/10.1037/a0033023

Rahman-Filipiak, A. A., & Woodard, J. L. (2013). Administration and environment considerations in computer-based sports-concussion assessment. *Neuropsychology Review, 23,* 314–334. http://dx.doi.org/10.1007/s11065-013-9241-6

Resch, J. E., McCrea, M. A., & Cullum, C. M. (2013). Computerized neurocognitive testing in the management of sport-related concussion: An update. *Neuropsychology Review, 23,* 335–349. http://dx.doi.org/10.1007/s11065-013-9242-5

Rimel, R. W., Giordani, B., Barth, J. T., & Jane, J. A. (1982). Moderate head injury: Completing the clinical spectrum of brain trauma. *Neurosurgery, 11,* 344–351. http://dx.doi.org/10.1227/00006123-198209000-00002

Schatz, P., & Glatts, C. (2013). "Sandbagging" baseline test performance on ImPACT, without detection, is more difficult than it appears. *Archives of Clinical Neuropsychology, 28,* 236–244. http://dx.doi.org/10.1093/arclin/act009

Schatz, P., & Maerlender, A. (2013). A two-factor theory for concussion assessment using ImPACT: Memory and speed. *Archives of Clinical Neuropsychology, 28,* 791–797. http://dx.doi.org/10.1093/arclin/act077

Schatz, P., Pardini, J. E., Lovell, M. R., Collins, M. W., & Podell, K. (2006). Sensitivity and specificity of the ImPACT Test Battery for concussion in athletes. *Archives of Clinical Neuropsychology, 21,* 91–99. http://dx.doi.org/10.1016/j.acn.2005.08.001

Schatz, P., & Putz, B. O. (2006). Cross-validation of measures used for computer-based assessment of concussion. *Applied Neuropsychology, 13,* 151–159. http://dx.doi.org/10.1207/s15324826an1303_2

Schatz, P., & Sandel, N. (2013). Sensitivity and specificity of the online version of ImPACT in high school and collegiate athletes. *The American Journal of Sports Medicine, 41,* 321–326. http://dx.doi.org/10.1177/0363546512466038

Schatz, P., Ybarra, V., & Leitner, D. (2015). Validating the accuracy of reaction time assessment on computer-based tablet devices. *Assessment, 22,* 405–410. http://dx.doi.org/10.1177/1073191114566622

Silverberg, N. D., Berkner, P. D., Atkins, J. E., Zafonte, R., & Iverson, G. L. (2016). Relationship between short sleep duration and preseason concussion testing. *Clinical Journal of Sport Medicine, 26,* 226–231. http://dx.doi.org/10.1097/JSM.0000000000000241

Tsushima, W. T., Shirakawa, N., & Geling, O. (2013). Neurocognitive functioning and symptom reporting of high school athletes following a single concussion. *Applied Neuropsychology: Child, 2,* 13–16. http://dx.doi.org/10.1080/09084282.2011.643967

Van Kampen, D. A., Lovell, M. R., Pardini, J. E., Collins, M. W., & Fu, F. H. (2006). The "value added" of neurocognitive testing after sports-related concussion. *The American Journal of Sports Medicine, 34,* 1630–1635. http://dx.doi.org/10.1177/0363546506288677

Woodard, J. L., Marker, C. D., Tabanico, F. E., Miller, S. K., Dorsett, E. S. W., Cox, L. R., . . . Bleiberg, J. (2002). A validation study of the automated neuropsychological assessment metrics (ANAM) in non-concussed high school football players. *Journal of the International Neuropsychological Society, 8,* 175.

Zhu, D. C., Covassin, T., Nogle, S., Doyle, S., Russell, D., Pearson, R. L., . . . Kaufman, D. I. (2015). A potential biomarker in sports-related concussion: Brain functional connectivity alteration of the default-mode network measured with longitudinal resting-state fMRI over thirty days. *Journal of Neurotrauma, 32,* 327–341. http://dx.doi.org/10.1089/neu.2014.3413

10

DO TRADITIONAL NEUROPSYCHOLOGICAL MEASURES ADD VALUE TO COMPUTERIZED TESTS FOR CONCUSSION ASSESSMENT IN COLLEGIATE ATHLETES?

JESSICA MEYER AND PETER A. ARNETT

Neuropsychological assessment has long been considered a cornerstone of concussion evaluations (McCrory et al., 2017). The development of the Sports Laboratory Assessment Model, in which athletes are tested at baseline and then again after a concussion, has allowed for an individualistic approach to concussion assessment in which athletes' postconcussion scores are compared with their own scores at baseline (Barth et al., 1989). Because of the idiosyncratic nature of the typical injury and its recovery trajectory, there is no standard expected profile of postconcussion cognitive functioning (Iverson, Brooks, Collins, & Lovell, 2006; McCrea et al., 2003). Neuropsychological assessments therefore are not used to assess for domain-specific expected declines but to address whether an athlete shows a decline in functioning in any cognitive domain.

The development of computerized neuropsychological assessments has led to a shift in how cognitive symptoms of sport-related concussions

http://dx.doi.org/10.1037/0000114-011
Neuropsychology of Sports-Related Concussion, P. A. Arnett (Editor)

are assessed. The widespread availability of computerized assessments in particular, compared with the availability of clinical neuropsychologists, has led many youth, high school, college, and professional organizations to rely on computerized testing rather than traditional paper-and-pencil testing (Covassin, Elbin, Stiller-Ostrowski, & Kontos, 2009; Meehan, d'Hemecourt, Collins, Taylor, & Comstock, 2012). The ImPACT (Immediate Post-Concussion Assessment and Cognitive Testing; Lovell, 2007), developed in the late 1990s, is the most widely used computerized assessment in concussion management (Meehan et al., 2012). It consists of background demographic information, self-reported symptoms, and a battery of computerized neurocognitive tests. The results of the neurocognitive tests are summarized in five composite scores: (a) Verbal Memory, (b) Visual Memory, (c) Visual Motor Speed, (d) Reaction Time, and (e) Impulse Control (Lovell, 2007). In this chapter, we will discuss the merits of computerized versus traditional neuropsychological tests in concussion assessment. Because of its widespread use, we will focus on the ImPACT and present some data from our laboratory that compare its sensitivity with that of traditional neuropsychological tests. We also present a case study that illustrates some issues raised by our data, provide three take-home points for clinicians and, finally, identify three key questions in this area of study that we feel are most pressing to be answered in the next 5 years.

STRENGTHS AND LIMITATIONS OF THE IMPACT

The popularity of computerized assessments such as the ImPACT stems from their accessibility and ease of administration and scoring. Computerized assessments can be administered in a group format and are scored automatically, thereby minimizing time and personnel requirements (Collie, Darby, & Maruff, 2001; Schatz & Zillmer, 2003). Computerized assessment additionally allows for more reliable standard administration of the tests. Stimulus presentation is automated, thereby limiting the effects of potential human variability or error (Collie, Maruff, McStephen, & Darby, 2003). In addition, response latencies can be assessed to the millisecond, allowing for detection of more subtle changes in reaction time (B. J. Allen & Gfeller, 2011; Lovell & Collins, 2002). When one follows the Sports Laboratory Assessment Model of concussion management, repeat test administrations are inevitable. The availability of equivalent alternate forms for consecutive testing sessions is imperative for the minimization of practice effects. Although the ImPACT's five alternate forms can be considered a strength of this method of assessment (Lovell, 2007), some research has indicated a lack of equivalence of these five composites (Resch, Macciocchi, & Ferrara, 2013). Nonequivalence of alternate forms decreases reliability and may negatively affect clinical decision making.

Although the ImPACT offers many advantages, questions have been raised surrounding compliance with test administration and interpretation guidelines (Covassin et al., 2009; Meehan et al., 2012; Resch, McCrea, & Cullum, 2013). In addition, although group administration minimizes time and personnel requirements, research has shown that athletes who complete their baseline assessments in a group format score lower across all cognitive indices on average and are more likely to produce invalid baselines (Moser, Schatz, Neidzwski, & Ott, 2011). Further discussion of these limitations is beyond the scope of this chapter; however, a more relevant question regarding the ImPACT is how sensitive it is to postconcussion cognitive changes when it is appropriately administered.

Construct Validity of the ImPACT

Several studies have evaluated the construct validity of the ImPACT by using traditional neuropsychological measures to establish convergent validity. The Visual Motor Speed composite and Reaction Time composite have been found to have moderate to high correlations with measures of processing speed (Symbol Digit Modalities Test [SDMT], Smith, 1982; Digit Symbol subtest of the Wechsler Adult Intelligence Scale, Wechsler, 1997), and executive functioning (Trails B, Iverson, Lovell, & Collins, 2005; Schatz & Putz, 2006; Strauss, Sherman, & Spreen, 2006). The ImPACT Visual Memory composite has been found to have moderate correlations with a visual memory composite score created from Trial 1, total learning Trials 1–3, and delayed recall on the Brief Visuospatial Memory Test—Revised (BVMT–R; $r = .59$; Maerlender et al., 2010) and with the BVMT–R Total Score ($r = .38$) and Delayed Recall ($r = .35$; B. J. Allen & Gfeller, 2011).

The Verbal Memory composite has been found to have low to moderate correlations with the California Verbal Learning Test—Second Edition (CVLT–II; Delis, Kramer, Kaplan, & Ober, 2000) and the Hopkins Verbal Learning Test—Revised (HVLT–R; B. J. Allen & Gfeller, 2011; Maerlender et al., 2010). Interestingly, the Verbal Memory composite has also been found to have moderate correlations with the BVMT–R (B. J. Allen & Gfeller, 2011; Maerlender et al., 2010). Factor analyses have revealed no differentiation between verbal and visual memory on the ImPACT, and researchers have suggested that this may be due to the visual presentation of the verbal stimuli (B. J. Allen & Gfeller, 2011).

Although the ImPACT has moderate convergent validity with traditional neuropsychological measures in the domains that it assesses, there are several domains of cognitive functioning that it does not capture. Auditory working memory and sustained attention, both of which are often compromised as the result of concussions, are not assessed by the ImPACT (Maerlender et al., 2010). Moreover, the memory tests on the ImPACT are in a recognition-only format, so there is no way to evaluate free recall, an objectively more difficult task that is likely to be more sensitive to changes in memory (De Marco & Broshek, 2016). The lack of free recall, in particular on the verbal memory tests, may account for its lower convergent validity with traditional verbal memory tests.

Test–Retest Reliability of the ImPACT

When assessing for clinically significant change, it is necessary to account for the test–retest reliability of the measure. In comparing athletes' post-concussion performance with their performance at baseline, the observed change must exceed that which can be explained by normal variability in performance at 2 time points. Studies evaluating the test–retest reliability of the ImPACT have yielded inconsistent results (Broglio, Macciocchi, & Ferrara, 2007; Iverson, Lovell, & Collins, 2003). Recently, when the test–retest reliability of the ImPACT was evaluated at several retest intervals (7 days, 14 days, 30 days, 44 days, and 198 days), the test–retest reliability values remained largely consistent across time intervals. Although consistent, only the Visual Motor Speed composite reached what is typically considered to be an adequate level of test–retest reliability for use in detecting clinically significant change ($r > .70$; Nelson et al., 2016). The low test–retest reliability of many indices of the ImPACT significantly limits the measure's ability to detect clinically significant change across 2 time points. Although other studies have yielded higher test–retest reliabilities for the ImPACT (Nakayama, Covassin, Schatz, Nogle, & Kovan, 2014), this has not been a consistent finding in the literature (Resch, Driscoll, et al., 2013).

SENSITIVITY OF THE IMPACT TO POSTCONCUSSION COGNITIVE CHANGES

The ImPACT's sensitivity to concussion has been reported to be between around 80% and 95% (79.2%, Broglio et al., 2007; 91.4%, Schatz & Sandel, 2013). These sensitivity reports, however, are based on all indices of the ImPACT, including the Symptom scale. Several studies have found significant impairments, relative to baseline, on cognitive indices of the ImPACT after concussion (Covassin, Elbin, & Nakayama, 2010; Iverson et al., 2006; McClincy, Lovell, Pardini, Collins, & Spore, 2006). It is important to note, however, that most of these impairments are demonstrated in the acute stages of concussion in athletes who are symptomatic.

In studies that have evaluated the sensitivity of the ImPACT over the course of recovery, a consistent finding has been that when athletes are asymptomatic, they rarely show declines from baseline on the cognitive indices of the ImPACT (Mayers & Redick, 2012; Nelson et al., 2016). Although evaluating cognitive changes in symptomatic athletes is important for monitoring recovery trajectories and for establishing cognitive changes of acute concussion, athletes often do not undergo cognitive testing until they are asymptomatic, because they will not be returning to play regardless of cognitive status if they are symptomatic (Randolph, McCrea, & Barr, 2005). Furthermore, there is evidence that the cognitive exertion involved in testing athletes may exacerbate concussion symptoms in a subset of athletes (Meyer & Arnett, 2015a). For these reasons, an important aspect of clinical utility of computerized assessments is their ability to detect neuropsychological deficits in asymptomatic athletes who are being tested to determine readiness for return-to-play procedures (Resch, McCrea, & Cullum, 2013).

Although research suggests a high sensitivity of the ImPACT to acute post-concussion changes in cognition (Iverson et al., 2006), the idiosyncratic and variable response to concussion suggests that a 20-min test battery may not be sufficient to capture all clinically significant changes. The ImPACT is marketed as a screening measure and is intended to be used by a qualified clinician in conjunction with other concussion assessment tools. As noted above, however, the ImPACT may not adequately assess all cognitive domains potentially affected by concussion (De Marco & Broshek, 2016; Maerlender et al., 2010). Thus, although the ImPACT may effectively screen for visual memory, reaction time, and processing speed deficits, it will not be able to detect deficits in domains such as sustained attention, auditory working memory, or free recall. Furthermore, its ability to screen for verbal memory is complicated by the visual presentation of verbal stimuli.

To our knowledge, one published study to date has directly compared the sensitivity of computerized and paper-and-pencil neuropsychological tests to concussion (Broglio et al., 2007). This study showed that computerized assessments had a sensitivity of 79% compared with 43% for paper-and-pencil measures. However, the authors included symptom report in the ImPACT sensitivity, but not the paper-and-pencil measures; still, the sensitivity of the ImPACT was still relatively high (62.5%) even after the symptom index was removed. Several noteworthy methodological considerations should be discussed. First, this study evaluated athletes within 24 hours of concussion; as discussed above, this is not the typical use of cognitive testing in concussion management. The increased sensitivity of the computerized assessments may be inflated by symptomatic athletes' response to engaging with a computer screen. Second, the authors defined *clinically significant change* as 1 SD or more decline from baseline. Although this method is quick and easy to implement, it does not consider factors such as the variable test–retest reliability of the measures. Last, this was a cross-sectional study with different athletes being administered either the paper-and-pencil battery or the ImPACT depending on the year in which they were tested, thereby leaving open the possibility of cohort effects.

With these considerations in mind, the study that we present in this chapter was aimed to evaluate the sensitivity of traditional neuropsychological measures in comparison to the ImPACT to postconcussive cognitive changes in the same group of athletes. The athletes involved in the study were being tested to determine their readiness to return to play. In this way, it is different than many studies evaluating sensitivity to postconcussion cognitive changes, because it includes both symptomatic and asymptomatic athletes and evaluates clinical sensitivity in an ecologically valid sample. The data presented in this chapter are new and have not been formally peer reviewed.

METHOD

Informed consent was obtained for all participants, and the study was approved by the Behavioral Committee of the Pennsylvania State University's institutional review board.

Research Participants and Procedure

The athlete sample was composed of 53 college athletes who were involved in a concussion program at a large Division I university between 2000 and 2013. These athletes were assessed before starting their sports participation at the university to determine their baseline level of cognitive functioning and were assessed again within 1 week after sustaining a concussion. Team physicians and athletic trainers referred athletes for postconcussion testing on the basis of the following definition of *concussion*: any alteration in mental status and/or postconcussion signs or symptoms at the time of injury, posttraumatic amnesia lasting less than 24 hours, and/or loss of consciousness lasting 30 minutes or less (Ruff et al., 2009). The timing of referrals to the concussion program depended on athletic trainers and team physicians. Referrals were made with the intention of testing to determine whether athletes were ready to return to play; some physicians and trainers wait until an athlete is completely asymptomatic before making the referral, but others do not. The athlete group of the present study included only athletes who were not yet cleared to return to play on the basis of the neuropsychological test results, the athlete's self-report of symptoms, and the results of a clinical interview. Each of these factors was considered when making return-to-play recommendations, and athletes who were positive on at least one factor were recommended not to return to play yet.

The sample was drawn from a group of 170 athletes who had completed postconcussion assessments through our concussion program between 2000 and 2013. Athletes who were tested outside of the 7-day postconcussion time range ($n = 64$) and those who did not complete a baseline evaluation ($n = 27$) were excluded. The Computerized Assessment of Response Bias (CARB; L. M. Allen, Conder, Green, & Cox, 1997) was used to detect suboptimal effort, and athletes who performed below 90% on this measure at baseline or postconcussion were excluded ($n = 2$). For participants who did not complete the CARB, a cutoff of 30 on the ImPACT Impulse Control composite was used to assess for suboptimal effort, and an additional 2 participants were excluded using this criterion. Last, participants who were cleared to return to play ($n = 22$) after neuropsychological assessment were excluded. This resulted in a final sample of 53.

The comparison group comprised 42 healthy college students recruited from the Department of Psychology subject pool, who were given credit for their psychology courses for participating in this study. These participants were tested during two sessions approximately 6 weeks apart. The battery of tests was the same as that administered to athletes through the concussion program. Demographic data for the athlete and comparison groups are presented in Table 10.1.

At each assessment the athletes and comparison group completed questionnaires focused on previous head injuries and demographic information and completed a neuropsychological assessment that included both paper-and-pencil and computerized neuropsychological measures. Baseline and postconcussion testing, as well as the testing of the comparison group, was administered by either a doctoral-level clinical neuropsychologist or by graduate or undergraduate assistants who were trained by the doctoral-level clinical neuropsychologist. All evaluations were conducted in small rooms free of distractions; all athletes and control participants were tested individually. The battery of questionnaires and neuropsychological tests took approximately 2 hours to complete. The measures administered are described below.

The test battery was standard for all participants and was administered in the following order: Rivermead Behavioral Memory Story Test Immediate Recall (Wilson, Cockburn, & Baddeley, 1991), the BVMT–R Trials 1–3, HVLT–R Trials 1–3, CARB, SDMT, Comprehensive Trail-making Test (Reynolds, 2002), Rivermead Behavioral Memory Story Test Delayed Recall (Wilson et al., 1991), HVLT–R Delayed Recall, BVMT–R Delayed Recall, Affective Word List Trials 1–3 (Meyer & Arnett, 2015b), Vigil Continuous Performance Test (Cegalis & Cegalis, 1994), Stroop Color–Word Test

TABLE 10.1
Demographic Information for the Athletes and Comparison Group

Variable	Athletes (n = 53)		Comparison group (n = 42)	
	M	SD	M	SD
Age	20.35	1.45	18.55	0.77
Days between testing	537.73	435.60	43.38	6.23
	n	%	n	%
Sex				
Male	46	87	21	50
Female	7	13	21	50
Race				
Caucasian	30	57	40	96
African American	18	34	0	0
Hispanic American	0	0	1	2
Asian American	0	0	1	2
Multiracial	4	8	0	0
Other	1	2	0	0
Concussion history				
0	26	50	31	74
1	17	33	11	26
2+	9	17	0	0
Sport				
Football	25	47		
Lacrosse	12	11		
Basketball	9	17		
Soccer	3	6		
Ice hockey	4	8		

(Trenerry, Crosson, DeBoe, & Leber, 1989), Pennsylvania State University (PSU) Cancellation Test (Echemendia & Julian, 2001), Affective Word List Delayed Recall, Controlled Oral Word Association Test (Goodglass, Kaplan, & Baressi, 2001), Shipley–2 Vocabulary (Zachary, 1986), Wechsler Test of Adult Reading (The Psychological Corporation, 2001), and the ImPACT. The CARB is a measure of effort and was therefore not included in sensitivity to concussion analyses. The Shipley–2 and Wechsler Test of Adult Reading are used to estimate premorbid functioning and would not be expected to change between baseline and after a concussion; thus, these were not included in the analyses. Athletes received different forms of the Comprehensive Trail-making Test at baseline and after a concussion and because not all of the different forms are comparable this measure was not included in the analyses. At baseline, each athlete was randomly assigned to receive one of four alternate forms of the HVLT–R, BVMT–R, SDMT, and PSU Cancellation Test. The same forms were always given together (e.g., HVLT–R Form 1,

BVMT–R Form 1, SDMT Form 1, and PSU Cancellation Test Form 1). Athletes received alternate forms after a concussion in the following order: 1–3, 2–4, 3–1, 4–2. For example, if athletes received Form 1 at Time 1, they would receive Form 3 at Time 2, and so on. All athletes completed Form 1 of the ImPACT Word List at baseline and completed form 2 at their first postconcussion assessment.

Measures

As described above, each participant completed an extensive battery of cognitive and affective measurements. The full ImPACT, including demographics, symptom report, and cognitive testing, was completed; however, the current study focused only on the analysis of the cognitive indices of the ImPACT.

Indices from the ImPACT analyzed in this study included the Verbal Memory, Visual Memory, Visual Motor Speed, and Reaction Time composites. The majority of athletes received Version 2.0 (Lovell, 2000) of the ImPACT, with three participants tested early in the enrollment period given Version 1.0 (Lovell, Collins, Podell, Powell, & Maroon, 2000).

In the administration of the HVLT–R, examinees are read a list of 12 words over three trials and asked to recall as many words as they can remember (Brandt & Benedict, 2001), followed by a delayed recall trial 20 to 25 minutes later. The total immediate recall and the delayed recall indices measured verbal learning and memory.

The BVMT–R consists of three learning trials in which examinees are presented a display of six figures for 10 s and are then asked to draw the figures from memory. After a 25-min delay, the examinees are asked to draw the figures again (Benedict, 1997). The total immediate recall and delayed recall indices measure visuospatial learning and memory.

In the PSU Cancellation Test, a measure of visual attention, participants are asked to cross out as many target symbols as possible in 90 s, working left to right across the rows. It has four equivalent forms (Echemendia, Putukian, Mackin, Julian, & Shoss, 2001). Total correct symbols marked is the primary index for this measure and serve as a measure of processing speed.

The SDMT is designed to assess speeded information processing and visual tracking (Lezak, Howieson, & Loring, 2005). It requires the participant to pair a number with a symbol based on a key at the top of the page, which has nine unique symbols paired with each of the nine numerals. The total number of correct responses, in 90s, is used in this study as a measure of visual processing speed.

The Stroop Neuropsychological Screening Test consists of two tasks; in the Color Task the examinee reads aloud a list of color names, and in the

Color–Word Task the examinee names the ink color in which the names of colors are printed (Trenerry et al., 1989). Scores for these tasks are presented as time (in seconds) to complete each task.

The Post-Concussion Symptom Scale (PCSS) is a 22-item self-report measure of post-concussive symptoms. Participants rate the extent to which they are experiencing each symptom on a 7-point Likert scale (0 = *none*–6 = *severe*). It is modeled after the Post-Concussion Scale (PCS), which was designed to measure post-concussive symptom severity in athletes (Lovell et al., 2006). This scale has been found to be a reliable measure of post-concussive symptoms, and variations of this scale have been used frequently in concussion research (Chen, Johnston, Collie, McCrory, & Ptito, 2007; Kontos et al., 2012; Lovell et al., 2006).

Analyses

Reliable change indices (RCIs) were calculated to establish clinically significant change. RCIs were calculated in accordance with guidelines by Speer (1992), which are summarized in Rosenbaum, Arnett, Bailey, and Echemendia (2006). Each measure was evaluated for regression to the mean using the method recommended by Speer. Edwards–Nunnally true score adjustments were calculated for measures where regression to the mean was present; RCIs calculated with a true-score adjustment are indicated with an asterisk in Table 10.2. Practice effects were accounted for by subtracting the mean difference between time points on each measure in the normative sample. These mean difference scores can be seen in Table 10.2.

The control group was used to calculate the necessary standard deviations for the RCI calculations. When possible, test manuals and empirical research studies were used to establish the test–retest reliabilities used in the calculations. ImPACT composite test–retest reliability scores were taken from Schatz and Ferris (2013). Although other studies have provided test–retest reliability data for the ImPACT over longer time periods, we chose to use the 1-month interval because this most resembled the test–retest intervals used in studies of the other measures in the present study and maximized test–retest reliability. Using lower test–retest reliabilities for the ImPACT would complicate interpretation of low sensitivity results because they could then be attributable to the low reliability instead of with the format and content of the test itself. Thus, maximizing the test–retest reliability allows for a fairer assessment of clinical sensitivity in comparison to other neuropsychological tests. Furthermore, Schatz and Ferris's study included participants who were administered the ImPACT individually or in pairs under supervision, thereby minimizing the potential for group administration to affect the validity of the results. The test–retest reliability coefficients used for all other measures are covered earlier in the chapter, as well as in Table 10.2.

TABLE 10.2

TABLE 10.2
Mean Values and Variables Used for Reliable Change Index (RCI) Calculations

Variable	Test–retest reliability	SE	S_{diff}	Baseline		After concussion		90% RCI cutoff	Practice effects adjustment
				M	SD	M	SD		
ImPACT Verbal Memory*	.66[a]	6.89	9.75	83.35	11.76	81.28	11.38	15.99	0.10
ImPACT Visual Memory*	.43[a]	10.11	14.30	76.62	13.24	74.50	12.20	23.44	-3.07
ImPACT Reaction Time	.63[a]	.05	.07	0.61	0.07	0.62	0.11	0.12	0.002
ImPACT VMS*	.78[a]	3.83	5.41	35.03	8.09	36.42	6.88	8.87	-0.02
HVLT–R TR*	.74[b]	2.06	2.91	26.57	4.00	25.64	4.25	4.77	-1.41
HVLT–R DR*	.66[b]	1.16	1.64	9.45	1.98	8.43	2.21	2.69	-0.12
BVMT–R TR*	.80[c]	2.41	3.40	27.80	5.59	27.52	5.49	5.58	-0.50
BVMT–R DR*	.79[c]	0.84	1.19	10.46	1.76	10.33	2.01	1.95	-0.19
SDMT*	.70[d]	6.53	9.24	57.96	12.44	58.44	13.80	15.15	-5.98
SNST Word Reading	.84[e]	3.69	5.22	51.41	8.20	55.14	10.11	8.56	0.89
SNST Color–Word	.84[e]	9.56	13.52	118.18	23.87	110.93	19.44	22.17	3.14
PSU*	.65	7.31	10.34	47.90	12.94	47.49	11.59	16.96	-1.83

Note. Asterisks denote tests that were corrected for regression to the mean in the RCI calculations. ImPACT = Immediate Post-Concussion Assessment and Cognitive Testing; VMS = Visual Motor Speed; HVLT–R = Hopkins Verbal Learning Test—Revised; TR = Total Recall; DR = Delayed Recall; BVMT–R = Brief Visuospatial Memory Test—Revised; SDMT = Symbol Digit Modalities Test; SNST = Stroop Neuropsychological Screening Test; PSU = PSU Cancellation Test. [a]Schatz and Ferris (2013). [b]Benedict, Schretlen, Groninger, and Brandt (1998). [c]Benedict (1997). [d]Smith (1982). [e]Dikmen, Heaton, Grant, and Temkin (1999).

A 90% cutoff was used to establish clinical significance (RCI = ± 1.64). Test–retest reliability mean scores at baseline and after a concussion, cut-off scores for reliable change, and practice effect adjustments are shown in Table 10.2. The cutoff scores included in this table reflect the minimum decrease in performance on each test necessary to reflect clinically significant change in individual participants.

RCIs were calculated for each participant on each measure, and the proportion of athletes and control participants showing reliable decline (based on the 90% cutoff values provided in Table 2) on the nine paper-and-pencil indices and the four ImPACT indices were calculated. To establish the clinical utility of each measure, the net detection rate was calculated by subtracting the false positive rate (proportion of control participants showing reliable decline) from the true positive rate (proportion of athletes showing a reliable decline).

To correct for different lengths of batteries (nine paper-and-pencil indices vs. four ImPACT composites), an additional analysis was run that included only four paper-and-pencil indices. The HVLT–R TR, BVMT–R TR, SDMT, and SNST Word Reading subtest were included in a battery that was most analogous to the ImPACT composites. McNemar's test was run to evaluate the difference between the proportion of athletes who showed decline on at least one ImPACT index and the proportion of athletes who showed a decline on at least one of these four paper-and-pencil indices. The same analysis was completed for the comparison group.

To evaluate the sensitivity of paper-and-pencil measures and the ImPACT to cognitive changes in athletes who reported low levels of symptoms after a concussion, the sample was divided into low- (M = 1.50, SD = 1.90) and high- (M = 20.64, SD = 14.68) symptom groups on the basis of the median postconcussion symptom score (Mdn = 5.00). The proportion of athletes in the low-symptom group showing reliable decline on the nine paper-and-pencil indices and the four ImPACT composites were calculated.

RESULTS

Overall, traditional paper-and-pencil measures appeared to be more sensitive to postconcussion cognitive changes than the ImPACT (see Table 10.3). This held true when accounting for false positive rates through calculating net detection rates (see Table 10.4). The HVLT–R was better able to capture deficits in verbal learning and memory (HVLT–R Total Recall net detection rate = 22.3%) than was the ImPACT Verbal Memory composite (net detection rate = 3.1%). The BVMT–R Delayed Recall yielded a net detection rate of 9.6%, however, neither the BVMT–R Total

TABLE 10.3
Reliable Change Index Calculations of Increase, Decrease, and No Change

Measure	Decrease *n* (%)	No change *n* (%)	Increase *n* (%)
ImPACT Verbal Memory	5/48 (10.4)	41/48 (85.4)	2/48 (4.2)
ImPACT Visual Memory	2/45 (4.4)	43/45 (95.6)	0/45 (0)
ImPACT Reaction Time	6/48 (12.5)	39/48 (81.3)	3/48 (6.3)
ImPACT VMS	2/48 (4.2)	43/48 (89.6)	3/48 (6.3)
HVLT–R TR	15/51 (29.4)	35/51 (68.6)	1/51 (2.0)
HVLT–R DR	10/51 (19.6)	39/51 (76.5)	2/51 (3.9)
BVMT–R TR	7/51 (13.7)	38/51 (74.5)	6/51 (11.8)
BVMT–T DR	6/51 (11.8)	41/51 (80.4)	4/51 (7.8)
SDMT	7/50 (14.0)	42/50 (84.0)	1/50 (2.0)
SNST Word Reading	12/50 (24.0)	37/50 (74.0)	1/50 (2.0)
SNST Color Word	5/49 (10.2)	37/49 (75.5)	7/49 (14.3)
PSU	5/48 (10.4)	40/48 (83.3)	3/48 (6.3)

Note. ImPACT = Immediate Post-Concussion Assessment and Cognitive Testing; VMS = Visual Motor Speed; HVLT–R = Hopkins Verbal Learning Test—Revised; TR = Total Recall; DR = Delayed Recall; BVMT–R = Brief Visuospatial Memory Test—Revised; SDMT = Symbol Digit Modalities Test; SNST = Stroop Neuropsychological Screening Test; PSU = PSU Cancellation Test.

TABLE 10.4
Net Detection Rates of Immediate Post-Concussion Assessment and Cognitive Testing (ImPACT) Indices and Paper-and-Pencil Measures

Measure	Net detection rate (hits–false positives)
ImPACT Verbal Memory	3.1
ImPACT Visual Memory	2.0
ImPACT Reaction Time	7.6
ImPACT VMSC	−0.7
HVLT–R TR	22.3
HVLT–R DR	14.8
BVMT–R TR	4.2
BVMT–R DR	9.4
SDMT	14.0
SNST Word Reading	21.6
SNST Color–Word	7.8
PSU	10.4

Note. ImPACT = Immediate Post-Concussion Assessment and Cognitive Testing; VMS = Visual Motor Speed; HVLT–R = Hopkins Verbal Learning Test—Revised; TR = Total Recall; DR = Delayed Recall; BVMT–R = Brief Visuospatial Memory Test—Revised; SDMT = Symbol Digit Modalities Test; SNST = Stroop Neuropsychological Screening Test; PSU = PSU Cancellation Test.

Recall (net detection rate = 4.2%) nor the ImPACT Visual Memory composite (net detection rate = 2.0%) was found to be sensitive to postconcussion cognitive changes. A higher proportion of participants in the control group demonstrated a decline on the ImPACT Visual Motor Speed composite than did postconcussion athletes tested (net detection rate = −0.7). As anticipated, the ImPACT Reaction Time composite was the most sensitive of the ImPACT indices to postconcussion cognitive change (net detection rate = 7.6%). However, paper-and-pencil processing speed measures yielded higher net detection rates (SDMT net detection rate =14%; SNST Word Reading subtest net detection rate = 21.6%). The HVLT–R, SNST Word Reading subtest, and SDMT were the most sensitive to postconcussion cognitive changes.

Results from RCI analyses of the healthy comparison group can be found in Table 10.5. The ImPACT yielded false positive rates of 2% to 7%, whereas the paper-and-pencil battery demonstrated false positive rates of 0% to 10%.

To compare sensitivity to cognitive changes on the ImPACT with a test battery of comparable length, the proportion of athletes and control participants who showed a reliable decline on at least one ImPACT composite was compared with the proportion of athletes and control participants who showed a decline on at least one of the following four paper-and-pencil measures that are most analogous to the ImPACT indices: HVLT–R Total Recall, BVMT–R Total Recall, SDMT, and SNST Word Reading (see Figure 10.1). A significantly greater proportion of athletes

TABLE 10.5
Reliable Change Index Calculations of Increase, Decrease, and No Change in Healthy Control Group

Measure	Decrease n (%)	No change n (%)	Increase n (%)
ImPACT Verbal Memory	3/41 (7.3)	38/41 (92.7)	0/41 (0)
ImPACT Visual Memory	1/41 (2.4)	40/41 (97.6)	0/41 (0)
ImPACT Reaction Time	2/41 (4.9)	39/41 (95.1)	0/41 (0)
ImPACT VMS	2/41 (4.9)	37/41 (90.2)	2/41 (4.9)
HVLT–R TR	3/42 (7.1)	37/42 (88.1)	2/42 (4.8)
HVLT–R DR	2/42 (4.8)	37/42 (88.1)	3/42 (7.1)
BVMT–R TR	4/42 (9.5)	36/42 (85.7)	2/42 (4.8)
BVMT–R DR	1/42 (2.4)	40/42 (95.2)	1/42 (2.4)
SDMT	0/42 (0)	41/42 (97.6)	1/42 (2.4)
SNST Word Reading	1/42 (2.4)	39/42 (92.9)	2/42 (4.8)
SNST Color–Word	1/42 (2.4)	40/42 (95.2)	1/42 (2.4)
PSU	0/42 (0)	42/42 (100)	0/42 (0)

Note. ImPACT = Immediate Post-Concussion Assessment and Cognitive Testing; VMS = Visual Motor Speed; HVLT–R = Hopkins Verbal Learning Test—Revised; TR = Total Recall; DR = Delayed Recall; BVMT–R = Brief Visuospatial Memory Test—Revised; SDMT = Symbol Digit Modalities Test; SNST = Stroop Neuropsychological Screening Test; PSU = PSU Cancellation Test.

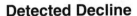

Detected Decline

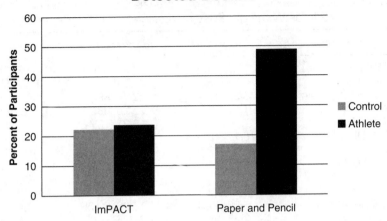

Figure 10.1. Comparison of the Immediate Post-Concussion Assessment and Cognitive Testing and the abbreviated paper-and-pencil battery on rates of reliable decline on at least one test in control and concussed athlete participants.

showed a decline on at least one of these paper-and-pencil measures in comparison with at least one ImPACT composite (McNemar's Test, $p = .008$). Notably, 31.9% of the athlete sample showed a decline on one of these four paper-and-pencil measures without showing a decline on any ImPACT composite (see Table 10.6).

The low- and high-symptom groups did not differ significantly on sex, ethnicity, days since baseline assessment, days since injury, or postconcussion symptoms reported at baseline. The pattern of results observed in the larger sample held when the sample was limited to the low-symptom group. Overall, the paper-and-pencil measures appeared to be more sensitive to postconcussion cognitive changes in athletes reporting low levels of postconcussion symptoms (see Table 10.7).

TABLE 10.6
Comparison of the Percentage of Athletes Showing a Reliable Decline
on at Least One Index of the Abbreviated Paper-and-Pencil Battery
and at Least One Index of the Immediate Post-Concussion Assessment
and Cognitive Testing (ImPACT)

| | ImPACT | |
Paper and pencil	Decline	No decline
Decline	17.0	31.9
No decline	6.4	44.7

TABLE 10.7
Reliable Change Index Calculations of Increase, Decrease, and No Change
in Athletes With Low Postconcussion Symptom Report

Measure	Decrease n (%)	No change n (%)	Increase n (%)
ImPACT Verbal Memory	1/25 (4)	23/25 (92)	1/25 (4)
ImPACT Visual Memory	1/22 (4.5)	21/2 (95.5)	0/22 (0)
ImPACT Reaction Time	3/25 (12)	22/25 (88)	0/25 (0)
ImPACT VMS	1/25 (4)	22/25 (88)	2/22 (8)
HVLT–R TR	7/27 (25.9)	19/27 (70.4)	1/27 (3.7)
HVLT–R DR	5/27 (18.5)	20/27 (74.1)	2/27 (7.4)
BVMT–R TR	5/27 (18.5)	18/27 (66.7)	4/27 (14.8)
BVMT–R DR	4/27 (14.8)	22/27 (81.5)	1/27 (3.7)
SDMT	2/26 (7.7)	24/26 (92.3)	0/26 (0)
SNST Word Reading	6/27 (22.2)	20/27 (74.1)	1/27 (3.7)
SNST Color–Word	3/26 (11.5)	18/26 (69.2)	5/26 (19.2)
PSU	2/25 (8)	21/25 (84)	2/25 (8)

Note. ImPACT = Immediate Post-Concussion Assessment and Cognitive Testing; VMS = Visual Motor Speed; HVLT–R = Hopkins Verbal Learning Test—Revised; TR = Total Recall; DR = Delayed Recall; BVMT–R = Brief Visuospatial Memory Test—Revised; SDMT = Symbol Digit Modalities Test; SNST = Stroop Neuropsychological Screening Test; PSU = PSU Cancellation Test.

DISCUSSION

The results of this study show that traditional neuropsychological measures are more sensitive than the ImPACT in detecting changes in cognitive functioning after an acute concussion. In each assessed domain, the traditional neuropsychological measures detected decline in more concussed athletes than did the ImPACT. The discrepancy in rates of decline on the measures of verbal and visual memory may be attributable to the recognition-only format of memory testing on the ImPACT. The relatively low sensitivity of the ImPACT Visual Motor Speed composite was a surprising finding in light of its reported strong convergent validity with traditional processing speed measures (Iverson et al., 2005). When we assessed a group of healthy control participants in our study, the ImPACT and traditional neuropsychological tests yielded similar patterns of results. Thus, the difference in rates of postconcussion decline in the present study cannot be attributed to the traditional measures being overly sensitive to normal fluctuations in cognition.

To compare rates of decline on the ImPACT to a paper-and-pencil battery of comparable length and content, we evaluated an abbreviated battery consisting of the HVLT–R, BVMT–R, SDMT, and the SNST Word Reading subtest. We found that significantly more athletes showed a decline on at least one paper-and-pencil measure (48.9%) than on at least one ImPACT composite (23.4%). Furthermore, 31.9% of athletes showed a decline on at least one of these four paper-and-pencil measures without showing a decline on any ImPACT composite. In comparison, only 6.4% of athletes declined on at least one ImPACT measure without showing a decline on any of these four paper-and-pencil measures (see Table 10.6). A similar evaluation of the healthy comparison group revealed comparable rates of decline on at least one ImPACT index (22%) and on at least one test in the paper-and-pencil battery index (17%). A comparable proportion of concussed athletes (23.4%) and healthy control participants (22%) showed a decline on at least one ImPACT composite (see Figure 10.1).

Over the past decade there has been a major shift in the management of sports-related concussions to rely on brief computerized neuropsychological testing instead of traditional paper-and-pencil measures. The most widely used computerized concussion assessment, the ImPACT, is currently used in a variety of professional sports (e.g., Major League Baseball, the National Hockey League, the National Football League, and World Wrestling Entertainment) and more than 7,400 high schools and over 1,000 colleges and universities (Lovell, 2007). The data presented in this chapter suggest that sole reliance on computerized tests in postconcussion cognitive assessment could put athletes at risk for being returned to play before they are truly back to their preinjury neurocognitive baseline. The ImPACT's concussion management model does include the step of determining whether more extensive neuropsychological assessment is necessary after the administration of the ImPACT (Lovell, 2007). However, it is unlikely that additional testing would be recommended in cases where no declines are detected on the ImPACT.

The results of this study raise concerns for sole reliance on the ImPACT for concussion management. The widespread availability and access to the ImPACT are marketed as major benefits of computerized assessments; however, overconfidence in the ImPACT may actually increase the risk of concussion mismanagement. Randolph (2011) previously critiqued the use of baseline testing, in particular computerized tests, partially because of the increased risk associated with the high false negative rates. In addition, the most recent consensus statement on concussions in sport highlights that brief computerized cognitive evaluation tools are not substitutes for complete neuropsychological assessments (McCrory et al., 2017).

CASE STUDY

Some of the original details of this case have been changed to protect the confidentiality of the individual tested.

The importance of not relying solely on the ImPACT for return-to-play decisions can be seen in the following case example of Ms. Z, a 21-year-old woman who plays on a collegiate soccer team. Ms. Z sustained a concussion when she was running during a soccer game and was struck either by an opponent's head or elbow on the right side of her chin. She was removed from play, running off the field of her own volition. Ms. Z remembered the impact, did not lose consciousness, and denied experiencing any retrograde amnesia. However, she reported experiencing a few seconds of anterograde amnesia and also noted that her visual field was completely white for a few seconds.

Immediately after her injury, Ms. Z reported experiencing the following symptoms, rated on a scale of 0 to 6 on which 0 indicates *no symptoms* and 6 represents *severe symptoms*: Disorientation (3), dizziness (4), balance problems (3), visual disturbance (6), mental fogginess (3), pressure in the head (3), problems concentrating (3), and headache (4). At 30 minutes after the injury, most of her symptoms had resolved, with the exception of pressure in the head, problems concentrating, and headache, which remained at comparable severity levels. By 2 hours after the injury, these latter symptoms persisted at similar levels. By 12 hours after the injury, she continued to experience problems concentrating (2) and headache (2). At the time of neuropsychological assessment, 3 days postinjury, Ms. Z reported only mild problems concentrating (1) but noted that she mostly felt back to her pre-injury self. She had been going to class and studying and had not noticed any increase in symptoms to cognitive exertion. She had avoided significant physical exertion since her injury.

Ms. Z's performance on neuropsychological testing was compared with her baseline evaluation, which was completed approximately 15 months before her injury. Results from both evaluations are presented in Table 10.8.

TABLE 10.8
Case Study: Ms. Z

Test	Baseline	Postconcussion	RCI value
ImPACT Verbal Memory	115.44	112.71	0.27
ImPACT Visual Memory	111.42	106.78	−0.09
ImPACT Reaction Time	95.31	100.94	0.82
ImPACT VMS	83.81	93.66	0.67
HVLT–R TR	120.93	101.03	−1.71*
HVLT–R DR	96.21	96.21	−0.19
BVMT–R TR	114.86	92.22	−2.21*
BVMT–R DR	104.35	95.47	−0.92
SDMT	88.46	85.81	−1.05
SNST Word Reading	98.21	101.92	0.28
SNST Color–Word	78.78	106.37	2.69
PSU–X	116.99	100.49	−0.92

Note. RCI = reliable change index; ImPACT = Immediate Post-Concussion Assessment and Cognitive Testing; VMS = Visual Motor Speed; HVLT–R = Hopkins Verbal Learning Test—Revised; TR = Total Recall; DR = Delayed Recall; BVMT–R = Brief Visuospatial Memory Test—Revised; SDMT = Symbol Digit Modalities Test; SNST = Stroop Neuropsychological Screening Test; PSU = PSU Cancellation Test.
*Indicates significant reliable decline.

Raw scores were converted to standard scores, based on normative data from a large sample of collegiate athletes. RCI values are also included in the table; A 90% cutoff was used to establish clinical significance (RCI = ±1.64).

If Ms. Z had only been administered the ImPACT, the evaluation of RCI scores would suggest that her neuropsychological functioning was back to her baseline, as she did not demonstrate any clinically significant change on the ImPACT indices. Evaluation of the paper-and-pencil test battery suggests that Ms. Z experienced a decline in immediate memory performance as indicated by the clinically significant decrease in performance on the HVLT–R Total Recall and BVMT–R Total Recall indices. This pattern of results may be attributable to the ImPACT's lack of free-recall memory indices. Free recall is objectively more difficult than recognition, and thus the ImPACT's recognition-only memory tests may not be adequately sensitive to changes in memory. If we had relied solely on the ImPACT scores for information on her neuropsychological functioning, she would have been cleared to begin return-to-play procedures prematurely because she would have appeared to be back to her baseline level of functioning.

LIMITATIONS

Our use of a clinical population without any adjustments to the clinical protocol allowed for a more ecologically valid assessment of test sensitivity; however, it also made it more difficult to determine whether all participants truly were experiencing any continued brain dysfunction at the time of the assessment and therefore whether there were any cognitive changes to be detected. Because of this limitation we cannot say with certainty that the observed cognitive changes are due to continued brain dysfunction related to their concussion rather than a result of our measures being overly sensitive. Still, if more athletes showed declines in performance from baseline on the paper-and-pencil measures compared with the ImPACT, what other explanation could there be? The "too sensitive" case would hold more weight if test results were being compared with normative data instead of participants' own baseline scores. Also, the traditional neuropsychological measures and the ImPACT showed similar rates of decline in a sample of healthy control participants.

The lack of established biomarkers in concussion has led to diagnoses being made primarily on the basis of self-reported symptoms (Jeter et al., 2013) and can be considered a limitation of all concussion studies. By including only athletes who were not yet returned to play, we aimed to circumvent this issue to the extent possible in the absence of established biomarkers.

CLINICAL TAKE-HOME POINTS

1. *Clinicians should exercise caution when using the ImPACT in isolation.* The results of the study presented in this chapter suggest that traditional tests were more sensitive than the ImPACT to postconcussion cognitive change. The risk in relying only on computerized tests is that their limited sensitivity may result in prematurely returning athletes to play and perhaps putting them at risk for injury before their brain functioning has returned to normal. If the findings presented in this chapter are replicated, then clinicians should consider supplementing computerized tests with more traditional neuropsychological measures. Previous authors have suggested that a "hybrid" approach of paper-and-pencil measures and computerized testing may allow for the maximization of the benefits of each approach (Iverson & Schatz, 2015).

2. *Consistent with prior work and recommendations made by others, in most sports concussion situations neuropsychological testing should not be conducted until athletes are mostly asymptomatic via their own self-report.* Because athletes will not be returned to play if they are symptomatic, neuropsychological testing is typically not needed until they report being asymptomatic relative to baseline (Randolph et al., 2005). Although a case can be made for neuropsychological testing in the acute phase postconcussion to track recovery in some cases (see Arnett et al., 2014), the sensitivity and specificity of both computerized and traditional neuropsychological tests in symptomatic athletes tested shortly after concussion may be less relevant for its clinical use.

3. *When resources are scarce, testing concussed athletes only after a concussion should be considered.* Given the time and personnel needs required to baseline test athletes at all levels of participation, this may not be a feasible approach for many athletic programs. In the absence of baseline data, clinicians can follow an evidence-based approach that incorporates base rates of impairment in interpreting the postconcussion data. Algorithms that allow for evidence-based evaluation of postconcussion cognitive functioning have been developed (Arnett, Meyer, Merritt, & Guty, 2016; Arnett, Rabinowitz, et al., 2014), and considering only postconcussion data can circumvent a number of problems associated with baseline testing (see Echemendia et al., 2012).

KEY ISSUES TO BE ADDRESSED IN THE NEXT 5 YEARS

1. *Can computerized tests such as the ImPACT be modified to increase their sensitivity?* One limitation that has been highlighted regarding the ImPACT and other computerized tests is that they do not adequately assess sustained attention, auditory working memory (Maerlender et al., 2010; Malojcic, Mubrin, Coric, Susnic, & Spilich, 2008; McAllister, Sparling, Flashman, Guerin, Mamourian, & Saykin, 2001), and free recall memory (De Marco & Broshek, 2016). Devising strategies that make it possible to assess these cognitive domains within the context of the efficient computerized format could greatly enhance the sensitivity of these tests.

2. *More research that compares computerized with traditional neuropsychological tests in the sports concussion context is needed.* The results of the study presented in this chapter provide compelling evidence that traditional neuropsychological tests are more sensitive than the ImPACT to postconcussion cognitive changes. However, more research is needed to replicate these findings before firm conclusions about clinical practice can be made.

3. *Additional research using neuropsychological batteries on concussed but now asymptomatic athletes prior to their return to play is needed.* In most clinical concussion contexts the neurocognitive assessment of athletes is not conducted until athletes are asymptomatic per their self-report. In our study, the evaluation of postconcussion change in athletes reporting low levels of postconcussion symptoms yielded results comparable to those found in the larger sample. Because many concussion programs do not complete neuropsychological testing until after an athlete is symptom free, it is important for neuropsychological tests to be able to detect cognitive changes in the absence of reported postconcussion symptoms.

The advantages of computerized assessments for accessibility and reliability of administration and scoring should not be overlooked. Neither should the demonstrated sensitivity of the ImPACT in acutely concussed symptomatic athletes. More research is necessary, however, to establish the ImPACT as a concussion screening measure in typical clinical populations. It may be that the recognition-only format of the memory tests significantly reduces the ImPACT's sensitivity to postconcussion cognitive changes. In its current form, users of the ImPACT should be aware of its limitations. If our findings are replicated by others, then clinicians relying on the ImPACT as a comprehensive postconcussion cognitive screen should be aware that it may not assess all domains possibly affected by concussion and may be less sensitive than traditional neuropsychological tests.

REFERENCES

Allen, B. J., & Gfeller, J. D. (2011). The Immediate Post-Concussion Assessment and Cognitive Testing battery and traditional neuropsychological measures: A construct and concurrent validity study. *Brain Injury, 25*, 179–191. http://dx.doi.org/10.3109/02699052.2010.541897

Allen, L. M., Conder, R. L., Green, P., & Cox, D. R. (1997). *CARB '97 manual for the Computerized Assessment of Response Bias.* Durham, NC: Cognisyst.

Arnett, P., Meyer, J., Merritt, V., & Guty, E. (2016). Neuropsychological testing in mild traumatic brain injury: What to do when baseline testing is not available. *Sports Medicine and Arthroscopy Review, 24*, 116–122. http://dx.doi.org/10.1097/JSA.0000000000000123

Arnett, P. A., Rabinowitz, A. R., Vargas, G. A., Ukueberuwa, D. M., Merritt, V. C., & Meyer, J. E. (2014). Neuropsychological testing in sports concussion management: An evidence-based model when baseline is unavailable. In S. M. Slobounov & W. J. Sebastianelli (Eds.), *Concussions in athletics: From brain to behavior* (pp. 35–48). New York, NY: Springer.

Barth, J. T., Alves, W. M., Ryan, T. V., Macciocchi, S. N., Rimel, R. W., Jane, J. A., & Nelson, W. E. (1989). Mild head injury in sports: Neuropsychological sequelae and recovery of function. In H. S. Levin, H. M. Eisenberg, & A. L. Benton (Eds.), *Mild head injury* (pp. 257–275). New York, NY: Oxford University Press.

Benedict, R. H. B. (1997). *Brief Visuospatial Memory Test—Revised: Professional manual.* Odessa, FL: Psychological Assessment Resources.

Benedict, R. H. B., Schretlen, D., Groninger, L., & Brandt, J. (1998). Hopkins Verbal Learning Test—Revised: Normative data and analysis of inter-form and test–retest reliability. *The Clinical Neuropsychologist, 12*, 43–55. http://dx.doi.org/10.1076/clin.12.1.43.1726

Brandt, J., & Benedict, R. H. B. (2001). *Hopkins Verbal Learning Test—Revised: Professional manual.* Odessa, FL: Psychological Assessment Resources.

Broglio, S. P., Macciocchi, S. N., & Ferrara, M. S. (2007). Sensitivity of the concussion assessment battery. *Neurosurgery, 60*, 1050–1058. http://dx.doi.org/10.1227/01.NEU.0000255479.90999.C0

Cegalis, J. A., & Cegalis, S. (1994). *The Vigil/W Continuous Performance Test manual.* New York, NY: ForThought.

Chen, J. K., Johnston, K. M., Collie, A., McCrory, P., & Ptito, A. (2007). A validation of the Post-Concussion Symptom Scale in the assessment of complex concussion using cognitive testing and functional MRI. *Journal of Neurology, Neurosurgery, and Psychiatry, 78*, 1231–1238. http://dx.doi.org/10.1136/jnnp.2006.110395

Collie, A., Darby, D., & Maruff, P. (2001). Computerised cognitive assessment of athletes with sports related head injury. *British Journal of Sports Medicine*, 35, 297–302. http://dx.doi.org/10.1136/bjsm.35.5.297

Collie, A., Maruff, P., McStephen, M., & Darby, D. G. (2003). Psychometric issues associated with computerised neuropsychological assessment of concussed athletes. *British Journal of Sports Medicine*, 37, 556–559. http://dx.doi.org/10.1136/bjsm.37.6.556

Covassin, T., Elbin, R. J., & Nakayama, Y. (2010). Tracking neurocognitive performance following concussion in high school athletes. *The Physician and Sportsmedicine*, 38, 87–93. http://dx.doi.org/10.3810/psm.2010.12.1830

Covassin, T., Elbin, R. J., III, Stiller-Ostrowski, J. L., & Kontos, A. P. (2009). Immediate Post-Concussion Assessment and Cognitive Testing (ImPACT) practices of sports medicine professionals. *Journal of Athletic Training*, 44, 639–644. http://dx.doi.org/10.4085/1062-6050-44.6.639

Delis, D. C., Kramer, J. H., Kaplan, E., & Ober, B. A. (2000). *California Verbal Learning Test—Second edition* (Adult version). Pearson Education.

De Marco, A. P., & Broshek, D. K. (2016). Computerized cognitive testing in the management of youth sports-related concussion. *Journal of Child Neurology*, 31, 68–75.

Dikmen, S. S., Heaton, R. K., Grant, I., & Temkin, N. R. (1999). Test–retest reliability and practice effects of expanded Halstead–Reitan Neuropsychological Test Battery. *Journal of the International Neuropsychological Society*, 5, 346–356. http://dx.doi.org/10.1017/S1355617799544056

Echemendia, R. J., Bruce, J. M., Bailey, C. M., Sanders, J. F., Arnett, P., & Vargas, G. (2012). The utility of post-concussion neuropsychological data in identifying cognitive change following sports-related MTBI in the absence of baseline data. *The Clinical Neuropsychologist*, 26, 1077–1091.

Echemendia, R. J., & Julian, L. J. (2001). Mild traumatic brain injury in sports: Neuropsychology's contribution to a developing field. *Neuropsychology Review*, 11(2), 69–88.

Echemendia, R. J., Putukian, M., Mackin, R. S., Julian, L., & Shoss, N. (2001). Neuropsychological test performance prior to and following sports-related mild traumatic brain injury. *Clinical Journal of Sport Medicine*, 11, 23–31. http://dx.doi.org/10.1097/00042752-200101000-00005

Goodglass, H., Kaplan, E., & Baressi, B. (2001). *Boston Diagnostic Aphasia Examination* (3rd ed.). San Antonio, TX: Psychological Corporation.

Iverson, G. L., Brooks, B. L., Collins, M. W., & Lovell, M. R. (2006). Tracking neuropsychological recovery following concussion in sport. *Brain Injury*, 20, 245–252. http://dx.doi.org/10.1080/02699050500487910

Iverson, G. L., Lovell, M. R., & Collins, M. W. (2003). Interpreting change on ImPACT following sport concussion. *The Clinical Neuropsychologist*, 17, 460–467. http://dx.doi.org/10.1076/clin.17.4.460.27934

Iverson, G. L., Lovell, M. R., & Collins, M. W. (2005). Validity of ImPACT for measuring processing speed following sports-related concussion. *Journal of Clinical and Experimental Neuropsychology, 27,* 683–689. http://dx.doi.org/10.1081/13803390490918435

Iverson, G. L., & Schatz, P. (2015). Advanced topics in neuropsychological assessment following sport-related concussion. *Brain Injury, 29,* 263–275. http://dx.doi.org/10.3109/02699052.2014.965214

Jeter, C. B., Hergenroeder, G. W., Hylin, M. J., Redell, J. B., Moore, A. N., & Dash, P. K. (2013). Biomarkers for the diagnosis and prognosis of mild traumatic brain injury/concussion. *Journal of Neurotrauma, 30,* 657–670. http://dx.doi.org/10.1089/neu.2012.2439

Kontos, A. P., Elbin, R. J., Schatz, P., Covassin, T., Henry, L., Pardini, J., & Collins, M. W. (2012). A revised factor structure for the Post-Concussion Symptom Scale: Baseline and postconcussion factors. *The American Journal of Sports Medicine, 40,* 2375–2384. http://dx.doi.org/10.1177/0363546512455400

Lezak, M. D., Howieson, D. B., & Loring, D. W. (2005). *Neuropsychological Assessment* (4th ed.). New York, NY: Oxford University Press.

Lovell, M. (2000). *ImPACT Version 2.0 clinical user's manual.* Retrieved from http://www.impacttest.com

Lovell, M. (2007). *Immediate Post-Concussion Assessment Testing (ImPACT) Test: Clinical interpretive manual.* Pittsburgh, PA: ImPACT Applications.

Lovell, M. R., & Collins, M. W. (2002). New developments in the evaluation of sports-related concussion. *Current Sports Medicine Reports, 1,* 287–292. http://www.ncbi.nlm.nih.gov/pubmed/12831691. http://dx.doi.org/10.1249/00149619-200210000-00006

Lovell, M. R., Collins, M. W., Podell, K., Powell, J., & Maroon, J. (2000). *ImPACT: Immediate Post-Concussion Assessment and Cognitive Testing.* Pittsburgh, PA: NeuroHealth Systems.

Lovell, M. R., Iverson, G. L., Collins, M. W., Podell, K., Johnston, K. M., Pardini, D., . . . Maroon, J. C. (2006). Measurement of symptoms following sports-related concussion: Reliability and normative data for the postconcussion scale. *Applied Neuropsychology, 13,* 166–174. http://dx.doi.org/10.1207/s15324826an1303_4

Maerlender, A., Flashman, L., Kessler, A., Kumbhani, S., Greenwald, R., Tosteson, T., & McAllister, T. (2010). Examination of the construct validity of ImPACT computerized test, traditional, and experimental neuropsychological measures. *The Clinical Neuropsychologist, 24,* 1309–1325. http://dx.doi.org/10.1080/13854046.2010.516072

Malojcic, B., Mubrin, Z., Coric, B., Susnic, M., & Spilich, G. J. (2008). Consequences of mild traumatic brain injury on information processing assessed with attention and short-term memory tasks. *Journal of Neurotrauma, 25,* 30–37. http://dx.doi.org/10.1089/neu.2007.0384

Mayers, L. B., & Redick, T. S. (2012). Clinical utility of ImPACT assessment for postconcussion return-to-play counseling: Psychometric issues. *Journal of Clinical and Experimental Neuropsychology, 34*, 235–242. http://dx.doi.org/10.1080/13803395.2011.630655

McAllister, T. W., Sparling, M. B., Flashman, L. A., Guerin, S. J., Mamourian, A. C., & Saykin, A. J. (2001). Differential working memory load effects after mild traumatic brain injury. *NeuroImage, 14*, 1004–1012. http://dx.doi.org/10.1006/nimg.2001.0899

McClincy, M. P., Lovell, M. R., Pardini, J., Collins, M. W., & Spore, M. K. (2006). Recovery from sports concussion in high school and collegiate athletes. *Brain Injury, 20*, 33–39. http://dx.doi.org/10.1080/02699050500309817

McCrea, M., Guskiewicz, K. M., Marshall, S. W., Barr, W., Randolph, C., Cantu, R. C., . . . Kelly, J. P. (2003). Acute effects and recovery time following concussion in collegiate football players: The NCAA Concussion Study. *JAMA, 290*, 2556–2563. http://dx.doi.org/10.1001/jama.290.19.2556

McCrory, P., Meeuwisse, W., Dvořák, J., Aubry, M., Bailes, J., Broglio, S., . . . Vos, P. E. (2017). Consensus statement on concussion in sport—The 5th International Conference on Concussion in Sport held in Berlin, October 2016. *British Journal of Sports Medicine, 51*, 838–847. http://dx.doi.org/10.1136/bjsports-2017-097699

Meehan, W. P., III, d'Hemecourt, P., Collins, C. L., Taylor, A. M., & Comstock, R. D. (2012). Computerized neurocognitive testing for the management of sport-related concussions. *Pediatrics, 129*, 38–44. http://dx.doi.org/10.1542/peds.2011-1972

Meyer, J. E., & Arnett, P. A. (2015a). Changes in symptoms in concussed and nonconcussed athletes following neuropsychological assessment. *Developmental Neuropsychology, 40*, 24–28. http://dx.doi.org/10.1080/87565641.2014.1001065

Meyer, J. E., & Arnett, P. A. (2015b). Validation of the Affective Word List as a measure of verbal learning and memory. *Journal of Clinical and Experimental Neuropsychology, 37*, 316–324.

Moser, R. S., Schatz, P., Neidzwski, K., & Ott, S. D. (2011). Group versus individual administration affects baseline neurocognitive test performance. *The American Journal of Sports Medicine, 39*, 2325–2330. http://dx.doi.org/10.1177/0363546511417114

Nakayama, Y., Covassin, T., Schatz, P., Nogle, S., & Kovan, J. (2014). Examination of the test–retest reliability of a computerized neurocognitive test battery. *The American Journal of Sports Medicine, 42*, 2000–2005. http://dx.doi.org/10.1177/0363546514535901

Nelson, L. D., LaRoche, A. A., Pfaller, A. Y., Lerner, E. B., Hammeke, T. A., Randolph, C., . . . McCrea, M. A. (2016). Prospective, head-to-head study of three computerized neurocognitive assessment tools (CNTs): Reliability and validity for the assessment of sport-related concussion. *Journal of the*

International Neuropsychological Society, 22, 24–37. http://dx.doi.org/10.1017/S1355617715001101

Randolph, C. (2011). Baseline neuropsychological testing in managing sport-related concussion: Does it modify risk? *Current Sports Medicine Reports, 10*, 21–26. http://dx.doi.org/10.1249/JSR.0b013e318207831d

Randolph, C., McCrea, M., & Barr, W. B. (2005). Is neuropsychological testing useful in the management of sport-related concussion? *Journal of Athletic Training, 40*, 139–152.

Resch, J., Driscoll, A., McCaffrey, N., Brown, C., Ferrara, M. S., Macciocchi, S., . . . Walpert, K. (2013). ImPACT test–retest reliability: Reliably unreliable? *Journal of Athletic Training, 48*, 506–511. http://dx.doi.org/10.4085/1062-6050-48.3.09

Resch, J. E., Macciocchi, S., & Ferrara, M. S. (2013). Preliminary evidence of equivalence of alternate forms of the ImPACT. *The Clinical Neuropsychologist, 27*, 1265–1280. http://dx.doi.org/10.1080/13854046.2013.845247

Resch, J. E., McCrea, M. A., & Cullum, C. M. (2013). Computerized neurocognitive testing in the management of sport-related concussion: An update. *Neuropsychology Review, 23*, 335–349. http://dx.doi.org/10.1007/s11065-013-9242-5

Reynolds, C. R. (2002). *Comprehensive Trail-Making Test*. Austin, TX: Pro-Ed.

Rosenbaum, A. M., Arnett, P. A., Bailey, C. M., & Echemendia, R. J. (2006). Neuropsychological assessment of sports-related concussion: Measuring clinically significant change. In S. M. Slobounov & W. J. Sebastianelli (Eds.), *Foundations of sport-related brain injuries* (pp. 137–169). New York, NY: Springer. http://dx.doi.org/10.1007/0-387-32565-4_7

Ruff, R. M., Iverson, G. L., Barth, J. T., Bush, S. S., Broshek, D. K., & the NAN Policy and Planning Committee. (2009). Recommendations for diagnosing a mild traumatic brain injury: A National Academy of Neuropsychology education paper. *Archives of Clinical Neuropsychology, 24*, 3–10. http://dx.doi.org/10.1093/arclin/acp006

Schatz, P., & Ferris, C. S. (2013). One-month test–retest reliability of the ImPACT test battery. *Archives of Clinical Neuropsychology, 28*, 499–504. http://dx.doi.org/10.1093/arclin/act034

Schatz, P., & Putz, B. O. (2006). Cross-validation of measures used for computer-based assessment of concussion. *Applied Neuropsychology, 13*, 151–159. http://dx.doi.org/10.1207/s15324826an1303_2

Schatz, P., & Sandel, N. (2013). Sensitivity and specificity of the online version of ImPACT in high school and collegiate athletes. *The American Journal of Sports Medicine, 41*, 321–326. http://dx.doi.org/10.1177/0363546512466038

Schatz, P., & Zillmer, E. A. (2003). Computer-based assessment of sports-related concussion. *Applied Neuropsychology, 10*, 42–47. http://dx.doi.org/10.1207/S15324826AN1001_6

Smith, A. (1982). *Symbol Digit Modalities Test*. Los Angeles, CA: Western Psychological Services.

Speer, D. C. (1992). Clinically significant change: Jacobson and Truax (1991) revisited. *Journal of Consulting and Clinical Psychology, 60*, 402–408. http://dx.doi.org/10.1037/0022-006X.60.3.402

Strauss, E., Sherman, E. M. S., & Spreen, O. (2006). *A compendium of neuropsychological tests: Administration, norms, and commentary* (3rd ed.). New York, NY: Oxford University Press.

The Psychological Corporation. (2001). *Wechsler Test of Adult Reading*. San Antonio, TX: Harcourt Assessment.

Trenerry, M., Crosson, B., DeBoe, J., & Leber, W. (1989). *Stroop neuropsychological screening manual*. Odessa, FL: Psychological Assessment Resources Inc.

Wechsler, D. (1997). *Wechsler Adult Intelligence Scale—III (WAIS–III)*. New York, NY: The Psychological Corporation.

Wilson, B., Cockburn, J., & Baddeley, A. (1991). *The Rivermead Behavioural Memory Test manual*. Bury St. Edmunds, Suffolk, England: Thames Valley Test Corporation.

Zachary, R. A. (1986). *Shipley Institute of Living Scale: Revised manual*. Los Angeles, CA: Western Psychological Services.

IV

SPECIALTY CONTRIBUTIONS TO SPORTS CONCUSSION

11

PROFESSIONAL SPORTS NEUROPSYCHOLOGY

RUBEN J. ECHEMENDIA, JARED M. BRUCE,
AND MORGAN GLUSMAN

It is critical that any neuropsychologist working with professional athletes is acutely aware of the context in which professional athletes play their sport. Although professional athletes typically play a sport they love, a sport that has been a central and consistent force throughout much of their lives, and which in many instances serves as the foundation for an athlete's self-image, once they become a professional it becomes "business." At the outset of this chapter, it is important to underscore the significant role of money and fame in the professional realm because their impact on sports has wide-reaching implications for the context in which these athletes live their lives and in turn have important implications for the practice of sports neuropsychology.

The meaning of the term *professional athlete* varies by country, culture, and sport. In the United States the primary distinction between amateur and professional athletes stems from the means and methods of remuneration.

http://dx.doi.org/10.1037/0000114-012

Neuropsychology of Sports-Related Concussion, P. A. Arnett (Editor)

Typically, professional athletes are paid for playing their sport, receiving payment or prize money based on contracts or performance incentives. In contrast, amateur athletes may receive nonmonetary compensation, such as scholarships, housing/travel/subsistence costs, or trust payments for later use, but they typically do not receive a salary or prize money.

Given the worldwide focus on sports, many athletes quickly become celebrities or role models. This elevated stature in the public eye is not reserved just for professional athletes. In the United States in particular, there is a very strong amateur cohort of athletes at the collegiate level whose celebrity status may often rival that of their professional counterparts. Indeed, in some sports, professional athletes are almost exclusively drawn from colleges and universities. Although there are many similarities between professional and amateur ranks, the focus of this chapter is on examining the unique context of professional sports.

Professional sports are a major economic force in the entertainment industry. They represent a multibillion dollar worldwide business, with projected revenues expected to exceed $90 billion by 2017. For example, the National Football League (NFL) had revenues of $13 billion in 2015; Major League Baseball had revenues of $9.5 billion; the National Basketball Association made $5.2 billion; and the National Hockey League (NHL) made $3.7 billion. At the international level, the Premier League had revenues of £3.4 billion (in 2015 values; Young, 2015), the Bundesliga earned €2.6 billion ("Bundesliga Report 2016," 2016), and Australia's National Rugby League grossed $374.1 million. It is not surprising that athletes are compensated at rates that reflect the earnings of their employers. For example, the NFL's minimum salary is $435,000 with a maximum of $24.2 million (*Mdn* = $860,000), whereas Major League Soccer minimum salary is $60,000 with a maximum at $7.17 million (*Mdn* = $110,000; "NFL Team Salary Cap Tracker," 2016, 2017). Most athletes have relatively brief professional careers, increasing the importance of quickly maximizing their earning potential. To achieve these ends, many professional athletes become businesses unto themselves, hiring agents, accountants, dietitians, masseuses, sports psychologists, and other staff. They frequently are members of unions that serve to collectively bargain terms of employment, even down to the amount and types of soap that must be in locker room showers. These extraordinary aspects of professional athletes' existence and lifestyles can create a sense of privilege that may at times cause tension in the relationships among players and medical staff. This tension is particularly noticeable when players are asked to engage in unpleasant or undervalued activities (e.g., baseline testing) or when they are removed from competition for medical reasons. As a consequence, instead of the customary role of a neuropsychologist being respected and valued as a medical professional, sports neuropsychologists may at times be viewed as a necessary evil (Bailey, Echemendia, & Arnett, 2006; Despres, Brady, & McGowan, 2008).

Professional athletes work under the spotlight of a critical media that observe their every move, dissecting their performance, behaviors, health, appearance, and personality, in and out of the playing environment. The media can lavish praise, or they can be cutting in their criticism. Although many athletes thrive under this pressure, the public spotlight can extract a psychological cost in the form of stress and anxiety, as well as the need to defend and protect one's self-image under such public scrutiny (Charbonneau & Garland, 2005).

Moreover, professional athletes are surrounded by groups of people who are important in their lives but may have inconsistent agendas. For example, athletes are surrounded by agents, families, friends, and business associates. The agents who represent them seek to protect the athlete and obtain the best deals by negotiating contracts, serving as liaisons or gatekeepers between the athlete and the general population, their sports team or organization, business associates and ventures, and sometimes even friends and family. Given that athletes typically pay their agents proportionately based on monies earned, the longer the athlete's career and the more money that he or she earns, the more money the agent makes. This interdependent relationship brings with it many of the benefits and challenges that are seen in any important relationship. Like nonathletes, professional athletes also have families who provide support, nurturance, and a grounding in reality, who are central to the athlete's life functioning. Families also require nurturance, attention, and support (emotional and financial). They too are affected by the fickle nature of that limelight. Importantly, injuries, whether concussion or musculoskeletal, affect not only the player but also his or her family more broadly. Friends, in particular those outside of the sport, are also an important source of emotional support and have relationships with the athlete that often predate and transcend their celebrity status. However, these friendships also need to be nurtured and often come with seemingly simple requests that may at times feel like oppressive demands (e.g., tickets to a big game). Rounding out the cadre of individuals involved with professional athletes are the venture capitalists, financial planners, attorneys, and business associates who seek to protect and grow the athlete's wealth. All of these groups, though well meaning and well intentioned, may lead the athlete to feel that "everyone wants a piece of me," which may in turn lead to both healthy and unhealthy levels of distrust or skepticism (Carlson & Donavan, 2013). It is not surprising, then, that sports teams and leagues in general sometimes exist in an encapsulated culture where you are either in the "family" or outside of the family.

THE PROFESSIONAL ATHLETE AND CONCUSSIONS

The international attention given to sport-related concussions (SRCs) has had a profound impact on professional sports. Much of the attention began when high-profile athletes cut their careers short, in part either because of persistent symptoms after concussions or concerns about possible long-term neurocognitive deficits after repetitive concussions (The Sports Xchange, 2017). The focus intensified with published cases of professional American football players who were diagnosed during autopsy with chronic traumatic encephalopathy (CTE; McKee, Alosco, & Huber, 2016). CTE is hypothesized to be a degenerative brain disease associated with repetitive head trauma. The intense media focus on CTE, which has often outpaced the scientific understanding of this pathological condition, elevated the perception of concussion from its previous position as a relatively benign and routine part of sports to a brain injury that needs to be promptly identified, evaluated, and managed appropriately.

Sports leagues, players' unions, and the medical community have responded by developing concussion protocols and approaches to better detect and manage the injury using the relatively scant data available for guidance. Given the amount of attention that has been focused on concussions, many individuals may be surprised to learn that the bulk of what we know about sports-related concussion has evolved from research conducted over the past 10 to 15 years. Indeed, it was only in 1997 that the NHL became the first professional league to mandate league-wide baseline and postinjury neuropsychological testing across all players. In the pages that follow we discuss concussion-related research as it relates to professional sports. However, because many of the issues related to professional athletes also intersect with athletes at all levels of play, pertinent research on SRC in nonprofessional athletes also is discussed.

Professional leagues have the resources, financial and medical, to deploy comprehensive concussion evaluation and management programs using the expertise of a broad range of health care disciplines. However, by the time athletes reach professional status, they have often experienced several concussions, with unknown levels of care and management, in particular those athletes who sustained injuries many years ago, when knowledge of concussions was in its infancy.

Professional athletes are not solely concerned about the effects of injury on their bodies and their subsequent ability to perform at elite skill levels; they are also concerned about the effects of injury on their "value" as a professional (Carless & Douglas, 2013). This is true for all injuries, not just concussions. However, in the absence of scientific data to inform clear-cut guidelines, the effect of concussions on an athlete's employability or value to an organization creates misinformation (Block, West, & Goldin, 2016) and anxiety and may affect the willingness of the athlete to seek medical attention or treatment (Williams, Langdon, McMillan, & Buckley, 2016). For example, the number of concussions an athlete is known to have had may reduce their perceived value as an athlete, decreasing the length and size of the contract that their agent can successfully negotiate. As such, monetary incentives may exist that pressure athletes to minimize their concussion symptoms and "play through" injury (Glick & Horsfall, 2005). Ironically, these very actions can worsen the injury and lead to more persistent symptoms that could eventually end a career (Caron, Bloom, Johnston, & Sabiston, 2013; Elbin et al., 2016). The hesitation that players sometimes feel to promptly identify this injury must be combated with early and consistent education about what we know from empirical studies and what we do not know. This education must also be widely disseminated—to the leagues, their executives, owners, managers, agents, coaches, and others—to limit misconceptions that can become barriers to best practices in care.

THE INTERDISCIPLINARY TEAM

Successful concussion management at the professional level involves an interdisciplinary team of health care professionals. The medical staff typically include a physician with expertise in primary care sports medicine, orthopedics, or both. The role of the team physician is to evaluate physical functioning and integrate information from a variety of specialists to inform treatment and return-to-play decision making. Athletic trainers and physiotherapists provide the foundation upon which the medical team is built. These professionals interact with the players on a daily basis, know them personally, and have the best understanding of the player's usual behavior patterns. They are the "eyes and ears" of the medical team and typically the first to respond to injury. They usually work closely with the team physician to coordinate medical care, and they play primary roles in acute evaluations, day-to-day symptom monitoring, and execution of stepwise exertion protocols. Depending on their individual health care needs, athletes may be referred to a wide range of specialists, including neurologists, vestibular therapists, ophthalmologists, dentists, and others. Psychologists and psychiatrists may treat behavioral disturbances, and sports psychologists may be used for performance enhancement.

It is important to note, however, that successful implementation of a concussion program at the professional level requires more than a strong interdisciplinary *medical* team. Coaches, league executives, athletes, and player representatives must strongly support best-practice clinical guidelines. Ideally, a committee composed of all stake holders will receive concussion education and commit themselves to improving concussion identification, assessment, and care within the bounds of their respective sports. The clinical neuropsychologist with research experience can play an important educational role that helps foster ongoing program evaluation and a top-down culture of scientifically supported concussion management (Moser et al., 2007).

PRACTICE CHALLENGES IN PROFESSIONAL SPORTS

Cultural Diversity

Professional sports leagues commonly have competitors who hail from around the globe. The major professional leagues in North America have contracted athletes from South America, North America, Europe, Africa, Asia, and Australia. Athletes from different parts of the world bring a unique set of languages, cultural beliefs, and values. It has been well documented that differences in language, culture, and education have a significant impact on the neuropsychological evaluation (Ardila, Rodriguez-Menendez, & Rosselli, 2002; Harris, Echemendia, Ardila, & Rosselli, 2001; Manly & Echemendia, 2007). For instance, although concussion awareness has grown considerably over the past 20 years in the United States, athletes with diverse cultural backgrounds may continue to view a concussion as an insignificant injury that athletes should play through. Differences in education and literacy rates are also notable, with some professional athletes having had very little access to formal or adequate schooling when compared to North American standards (Echemendia, 2004). Access to medical facilities and awareness of neuro-psychological tests and practices also vary by country and socioeconomic status, with some professional athletes having little or no experience with standardized testing. Some professional athletes also have limited computer literacy. These cultural and linguistic differences may lead to misunderstandings about the role of neuropsychologists and the purpose of testing, with some athletes incorrectly believing that the tests are being used to evaluate their fitness to join the team (Echemendia, 2004).

Language differences present unique challenges given that many of the most sensitive neuropsychological tests (Daugherty, Puente, Fasfous, Hidalgo-Ruzzante, & Perez-Garcia, 2017) used in the sports domain are language dependent (Jones et al., 2014; Shuttleworth-Edwards, Whitefield-Alexander, Radloff, Taylor, & Lovell, 2009), most notably tests of verbal learning and memory. Unfortunately, large-scale normative neuropsychological data for use with concussed athletes from varying language backgrounds are not commercially available. As such, language-specific normative data are best obtained by means of coordinated league-wide efforts to obtain test data using a standardized battery of instruments that have appropriate translations, minimal language demands, or both. Moreover, best practices would dictate the use of a translator or perhaps translated handouts to aid the clinical interview and consent process when necessary.

Decades of research indicate that cultural factors influence performance on standardized and neuropsychological tests. Although some tests are, or have been, described as being free of cultural bias, it is now widely held that there are no culture-free tests (Glymour, Weuve, & Chen, 2008; Lim et al., 2009; Pedraza & Mungas, 2008). As a consequence, neuropsychologists who work with international athletes are encouraged to learn about their patients' cultures, adapt testing as needed, and interpret findings with an awareness of the limitations that exist when working with individuals whose backgrounds and history are different from those of the majority culture.

Time Pressures

Traditional neuropsychological assessments can take months to schedule, up to 8 hours to complete, and weeks to provide results. Evaluation of professional athletes is, by necessity, flexible and brief (Echemendia, 2006). Time is at a premium for athletes and their teams. For instance, during the preseason athletes must complete a laundry list of tasks (e.g., publicity pictures, equipment, media interviews, coaches' meetings, medical evaluations). In addition, they are frequently given a comprehensive medical evaluation at the outset of their competitive season. Baseline neuropsychological evaluation is only one part of this evaluation. Given the limited amount of time for medical evaluations (often dictated by collective bargaining agreements between league and union representatives) and the large number of players to be tested, baseline evaluations typically include a short battery of computerized neuropsychological or traditional tests, or both, administered as part of the preseason medical evaluation (usually 30 minutes and no more than 1 hour). Postinjury assessment requires scheduling flexibility because athletic trainers and team physicians frequently do not have notice as to when a player is ready for testing and often ask for an assessment with less than 48 hours' notice. Neuropsychological interview and testing usually lasts approximately 2 hours. Moreover, because results are provided the same day as the evaluation, reports are brief, often no more than one page.

Effort, Sandbagging, and Test Validity

Return-to-play decision making relies, in part, on baseline and post-concussion neuropsychological test comparisons. These results can inform postinjury deficits and aid in tracking recovery. However, the clinical utility of pre- to postinjury test comparisons can be limited if athletes exert suboptimal effort during baseline testing. In addition to concerns about suboptimal baseline effort, some players may try to outright game the system. Commonly referred to as *sandbagging*, this strategy has been anecdotally reported among players across many leagues who admit to purposefully performing poorly on baseline cognitive tests to ensure a quick return to play (Pennington, 2013). Although neuropsychological tests aim to detect malingering, suboptimal effort, and false reporting, problems with test validity persist. Commonly used neuropsychological assessments include free-standing and embedded validity measures to detect suboptimal effort (Lezak, Howieson, Bigler, & Tranel, 2012). However, the sensitivity of these measures has not been established among professional athletes. At present, clinicians are advised to create an environment that minimizes the risk of suboptimal effort by testing players individually or in small groups, providing education on the importance of the tests and the need for valid baseline data and requiring a player to repeat any test that is suspicious in regard to suboptimal performance.

Practice Effects and Testing Frequency

The traditional sports career is 4 years in both high school and collegiate play. Most amateur programs provide baseline testing on entry to the league with the assumption that these tests will remain valid throughout the athlete's playing career. Although the average professional career is relatively brief, some professional athletes remain active for decades. This begs the question: How long are baselines valid, and how many times does a baseline need to be repeated? Several investigators now question the long-term reliability of computerized testing (Bruce et al., 2016; Echemendia et al., 2016; Lezak et al., 2012; Odom et al., 2016; Putukian et al., 2015). Researchers have found that shorter time intervals between tests lead to better test–retest reliability (Moser, Schatz, Grosner, & Kollias, 2017; Randolph, McCrea, & Barr, 2005), which increases test sensitivity to cognitive perturbation. Many professional sports leagues have resources that allow for yearly testing; however, yearly testing is time consuming and expensive, and it raises the concern of practice effects due to a limited number of alternative test forms. No clear consensus has emerged regarding the absolute number of baselines required to maintain adequate test–retest reliability over longer careers.

Practice effects have widely been viewed as a measure of test error that helps lower the temporal stability of test scores. Although true, if practice effects are known through repeated testing of injured athletes these practice effects can be incorporated into interpretive algorithms using reliable change indices. Furthermore, the absence of practice effects in situations where practice effects are expected may be clinically useful in detecting subtle changes in learning and memory (Echemendia, Putukian, Mackin, Julian, & Shoss, 2001).

CURRENT PRACTICES IN ASSESSMENT OF PROFESSIONAL ATHLETES

Baseline Evaluation

Although some research has questioned the utility of the baseline–retest approach over standard normative approaches (Echemendia et al., 2012; Louey et al., 2014; McCrory, Makdissi, Davis, & Collie, 2005; Schatz & Robertshaw, 2014), obtaining baselines remains a cornerstone of neuropsychological assessment programs in professional sports. Obtaining baselines allows for the creation of population-specific norms that can be corrected for language and culture. Providing re-baselines for a large sample of professional athletes also facilitates the construction of population-specific reliable change indices, which allows for more accurate pre- and postinjury self-comparison.

Despite the widespread use of the within-patient baseline–postinjury approach, questions have been raised about the long-term test–retest reliability of commonly used neuropsychological measures at all levels of play (Broglio, Ferrara, Macciocchi, Baumgartner, & Elliott, 2007; Resch, McCrea, & Cullum, 2013). For instance, in a sample of professional athletes, Bruce and colleagues (2016) found low 1-year test–retest reliability for multiple language versions of Immediate Post-Concussion Assessment and Cognitive Testing (ImPACT), the most commonly used computerized battery in professional sports (Bruce, Echemendia, Meeuwisse, Comper, & Sisco, 2014). Similarly, Echemendia and colleagues (2016) found low 2-, 3-, and 4-year test–retest reliability of ImPACT among samples of English-speaking professional hockey players. Poor reliability reduces the sensitivity of a measure, increasing the likelihood that an athlete may return to play before full cognitive recovery.

Evidence indicates that the reliability of ImPACT can be improved by using alternative approaches of test administration and interpretation. Replicating Schatz and colleagues' findings among collegiate athletes, improved reliability has been demonstrated using a two-factor (Memory and Processing Speed) version of ImPACT in professional hockey (Bruce et al., 2016; Echemendia et al., 2016; Schatz & Maerlender, 2013). Despite converging evidence that the two-factor solution of ImPACT improves reliability, it is not available for commercial use. Consistent with classical test theory, Bruce and colleagues (2016) also demonstrated improved reliability of ImPACT using an aggregate baseline approach. Using the average of two baseline tests and the two-factor solution provided adequate or better long-term reliability in professional hockey. More research is needed to determine whether additional baselines (e.g., two or four) further improve reliability and clinical sensitivity to the cognitive effects of concussion.

Given time constraints for baseline testing as part of the preseason medical evaluation, as well as the considerable resources required for traditional neuropsychological evaluation, paper-and-pencil baseline tests are seldom given to all athletes. Instead, the hybrid testing model has been widely adopted. Using this model, in addition to repeat computerized testing, concussed athletes are given a short battery of traditional neuropsychological tests that is tailored to their language and cultural background. Because athletes with a history of concussion are at increased risk of concussion in the future, they also receive a baseline evaluation using a core battery of traditional paper-and-pencil tests at the outset of the next season. Should another concussion occur, neuropsychologists can use the baseline–retest approach when interpreting both computerized and traditional neuropsychological tests.

Acute Evaluation

In all professional sports, an athletic trainer and/or team physician will conduct an acute evaluation in the game setting. The nature and extent of the evaluation are sports specific given the variability in substitution rules. For example, the Fédération Internationale de Football Association (FIFA) only allows three substitutions per game, and pitch-side assessments typically cannot exceed 3 minutes. Pitch-side assessments that do exceed 3 minutes either require the team to play down one player or use a substitute, which is a clear disincentive to an adequate evaluation. In contrast, most other professional sports allow for game stoppage and evaluation of players without a substitution penalty. If a concussion is suspected after a sideline evaluation the medical team will proceed to a more comprehensive acute evaluation, usually modeled on the Sport Concussion Assessment Tool 5th Edition (SCAT5), a consensus-based standardized concussion evaluation that assesses self-reported symptoms, motor/vestibular functions, orientation, neurologic signs, and cognition (Echemendia et al., 2017; Yengo-Kahn et al., 2016). Briefer measures are sometimes used for sideline concussion screenings, including the Standardized Assessment of Concussion, which tests orientation and basic cognitive functions and is incorporated in the SCAT5 (McCrea et al., 1998; Yengo-Kahn et al., 2016); and the King–Devick (a visual measure of speeded information processing; Galetta et al., 2011). The SCAT5 typically is accompanied by a clinical examination by a team physician that includes evaluation of the cervical spine and neurological functioning. Checklists, such as those used in the Auckland (New Zealand) Rugby League and the National Rugby League, also may be used.

Athletes who are suspected of having a concussion often continue to play, which risks additional injury and prolonged recovery (Asken, McCrea, Clugston, et al., 2016; Elbin et al., 2016; Fraas, Coughlan, Hart, & McCarthy, 2014; McCrea, Hammeke, Olsen, Leo, & Guskiewicz, 2004; Meehan, Mannix, O'Brien, & Collins, 2013; Terwilliger, Pratson, Vaughan, & Gioia, 2016). As such, most professional leagues aim to identify concussed athletes promptly when a concussion is suspected. The identification of athletes with possible concussion typically involves the observation of visible signs of concussion (e.g., loss of consciousness, vacant look, motor incoordination, or balance problems) and/or self-reported symptoms. Observation of visible signs is typically conducted by medical staff and coaches, although some leagues (including the NFL and NHL) also employ spotters whose job it is to scan the playing environment for any visible signs of concussion and notify medical personnel promptly. Research examining the added clinical value of these approaches is currently underway.

Postinjury Evaluation

Postinjury assessment includes regular evaluation of symptoms when the athlete is at rest and, eventually, as part of a stepwise exertion protocol. Neuropsychological testing is typically ordered, either after symptoms have resolved or while the athlete is in the process of recovery, to assist the team physician with return-to-play decisions. Referrals to neuropsychology professionals are also often made to assist with complicated diagnoses, track recovery, and help in the evaluation of persisting symptoms.

The role of neuropsychologists is to integrate information from clinical interviews; test data; and the athlete's medical, academic, and social history. Common domains assessed as part of a focused neuropsychological clinical interview typical in a professional sports concussion assessment are shown in Table 11.1. There are different approaches to the selection of neuropsychological test instruments. Some leagues mandate a standardized core neuropsychological battery that serves as the minimum set of tests that should be administered to all players, although individual tests may be removed or added on the basis of clinical and cultural presentation. For instance, athletes who report significant emotional distress may be given validated self-report measures and semistructured diagnostic interviews to aid with diagnosis and treatment of possible psychopathology. When testing athletes who speak English as a second language, neuropsychologists may select tests on the bases of language demands, the existence of a comparative baseline, and the availability of appropriate normative data. In some instances, leagues do not dictate the specific tests that should be administered, leaving the decision to be made at the discretion of the neuropsychologist. Standardization of

TABLE 11.1

Common Components of a Clinical Interview

Area	Topics addressed
Demographics	Name, sex, age (DOB), education, acculturation, and language
Concussion	Date, mechanism, events, LOC, retrograde, anterograde, and symptoms (presence, length of time experienced, severity, changes in symptoms)
Current symptoms	Changes in cognition, mood, balance, sensory, and neurologic function at rest and during exertion
Concussion history	Date, LOC, amnesia, imaging, and length/type/severity of past symptoms
Medical/psychiatric history	Developmental (birth, milestones, childhood illnesses, learning disability, attention-deficit/hyperactivity disorder), neurologic, psychiatric (mood—specifically anxiety and/or depression, substance use), sleep, migraine, allergies, cardiovascular, surgical, and current medications

Note. DOB = date of birth; LOC = loss of consciousness.

test batteries within a league has the advantage of providing consistency of care for players across all teams in the league and allows for the development of sport-specific comprehensive normative data. However, as noted above, allowances for individual differences must be made for a broad range of clinical, cultural, educational, and linguistic presentations.

Providing Feedback and Counseling

Feedback is not typically given after baseline evaluation—unless it is requested by the athlete or when a test is invalid and repeat baseline testing is required. In contrast, feedback is typically given to both the medical staff and the concussed athlete immediately after the injury. The relationship among the neuropsychologist, the sports team, the team medical staff, and the individual athlete can be a source of ethical tension, as discussed by Echemendia and Bauer (2015). The team physician typically integrates information from various members of the interdisciplinary medical team and makes the ultimate determination regarding return to play. Therefore, consulting neuropsychologists working with professional teams generally restrict their feedback to whether the athlete has returned to baseline functioning. Neuropsychologists provide additional recommendations (e.g., cognitive-behavioral interventions) depending on the player's clinical presentation and the nature of the neuropsychologist's role as a member of the treatment team. It has also become increasingly common that athletes ask questions about possible neurocognitive effects of playing sports and seek advice. In these instances, it is incumbent on the neuropsychologist to provide information to the extent that he or she is comfortable and well versed in the current literature. It is also important to encourage athletes to speak with their team physicians about their concerns and to arrange for referrals as needed.

Education and prompt intervention have been shown to reduce the likelihood of a prolonged recovery (Silverberg et al., 2013; Zhang, Sing, Rugg, Feeley, & Senter, 2016). In professional arenas, educational programs designed to promote concussion awareness are becoming more commonplace (Lawrence, Comper, & Hutchison, 2016). Although the effectiveness of such programs is not fully understood, research suggests that education among coaching staff, trainers, and referees is beneficial (Fraas & Burchiel, 2016; Kroshus, Baugh, & Daneshvar, 2016). Neuropsychologists commonly counsel athletes regarding the typical symptoms that are associated with concussion and the typical course of recovery after concussion. As mentioned earlier, in light of recent significant media attention, many professional athletes also express concern about the possibility of CTE. To date, CTE can be diagnosed only postmortem by the identification of an agreed-on pattern of p-tau deposition. As a result of concerns about the possible long-term effects of concussion and subconcussive blows, neuropsychologists are increasingly educating athletes about the risks of repetitive brain trauma, distinguishing media and interpersonal speculation from scientific knowns and unknowns. For instance, the Sports Neuropsychological Society recently drafted a brief consensus educational document that can be used with players, coaches, and medical staff (Sports Neuropsychology Society, 2015). There is a growing literature on CTE and other neurodegenerative disorders as they relate to professional sports. Adequately covering this complex area is beyond the scope of this chapter (Alosco et al., 2017; Asken, Sullan, Snyder, et al., 2016; Iverson, Gardner, McCrory, Zafonte, & Castellani, 2015; Meehan, Mannix, Zafonte, & Pascual-Leone, 2015; Shetty, Raince, Manning, & Tsiouris, 2016).

FUTURE DIRECTIONS FOR NEUROPSYCHOLOGICAL RESEARCH AND PRACTICE

Development of a Best Practice Battery

In light of the limited time for baseline and postinjury assessments in the context of professional sports, the development of an evidence-based best practice test battery could help ensure that professional athletes are receiving the most efficient and effective evaluations. Delivery of evidence-based best practice batteries would, in turn, increase player safety and reduce the chance of premature return to play. Although the computerized and traditional tests commonly given as part of the postconcussion neuropsychological battery have each shown value in differentiating concussed athletes from nonconcussed controls, the unique value of each test when given in combination is unknown. As a result, it is possible that a shorter battery of highly sensitive tests would differentiate concussed from nonconcussed athletes as well or better than (due to reduced risk of Type I error) a longer battery that includes tests with no unique predictive ability. Removing tests that do not provide added value would free up assessment time, which may allow neuropsychologists to more thoroughly assess emotional functioning, motivation, or other domains of cognition that may improve diagnostic clarity and treatment.

Advancing Computerized Testing and Technology

Computerized testing offers several practical and clinical benefits. Administration is standardized and can be presented in multiple languages. Scoring is automated, and reaction time is generally more precise than manual timing. Nevertheless, there is significant room for improvement.

Memory Assessment

The most commonly used commercially available computerized measures do not assess free recall. Instead, these software platforms assess visual and verbal recognition memory, tasks that are typically less challenging and rely on different brain networks. This shortcoming is largely due to historical programming limitations in automated voice recognition and platform limitations that could not accurately capture and score patients' drawings. However, given substantial advances in voice recognition technologies and touchscreen interfaces that allow drawing with semiautomated scoring of recalled figures, it should be possible to capture these domains using computerized platforms. In addition to improving the sensitivity of computerized tests, incorporating these advances would allow for more thorough neuropsychological evaluations among professional athletes who do not fluently read or speak English.

Improved Reliability

Several studies have suggested that many automated tests have suboptimal test–retest reliability for time intervals commonly encountered in sports neuropsychology (Broglio et al., 2007; Bruce, Echemendia, Meeuwisse, et al., 2014; Bruce, Echemendia, Tangeman, et al., 2016; Echemendia et al., 2012; Iverson, Lovell, & Collins, 2003). Advances in computerized testing could make use of real-time automated feedback systems that could assess internal reliability and adjust testing accordingly. Professional athletes who demonstrate more inter- and intratest variability could receive tailored, longer, or split versions of the test that could more precisely measure their true ability. For example, if an athlete produced widely discrepant performances on two memory tests used to form a single general memory composite, then additional tests, alternate forms, or additional items could be automatically administered to clarify the athlete's estimated baseline abilities. This theoretically more accurate estimate of the athlete's baseline abilities could be used in combination with a regression-based formula to improve test–retest reliability. Higher reliability improves a test's ability to detect subtle cognitive deficits, providing additional protections to professional athletes who may be at increased risk for long-term cognitive changes. This tailored approach could also have additional benefits. For example, it is possible that test-taking motivation would improve if professional players were informed that consistent accurate responding could reduce exam time.

Real-Time Normative Data Development

One advantage of the baseline–postinjury approach is the use of automated scoring; however, additional advances in scoring could be made. To be specific, given the large number of baseline tests administered in sports neuropsychology, it would be possible to develop automated norms that update on a regular basis. In addition to reducing Flynn effects (the gradual improvement of normative test scores with increased societal industrialization; Hiscock, 2007; Russell, 2010), this would allow for the continual accrual of normative and reliable change data. Automated norming could foster further innovation, allowing for incremental software updates and the expansion of norms for non-English speakers and other traditionally underrepresented samples who are more commonly seen in professional sports.

Caveats to Advances in Computerized Assessment

Despite their clear benefits, computerized assessments and automated scoring reports can be easily misused by naïve but well-meaning health care professionals. Automated cognitive test results can be misleading, especially when interpreted by clinicians without adequate training in brain–behavior relationships and psychometric practice and theory. Competent interpretation of cognitive test results requires a detailed understanding of environmental, social, biological, and psychological factors that influence effort, motivation, and cognition (Echemendia, Herring, & Bailes, 2009). For example, use of these instruments by health care professionals without specialized training in these areas would jeopardize the validity of automated norm development. Improper interpretation of these data would also expose professional athletes to significant clinical risks. For instance, failing to properly assess for social, psychiatric, medical, and developmental history could lead an inexperienced clinician to erroneously ascertain that cognitive difficulties are due to concussion, leading to unwarranted treatments, increased emotional distress, and, possibly, curtailment of an athlete's career. Clinical neuropsychologists are best positioned to oversee the administration, scoring, and interpretation of neuropsychological tests at amateur and professional levels. Moreover, given advances in telemedicine and remote computerized assessment, we would expect improvements in access to this expertise in underserved areas.

ADVANCES IN MOTIVATION DETECTION

As noted above, media reports suggest that some professional athletes purposefully score poorly on baseline testing to make it easier to return to play with suboptimal cognitive performance postconcussion (Bailey et al., 2006). Many computerized and traditional cognitive batteries have embedded test validity measures. Although they likely are sensitive to grossly fabricated impairments that would typically be noted among samples of malingerers, these measures may not be sensitive to subtler motivational decrements typically seen in the sports context. Additional research to identify effective and accurate ways to detect poor motivation and ensure maximal effort during baseline testing at the professional level is needed. As noted above, one means of increasing test-taking motivation may be to provide external incentives (e.g., shorter testing sessions in exchange for adequate effort). In addition to using forced-choice measures, detection of poor effort may also benefit from the development of algorithms that compare performance with estimated premorbid abilities and examine abnormal inter- and intratest variability.

Incorporating Psychological Factors

It is well established that concussion can cause increased anxiety and depressed mood. Moreover, athletes with these symptoms are more likely to have prolonged symptoms with complicated recovery. Determining how to best assess these constructs in the setting of professional sports is challenging. Most assessments of mood and anxiety rely on self-report. Professional athletes may minimize their report of emotional symptoms because of both cultural stigma and the desire to compete. Additional research may wish to investigate objective means of assessing emotional change from pre- to postinjury. Alternatively, inclusion of self-report questionnaires with embedded symptom validity measures may help clinicians detect symptom minimization. For a more detailed discussion of these issues, see Chapter 8, this volume.

CASE STUDY

Some of the original details of this case have been changed to protect the confidentiality of the individual tested.

As noted above, professional athletes share many commonalities with other athletes, but they differ from amateur athletes in many important ways. There is considerable variability within and between the ranks of professional sports. Some marquee sports bring the promise of very lucrative salaries, the support of professional unions, and comprehensive medical coverage. Other professional sports are not as well developed. The case study we present is a fictionalized account of an athlete evaluated and managed by the lead author. We chose this case because the sport involved is not common and does not have a defined concussion protocol. However, the case highlights many of the issues faced by professional athletes and the role that neuropsychologists may play in their care.

Frank is an action sports athlete in his 30s who has been competing at the professional level since his late teenage years. He started in the sport at age 8. He has achieved a high level of success, winning several gold medals in international competitions. He has a large, dedicated fan base, but this sport has not developed the level of professionalism seen in other popular national leagues. Although earnings from competitions and sponsorships can be substantial, they do not rival the rarified levels of the major sports leagues. There are no unions, medical staffs, concussion protocols, equipment standards, or even teammates. Every athlete competes for him- or herself, with no collective bargaining. Like many professional sports, equipment and apparel manufacturers are eager to enter into sponsorship arrangements that can yield substantial revenue streams, typically negotiated on a year-to-year basis. To borrow a common phrase, these athletes "eat what they kill." They typically pay their own travel expenses to competitions, often to foreign countries, and get paid only if they place "in the money," usually the top five competitors. There is no guaranteed income. If injured, they cannot compete and hence will not be paid unless they have a disability policy, which are often exorbitantly priced. Although not quantified by any empirical study or sport injury surveillance program, Frank's sport is at high risk for SRC and musculoskeletal injuries. Like many action sports, this sport requires speed and the ability to execute complex "tricks," often at significant heights.

Frank first scheduled an appointment because he was concerned about the possible effects of repetitive head injuries. A related concern was that he and his ex-wife were involved in a bitter custody dispute and she was claiming that his repetitive head injuries caused him to be paranoid and dangerous even though no such allegations had been made previously and he had no history of aggressive or acting-out behaviors toward anyone. By his own account, and later substantiated by medical records, Frank had 12 documented SRCs, with two causing brief loss of consciousness, and several leading to both posttraumatic and retrograde amnesia. He completed high school with good grades. He did not have a history of learning disorders, attention-deficit/hyperactivity disorder, alcohol dependence or clinically significant use of recreational drugs. Frank reported that he had "broken every bone in [his] body" and had a history of multiple surgeries for orthopedic injuries. Despite his history, he had never come to the attention of a neuropsychologist, nor had he received any type of cognitive testing.

Because of Frank's history and his reasons for requesting an evaluation, a comprehensive neuropsychological evaluation was completed, including a magnetic resonance image (MRI). His brain MRI was completely normal. He was not complaining of any concussion symptoms at rest or after vigorous physical exercise; he was continuing to train and compete. Although there were no baseline data, the results of a comprehensive battery of traditional neuropsychological tests revealed scores within the average to high average range, consistent with psychometrically derived premorbid estimates. Standardized measures of psychological functioning revealed no evidence of clinically significant psychopathology, although there were indications of situational anxiety due to the family dynamics. In short, despite a history of repeated, and at times dramatic, head injuries, Frank was "normal" from a neuropsychological standpoint.

Although all clinical information suggested that he was not exhibiting any signs of neurocognitive dysfunction, his history of SRCs was clearly worrisome. Many important questions surfaced, including whether he should continue competing. He felt "fine" and looked "fine," but what about the next concussion? Would deficits show up later in life? Although there was no evidence to recommend immediate retirement, and he had no plans to walk away from his sport, we began the process of talking about retirement. The term *process* is emphasized here to differentiate it from a solitary decision in a moment in time. Unless faced with a career-ending injury, professional athletes typically undergo a process by which they assess their playing careers, their current status, and their hopes for the future outside of sport. Frank had to deal with important questions/concerns:

- When do I know it's time to stop?
- What would I do—this is all I know how to do.
- I like feeling unique, being in the spotlight.
- Can I afford to retire?
- How will people view me?
- I'm not a quitter.

He came to the decision that he wanted and needed "a few more years." Approximately 2 years later he sustained another concussion during a routine practice, this time with a 4- to 6-minute loss of consciousness. He sustained multiple facial fractures and had significant vestibular issues. His brain MRI was again normal. Neuropsychological testing using a hybrid sports battery was initially impaired but returned to baseline in 3 weeks. Vestibular functioning was restored without active treatment.

Again, the issue of retirement was raised. Frank agreed to enroll in college and explore options in business or broadcasting/color commentary. The decision to actively explore retirement options was also influenced by declining sponsorship funds because of the economy and time away from sport due to injuries. Opportunities to compete or perform in events were reduced because of realignment of the industry.

Nonetheless, Frank wanted one more opportunity for a gold medal: "I want to go out on top." Unfortunately, during the last event he fell and sustained multiple, very significant orthopedic fractures. The need to retire seemed clear, but he continued to vacillate through his rehabilitation. Over a period of approximately 6 months of consistent appointments Frank decided to retire. Ironically, it was Frank's orthopedic injuries that finally caused him to retire. He is now in the business world, remarried, and doing well.

This case brings to light several issues that are critical in sports neuropsychology. First and foremost, sports neuropsychologists have a unique combination of neurological and psychological training. For Frank, both elements were crucial in identifying possible neurocognitive sequela from his injuries and concurrently dealing with the life issues and critical questions involved in facilitating his retirement. Even though it was ultimately an orthopedic injury that led Frank to retire, he was prepared to do so and did not suffer from the depression and anxiety that often surface in less prepared athletes. Second, as sports neuropsychologists we are often asked questions for which there is scant empirical evidence (e.g., "How will I know when it's time to retire?" "Will my next concussion cause permanent damage?"). We need to be clear about the limits of our science while also providing our best clinical opinion. Third, we frequently do not have baseline data, and the athletes we see are not part of a standardized concussion protocol. As sports neuropsychologists we need to adapt, using our training to create the most appropriate evaluation that we can provide. We also need to learn about a variety of sports, understand their unique cultures, and clarify the unique challenges these professional athletes face. Last, this case underscored a professional athlete's desire to compete despite very significant injuries that require months of painful rehabilitation. We need to respect and support this drive to compete, but we also must be willing to challenge this view when it places athletes at risk for additional, possibly life-altering, difficulties.

CLINICAL TAKE-HOME POINTS

1. *Sports-related concussions among professional athletes present a unique challenge to the sports medicine team because of their complex admixture of cognitive, psychological, and neurological symptoms.* Clinicians must be attuned to, and knowledgeable of, the complexities in identifying and managing this injury.

2. *Concussions are treatable injuries that require active rehabilitation, including education of the player and families, from the very start of the injury.* Given the complexities of this injury, the possible significant effects on a professional athlete's career, and the resources available in professional sports, an interdisciplinary approach to treatment and management is critical.

3. *The return-to-play decision after concussion is dynamic and reflects the complexity of the biopsychosocial nature of the injury itself.* Multiple factors, including whether the player desires to return to sport, must be weighed in reaching an informed decision.

4. *The retirement decision for a professional athlete is a process, not an isolated event, that requires careful consideration of the athlete's psychological functioning throughout the entire process.*

KEY QUESTIONS TO BE ADDRESSED IN THE NEXT 5 YEARS

1. *Is there a specific number of concussions that warrant retirement from play?* If no specific number exists, are there characteristics of the concussion (e.g., symptom burden, symptom severity, symptom duration, temporal sequencing of concussions) that provide clear indications for cessation of sports activity?

2. *Are there any biomarkers that definitively indicate the presence (or absence) of concussion?*

3. *Does physiological recovery extend beyond clinical recovery and, if so, does physiological recovery have implications for physical or cognitive functioning?*

4. *What, if any, associations exist between playing contact and collision sports and long-term neuropsychological, psychological, and physical functioning?*

REFERENCES

Alosco, M. L., Mez, J., Kowall, N. W., Stein, T. D., Goldstein, L. E., Cantu, R. C., . . . McKee, A. C. (2017). Cognitive reserve as a modifier of clinical expression in chronic traumatic encephalopathy: A preliminary examination. *The Journal of*

Neuropsychiatry and Clinical Neurosciences, 29, 6–12. http://dx.doi.org/10.1176/appi.neuropsych.16030043

Ardila, A., Rodriguez-Menendez, G., & Rosselli, M. (2002). Current issues in neuropsychological assessment with Hispanics/Latinos. In R. Ferraro (Ed.), *Minority and cross-cultural aspects of neuropsychological assessment* (pp. 161–179). Lisse, The Netherlands: Swets & Zeitlinger.

Asken, B. M., McCrea, M. A., Clugston, J. R., Snyder, A. R., Houck, Z. M., & Bauer, R. M. (2016). "Playing through it": Delayed reporting and removal from athletic activity after concussion predicts prolonged recovery. *Journal of Athletic Training, 51*, 329–335. http://dx.doi.org/10.4085/1062-6050-51.5.02

Asken, B. M., Sullan, M. J., Snyder, A. R., Houck, Z. M., Bryant, V. E., Hizel, L. P., . . . Bauer, R. M. (2016). Factors influencing clinical correlates of chronic traumatic encephalopathy (CTE): A review. *Neuropsychology Review, 26*, 340–363. http://dx.doi.org/10.1007/s11065-016-9327-z

Bailey, C. M., Echemendia, R. J., & Arnett, P. A. (2006). The impact of motivation on neuropsychological performance in sports-related mild traumatic brain injury. *Journal of the International Neuropsychological Society, 12*, 475–484. http://dx.doi.org/10.1017/S1355617706060619

Block, C. K., West, S. E., & Goldin, Y. (2016). Misconceptions and misattributions about traumatic brain injury: An integrated conceptual framework. *PM&R, 8*, 58–68. http://dx.doi.org/10.1016/j.pmrj.2015.05.022

Broglio, S. P., Ferrara, M. S., Macciocchi, S. N., Baumgartner, T. A., & Elliott, R. (2007). Test–retest reliability of computerized concussion assessment programs. *Journal of Athletic Training, 42*, 509–514.

Bruce, J., Echemendia, R., Meeuwisse, W., Comper, P., & Sisco, A. (2014). 1 year test–retest reliability of ImPACT in professional ice hockey players. *The Clinical Neuropsychologist, 28*, 14–25. http://dx.doi.org/10.1080/13854046.2013.866272

Bruce, J., Echemendia, R., Tangeman, L., Meeuwisse, W., Comper, P., Hutchison, M., & Aubry, M. (2016). Two baselines are better than one: Improving the reliability of computerized testing in sports neuropsychology. *Applied Neuropsychology: Adult, 23*, 336–342. http://dx.doi.org/10.1080/23279095.2015.1064002

Bundesliga Report 2016. (2016). *Frankfurt, Germany: DFL Deutsche FuBball Liga GmbH* [The 2014–15 season at a glance]. Retrieved from https://www.bundesliga.com/en/media-service/report/

Carless, D., & Douglas, K. (2013). Living, resisting, and playing the part of athlete: Narrative tensions in elite sport. *Psychology of Sport and Exercise, 14*, 701–708. http://dx.doi.org/10.1016/j.psychsport.2013.05.003

Carlson, B. D., & Donavan, D. T. (2013). Human brands in sport: Athlete brand personality and identification. *Journal of Sport Management, 27*, 193–206. http://dx.doi.org/10.1123/jsm.27.3.193

Caron, J. G., Bloom, G. A., Johnston, K. M., & Sabiston, C. M. (2013). National Hockey League players' experiences with career-ending concussions. *British Journal of Sports Medicine, 47*(5), e1. http://dx.doi.org/10.1136/bjsports-2012-092101.43

Charbonneau, J., & Garland, R. (2005). Talent, looks or brains? New Zealand advertising practitioners' views on celebrity and athlete endorsers. *Marketing Bulletin, 16*, 1–10.

Daugherty, J. C., Puente, A. E., Fasfous, A. F., Hidalgo-Ruzzante, N., & Perez-Garcia, M. (2017). Diagnostic mistakes of culturally diverse individuals when using North American neuropsychological tests. *Applied Neuropsychology: Adult, 24*, 16–22.

Despres, J., Brady, F., & McGowan, A. S. (2008). Understanding the culture of the student–athlete: Implications for college counselors. *The Journal of Humanistic Counseling, Education and Development, 47*, 200–211. http://dx.doi.org/10.1002/j.2161-1939.2008.tb00058.x

Echemendia, R. J. (2004). Cultural aspects of neuropsychological evaluation in sports. In M. Lovell, R. Echemendia, J. Barth, & M. Collins (Eds.), *Traumatic brain injury in sports: An international neuropsychological perspective* (pp. 435–443). Lisse, The Netherlands: Swets & Zeitlinger.

Echemendia, R. J. (2006). *Sports neuropsychology: Assessment and management of traumatic brain injury.* New York, NY: Guilford Press.

Echemendia, R. J., & Bauer, R. M. (2015). Professional ethics in sports neuropsychology. *Psychological Injury and Law, 8*, 289–299. http://dx.doi.org/10.1007/s12207-015-9241-3

Echemendia, R. J., Bruce, J. M., Bailey, C. M., Sanders, J. F., Arnett, P., & Vargas, G. (2012). The utility of post-concussion neuropsychological data in identifying cognitive change following sports-related MTBI in the absence of baseline data. *The Clinical Neuropsychologist, 26*, 1077–1091. http://dx.doi.org/10.1080/13854046.2012.721006

Echemendia, R. J., Bruce, J. M., Meeuwisse, W., Comper, P., Aubry, M., & Hutchison, M. (2016). Long-term reliability of ImPACT in professional ice hockey. *The Clinical Neuropsychologist, 30*, 311–320. http://dx.doi.org/10.1080/13854046.2016.1158320

Echemendia, R. J., Herring, S., & Bailes, J. (2009). Who should conduct and interpret the neuropsychological assessment in sports-related concussion? *British Journal of Sports Medicine, 43*(Suppl. 1), i32–i35. http://dx.doi.org/10.1136/bjsm.2009.058164

Echemendia, R. J., Meeuwisse, W., McCrory, P., Davis, G. A., Putukian, M., Leddy, J., . . . Herring, S. (2017). The Sport Concussion Assessment Tool 5th Edition (SCAT5): Background and rationale. *British Journal of Sports Medicine, 51*, 848–850. http://dx.doi.org/10.1136/bjsports-2017-097506

Echemendia, R. J., Putukian, M., Mackin, R. S., Julian, L., & Shoss, N. (2001). Neuropsychological test performance prior to and following sports-related mild traumatic brain injury. *Clinical Journal of Sport Medicine, 11*, 23–31. http://dx.doi.org/10.1097/00042752-200101000-00005

Elbin, R. J., Sufrinko, A., Schatz, P., French, J., Henry, L., Burkhart, S., . . . Kontos, A. P. (2016). Removal from play after concussion and recovery time. *Pediatrics,*

138(3), e20160910. Advance online publication. http://dx.doi.org/10.1542/peds.2016-0910

Fraas, M. R., & Burchiel, J. (2016). A systematic review of education programmes to prevent concussion in rugby union. *European Journal of Sport Science, 16*, 1212–1218. http://dx.doi.org/10.1080/17461391.2016.1170207

Fraas, M. R., Coughlan, G. F., Hart, E. C., & McCarthy, C. (2014). Concussion history and reporting rates in elite Irish rugby union players. *Physical Therapy in Sport, 15*, 136–142. http://dx.doi.org/10.1016/j.ptsp.2013.08.002

Galetta, K. M., Brandes, L. E., Maki, K., Dziemianowicz, M. S., Laudano, E., Allen, M., . . . Balcer, L. J. (2011). The King–Devick test and sports-related concussion: Study of a rapid visual screening tool in a collegiate cohort. *Journal of Neurological Science, 309*, 34–39.

Glick, I. D., & Horsfall, J. L. (2005). Diagnosis and psychiatric treatment of athletes. *Clinics in Sports Medicine, 24*, 771–781. http://dx.doi.org/10.1016/j.csm.2005.03.007

Glymour, M. M., Weuve, J., & Chen, J. T. (2008). Methodological challenges in causal research on racial and ethnic patterns of cognitive trajectories: Measurement, selection, and bias. *Neuropsychology Review, 18*, 194–213. http://dx.doi.org/10.1007/s11065-008-9066-x

Harris, J., Echemendia, R. J., Ardila, A., & Rosselli, M. (2001). Cross-cultural cognitive and neuropsychological assessment. In H. J. J. Andrews & D. Saklofske (Eds.), *Handbook of psychoeducational assessment* (pp. 391–414). San Diego, CA: Academic Press. http://dx.doi.org/10.1016/B978-012058570-0/50015-X

Hiscock, M. (2007). The Flynn effect and its relevance to neuropsychology. *Journal of Clinical and Experimental Neuropsychology, 29*, 514–529. http://dx.doi.org/10.1080/13803390600813841

Iverson, G. L., Gardner, A. J., McCrory, P., Zafonte, R., & Castellani, R. J. (2015). A critical review of chronic traumatic encephalopathy. *Neuroscience and Biobehavioral Reviews, 56*, 276–293. http://dx.doi.org/10.1016/j.neubiorev.2015.05.008

Iverson, G. L., Lovell, M. R., & Collins, M. W. (2003). Interpreting change on ImPACT following sport concussion. *The Clinical Neuropsychologist, 17*, 460–467. http://dx.doi.org/10.1076/clin.17.4.460.27934

Jones, N. S., Walter, K. D., Caplinger, R., Wright, D., Raasch, W. G., & Young, C. (2014). Effect of education and language on baseline concussion screening tests in professional baseball players. *Clinical Journal of Sport Medicine, 24*, 284–288. http://dx.doi.org/10.1097/JSM.0000000000000031

Kroshus, E., Baugh, C. M., & Daneshvar, D. H. (2016). Content, delivery, and effectiveness of concussion education for US college coaches. *Clinical Journal of Sport Medicine, 26*, 391–397. http://dx.doi.org/10.1097/JSM.0000000000000272

Lawrence, D. W., Comper, P., & Hutchison, M. G. (2016). Influence of extrinsic risk factors on National Football League injury rates. *Orthopaedic Journal of Sports Medicine, 4*. Advance online publication. http://dx.doi.org/10.1177/2325967116639222

Lezak, M., Howieson, D., Bigler, E., & Tranel, D. (2012). *Neuropsychological assessment* (5th ed.). New York, NY: Oxford University Press.

Lim, Y. Y., Prang, K. H., Cysique, L., Pietrzak, R. H., Snyder, P. J., & Maruff, P. (2009). A method for cross-cultural adaptation of a verbal memory assessment. *Behavior Research Methods, 41,* 1190–1200. http://dx.doi.org/10.3758/BRM.41.4.1190

Louey, A. G., Cromer, J. A., Schembri, A. J., Darby, D. G., Maruff, P., Makdissi, M., & Mccrory, P. (2014). Detecting cognitive impairment after concussion: Sensitivity of change from baseline and normative data methods using the CogSport/Axon cognitive test battery. *Archives of Clinical Neuropsychology, 29,* 432–441. http://dx.doi.org/10.1093/arclin/acu020

Manly, J. J., & Echemendia, R. J. (2007). Race-specific norms: Using the model of hypertension to understand issues of race, culture, and education in neuropsychology. *Archives of Clinical Neuropsychology, 22,* 319–325. http://dx.doi.org/10.1016/j.acn.2007.01.006

McCrea, M., Hammeke, T., Olsen, G., Leo, P., & Guskiewicz, K. (2004). Unreported concussion in high school football players: Implications for prevention. *Clinical Journal of Sport Medicine, 14,* 13–17. http://dx.doi.org/10.1097/00042752-200401000-00003

McCrea, M., Kelly, J. P., Randolph, C., Kluge, J., Bartolic, E., Finn, G., & Baxter, B. (1998). Standardized Assessment of Concussion (SAC): On-site mental status evaluation of the athlete. *The Journal of Head Trauma Rehabilitation, 13,* 27–35. http://dx.doi.org/10.1097/00001199-199804000-00005

McCrory, P., Makdissi, M., Davis, G., & Collie, A. (2005). Value of neuropsychological testing after head injuries in football. *British Journal of Sports Medicine, 39*(Suppl. 1), i58–i63. http://dx.doi.org/10.1136/bjsm.2005.020776

McKee, A. C., Alosco, M. L., & Huber, B. R. (2016). Repetitive head impacts and chronic traumatic encephalopathy. *Neurosurgery Clinics of North America, 27,* 529–535. http://dx.doi.org/10.1016/j.nec.2016.05.009

Meehan, W. P., III, Mannix, R. C., O'Brien, M. J., & Collins, M. W. (2013). The prevalence of undiagnosed concussions in athletes. *Clinical Journal of Sport Medicine, 23,* 339–342. http://dx.doi.org/10.1097/JSM.0b013e318291d3b3

Meehan, W. P., III, Mannix, R., Zafonte, R., & Pascual-Leone, A. (2015). Chronic traumatic encephalopathy and athletes. *Neurology, 85,* 1504–1511.

Moser, R. S., Iverson, G. L., Echemendia, R. J., Lovell, M. R., Schatz, P., Webbe, F. M., . . . Silver, C. H. (2007). Neuropsychological evaluation in the diagnosis and management of sports-related concussion. *Archives of Clinical Neuropsychology, 22,* 909–916. http://dx.doi.org/10.1016/j.acn.2007.09.004

Moser, R. S., Schatz, P., Grosner, E., & Kollias, K. (2017). One year test–retest reliability of neurocognitive baseline scores in 10- to 12-year-olds. *Applied Neuropsychology: Child, 6,* 166–171. http://dx.doi.org/10.1080/21622965.2016.1138310

NFL Team Salary Cap Tracker. (2016). Retrieved from http://www.spotrac.com/nfl/cap/

NFL Team Salary Cap Tracker. (2017). Retrieved from http://www.spotrac.com/nfl/cap/

Odom, M. J., Lee, Y. M., Zuckerman, S. L., Apple, R. P., Germanos, T., Solomon, G. S., & Sills, A. K. (2016). Balance assessment in sports-related concussion: Evaluating test–retest reliability of the equilibrate system. *Journal of Surgical Orthopaedic Advances, 25*, 93–98.

Pedraza, O., & Mungas, D. (2008). Measurement in cross-cultural neuropsychology. *Neuropsychology Review, 18*, 184–193. http://dx.doi.org/10.1007/s11065-008-9067-9

Pennington, B. (2013, May 5). Flubbing a baseline test on purpose is often futile. *The New York Times*. Retrieved from https://mobile.nytimes.com/2013/05/06/sports/sandbagging-first-concussion-test-probably-wont-help-later.html

Putukian, M., Echemendia, R., Dettwiler-Danspeckgruber, A., Duliba, T., Bruce, J., Furtado, J. L., & Murugavel, M. (2015). Prospective clinical assessment using Sideline Concussion Assessment Tool–2 testing in the evaluation of sport-related concussion in college athletes. *Clinical Journal of Sport Medicine, 25*, 36–42. http://dx.doi.org/10.1097/JSM.0000000000000102

Randolph, C., McCrea, M., & Barr, W. B. (2005). Is neuropsychological testing useful in the management of sport-related concussion? *Journal of Athletic Training, 40*, 139–152.

Resch, J. E., McCrea, M. A., & Cullum, C. M. (2013). Computerized neurocognitive testing in the management of sport-related concussion: An update. *Neuropsychology Review, 23*, 335–349. http://dx.doi.org/10.1007/s11065-013-9242-5

Russell, E. W. (2010). The "obsolescence" of assessment procedures. *Applied Neuropsychology, 17*, 60–67. http://dx.doi.org/10.1080/09084280903297917

Schatz, P., & Maerlender, A. (2013). A two-factor theory for concussion assessment using ImPACT: Memory and speed. *Archives of Clinical Neuropsychology, 28*, 791–797. http://dx.doi.org/10.1093/arclin/act077

Schatz, P., & Robertshaw, S. (2014). Comparing post-concussive neurocognitive test data to normative data presents risks for under-classifying "above average" athletes. *Archives of Clinical Neuropsychology, 29*, 625–632. http://dx.doi.org/10.1093/arclin/acu041

Shetty, T., Raince, A., Manning, E., & Tsiouris, A. J. (2016). Imaging in chronic traumatic encephalopathy and traumatic brain injury. *Sports Health, 8*, 26–36. http://dx.doi.org/10.1177/1941738115588745

Shuttleworth-Edwards, A. B., Whitefield-Alexander, V. J., Radloff, S. E., Taylor, A. M., & Lovell, M. R. (2009). Computerized neuropsychological profiles of South African versus U.S. athletes: A basis for commentary on cross-cultural norming issues in the sports concussion arena. *The Physician and Sportsmedicine, 37*, 45–52. http://dx.doi.org/10.3810/psm.2009.12.1741

Silverberg, N. D., Hallam, B. J., Rose, A., Underwood, H., Whitfield, K., Thornton, A. E., & Whittal, M. L. (2013). Cognitive–behavioral prevention of post-concussion syndrome in at-risk patients: A pilot randomized controlled trial. *The*

Journal of Head Trauma Rehabilitation, 28, 313–322. http://dx.doi.org/10.1097/ HTR.0b013e3182915cb5

Sports Neuropsychology Society. (2015). *Chronic traumatic encephalopathy: A Q and A fact sheet.* Retrieved from http://www.sportsneuropsychologysociety.com/ wp-content/uploads/2018/05/CTE-Fact-Sheet-2018.pdf

Terwilliger, V. K., Pratson, L., Vaughan, C. G., & Gioia, G. A. (2016). Additional post-concussion impact exposure may affect recovery in adolescent athletes. *Journal of Neurotrauma, 33,* 761–765. http://dx.doi.org/10.1089/neu.2015.4082

The Sports Xchange. (2017, February 8). *Green Bay Packers release CB Sam Shields after multiple concussions.* Retrieved from http://www.upi.com/Sports_News/ NFL/2017/02/08/Green-Bay-Packers-release-CB-Sam-Shields-after-multiple-concussions/6481486582785/

Williams, J. M., Langdon, J. L., McMillan, J. L., & Buckley, T. A. (2016). English professional football players concussion knowledge and attitude. *Journal of Sport and Health Science, 5,* 197–204. http://dx.doi.org/10.1016/ j.jshs.2015.01.009

Yengo-Kahn, A. M., Hale, A. T., Zalneraitis, B. H., Zuckerman, S. L., Sills, A. K., & Solomon, G. S. (2016). The Sport Concussion Assessment Tool: A systematic review. *Neurosurgical Focus, 40,* E6. http://dx.doi.org/10.3171/ 2016.1.FOCUS15611

Young, E. (2015). *The economic impact of the Premier League.* London, England: Ernst & Young.

Zhang, A. L., Sing, D. C., Rugg, C. M., Feeley, B. T., & Senter, C. (2016). The rise of concussions in the adolescent population. *Orthopaedic Journal of Sports Medicine, 4.* Advance online publication. http://dx.doi.org/10.1177/2325967116662458

12

APPLICATION OF VIRTUAL REALITY IN ASSESSMENT AND TREATMENT OF CONCUSSION

ALEXA E. WALTER AND SEMYON M. SLOBOUNOV

Mild traumatic brain injury has recently become a public concern because of its high prevalence in sports, affecting anywhere from 1.6 to 3.8 million Americans a year (Langlois, Rutland-Brown, & Wald, 2006). Mild traumatic brain injuries, or concussions, are still not well understood because of their individual natures; no two injuries are alike in mechanism, symptomology, or resolution. There is also still no agreed-on diagnosis or treatment for this injury, so in this chapter we explore the use of virtual reality (VR) as a potential clinical option.

Concussion is loosely defined as a disturbance of neural functions induced by a sudden acceleration or deceleration of the head (Trotter, 1924). Some mechanical trauma exposes the brain to various linear and rotational forces that results in a complex pathophysiological response (Barkhoudarian, Hovda, & Giza, 2011). On impact, cellular damage occurs when neurometabolic changes cause an inflammatory response and decreased cerebral blood flow. These changes to the brain chemistry can cause various acute and chronic

http://dx.doi.org/10.1037/0000114-013
Neuropsychology of Sports-Related Concussion, P. A. Arnett (Editor)

symptoms that typically affect neurocognitive, motor, and executive functioning. Acute (short term, within 7–10 days after the injury) and chronic (those persisting 6 months or longer after the injury) symptoms can include loss of consciousness, headache, nausea, dizziness, vomiting, changes in mood, sensitivity to noise and light, problems with sleep, and difficulty concentrating and remembering. Most concussions resolve spontaneously within 10 days of the injury, but there is a subset of concussive injuries that can persist for months to years after the injury. Underlying mechanisms and predisposing factors for differential clinical recovery after concussive injury are still unknown. Because of the growing clinical concerns over the immediate and long-term effects of multiple and frequent concussive blows, much research has been dedicated to various tools to study these impacts and their structural and functional effects.

In general, acute and chronic alterations after concussion have been documented in neurocognitive (Nauman et al., 2015), working memory (Talavage et al., 2014), biochemistry (Poole et al., 2014), white matter (Chun et al., 2015), brain networking (Abbas et al., 2015), cerebrovascular reactivity (Svaldi et al., 2015), and microhemorrhaging (Kou et al., 2013) studies. In addition, biomarkers, specifically serum and cerebral spinal fluid, have been used to examine tau (Gatson & Diaz-Arrastia, 2014), S100 calcium-binding protein B (Schulte, Podlog, Hamson-Utley, Strathmann, & Strüder, 2014), and glial fibrillary acidic protein (Papa et al., 2014) for use as a potential diagnostic tool. Also, the possibility of a genetic link has been explored, with promising results seen in apolipoprotein E (*APOE*; Terrell et al., 2014) and variable number tandem repeats (McDevitt et al., 2014). Recently, it has been reported that *APOE ε4* is associated with increased symptom reporting (Merritt & Arnett, 2016) and headache (Merritt, Ukueberuwa, & Arnett, 2016) after sports-related concussions.

Within magnetic resonance imaging (MRI), many sequences have been used to show structural changes due to concussion. Positron emission tomography (Chang, Ramirez, Herbst, & Coris, 2009; Radanov, 2001), magnetic resonance spectroscopy (Gardner, Iverson, & Stanwell, 2014), diffusion tensor imaging (Luther et al., 2012; Gardner et al., 2012), arterial spin labeling (Meier et al., 2015; Wang et al., 2015), resting state functional MRI (Chong & Schwedt, 2015; Slobounov, Gay, et al., 2011), and others have all shown various alterations in brain structure and function across acute, subacute, and chronic concussions. Details of these neuroimaging studies can be found elsewhere in this volume in Chapter 5.

Because of the controversy over concussions and their lasting effects, baseline testing has become implemented in many high school and collegiate sports. Computerized neuropsychological testing, including ImPACT (Lovell, Collins, & Bradley, 2004), is commonly used because of its ease of administration and the ability to administer it to large numbers quickly. However, conventional neuropsychological tests can be problematic because they are not designed to assess complex pathophysiological effects of a concussion. They also can have practice effect problems (Bartels, Wegrzyn, Wiedl, Ackermann, & Ehrenreich, 2010). There is a concern with athletes purposely manipulating their baseline results, and the possibility that lengthy neuropsychological testing can induce mental fatigue, especially in injured athletes (Barwick, Arnett, & Slobounov, 2012). However, one concern is that conventional neuropsychological testing may sometimes lack ecological validity and transferability to real-life situations. Therefore, advanced technologies, including VR, may partly address these concerns.

VR is an interactive, computer-generated three-dimensional (3D) environment that can simulate real-world environments and provide a sensation of immersion in the subjects. It can be programmed to be used as an assessment tool that can examine neurocognitive, executive, and motor functions. VR can also be used as a tool for the accurate assessment of the damage due to a concussive blow. The Berlin consensus statement on concussion in sport (McCrory et al., 2017) identified VR among the key areas of future research and possible clinical application. At present, VR is implemented into many therapies and can be used in the assessment and treatment of many medical conditions, including, but not limited to, neurological diseases, including stroke and cerebral palsy. In many cases, the use of VR results in improved functioning among these populations. In addition, many occupations, including the medical and military fields, use VR for training purposes; however, more implementation in clinical and research practices is needed.

USE OF VIRTUAL REALITY GRAPHICS IN THE ASSESSMENT OF CONCUSSION

Vision, in conjunction with other somatosensory systems, is heavily involved in most aspects of daily functioning both in and far beyond the athletic environment. After a concussion, abnormal balance is a common symptom and is most evident during dynamic postural tasks when vision is compromised (Thompson, Sebastianelli, & Slobounov, 2005). Compromised vision can lead to a destabilizing effect due to the involvement of vision in maintaining balance, optic flow, and visual field motion (Keshner & Kenyon, 2000). VR has the ability, through the use of programmable graphics, to induce *egomotion*, the actual body motion in response to optic flow (Slobounov, Slobounov, & Newell, 2006) which can be induced in subjects by exposing them to continuous and changing visual fields. Slobounov et al. (2006), tested 55 subjects on their postural response to visual field motion by using a VR environment, force platform, and a motion tracking (flock of birds) system. Subjects who had received a concussion during the season ($n = 10$) were tested again at 3 days, 10 days, and 30 days after the injury. The results showed that nonconcussed subjects could adapt to the visual field disruption, demonstrating an intact perceptual-motion integration network. However, no concussed subjects were able to preserve their balance while viewing a moving room at 3 days after the injury. At 10 days, the concussed subjects still had a significantly lower coherence than controls and it remained decreased at 30 days. This study demonstrated the use of VR graphics to examine the effects of visual field motion on balance, especially in a concussed population.

VR graphics can also be incorporated with electroencephalography (EEG) to examine brain activation patterns while subjects perform various postural or cognitive tasks; specifically, it can be used to look at patterns preceding a loss of stability induced by the moving-room VR task. In another study by Slobounov, Sebastianelli, and Newell (2011), 15 nonconcussed subjects and 14 concussed subjects were tested using VR with a force platform and body motion tracking system, along with a 64-channel EEG. Nonconcussed subjects were again able to adapt to the changing visual field motion, demonstrating they had intact visual–kinesthetic integration in their control of balance. Most important, the concussed subjects had an absence of enhanced central–frontal theta. In conjunction with their balance problems, this could also indicate impaired neural substrates related to focused attention when more challenging postural stances are required. VR has a unique ability to allow for the control and manipulation of movement while creating a sense of self-motion.

Virtual Reality Hardware Solutions

There are many different options available to implement VR technology in a research and clinical setting, including stationary (laboratory oriented; see Figure 12.1) or portable (oculus; see Figure 12.2) or head mount display (see Figure 12.3) systems. These systems allow the following modules, outlined in the next section, to be implemented in a laboratory, an athletic training setting, or on the sideline.

Virtual Reality Methods and Procedures

Spatial Navigation Task

This task assesses memory function (specifically spatial memory) using a 3D representation of a visual corridor (see Figure 12.4). The subjects are shown a route to and from a door (encoding stage) then immediately are asked to navigate the same route using a joystick. Subjects are able to move

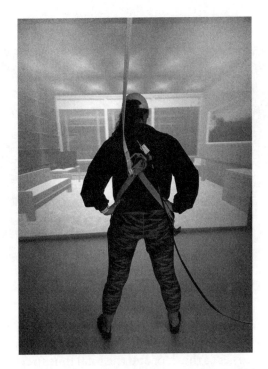

Figure 12.1. Stationary system. Photo courtesy of Alexa E. Walter.

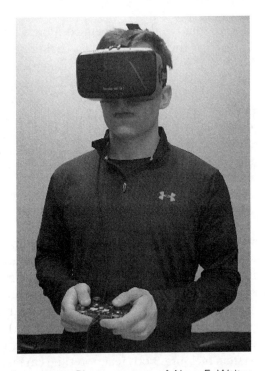

Figure 12.2. Oculus system. Photo courtesy of Alexa E. Walter.

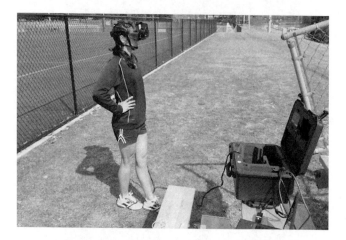

Figure 12.3. Head mount display system. Photo courtesy of Alexa E. Walter.

in a forward, backward, left, and right direction. A total of three trials are allowed to successfully complete the pathway. The system measures how many errors it takes to get to the door and the total time to complete the task.

Balance Task

Subjects are asked to stand in the Romberg position, with either foot in the front, and with hands on their hips. The first trial presents a stationary virtual room (see Figure 12.5) to obtain a baseline balance score. The remaining six to nine trials involve the room moving in the following five directions: (a) forward–backward oscillatory translation, (b) roll around heading y-axis between 10° and 30° at 0.2 Hz, (c) pitch around interaural x-axis between 10° and 30° at 0.2 Hz, (d) yaw around vertical z-axis between 10° and 30° at 0.2 Hz, and (e) translation along x-axis within 18 cm displacement at 0.2 Hz. The system measures the position and orientation in yaw, pitch, and roll directions.

Reaction Time Task

In this task, which focuses on executive functioning specifically, reaction times are measured. This module was designed to measure the full body response to unpredictable manipulation of optic flow (see Figure 12.6). The subject is asked to sway forward and backward (anterior–posterior) with the movement of the room. At a randomized point during each trial, an unpredictable change to the left or right (medial–lateral direction) is introduced. The subject is asked to respond to this change of direction with a whole-body motion. The system measures both reaction time (in ms) and errors of anticipation (wrong direction of response).

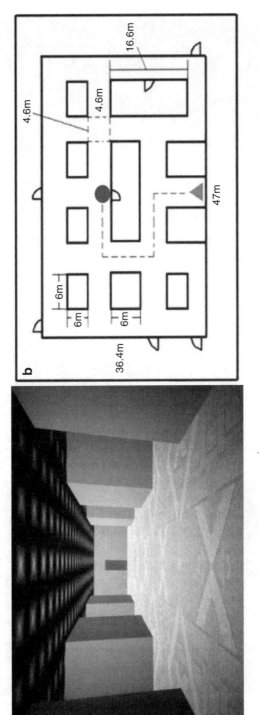

Figure 12.4. View of (a) the corridor as it would appear to the participant and (b) the floor plan and sample route of one of the trials. Subjects are shown the route from the triangle to the circle and then from the circle to the triangle and asked to reproduce the exact route. Copyright 2018 by HeadRehab, Inc.

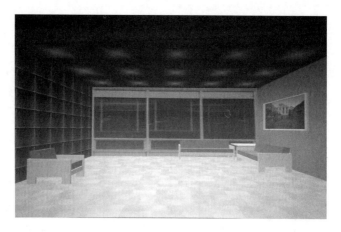

Figure 12.5. The room the participant is in for all balance scenarios. Copyright 2018 by HeadRehab, Inc.

Attention Task

In this task, participants are placed in an elevator to test various levels of attention. The elevator moves up (Floor 1–Floor 12) and down (Floor 12–Floor 1) with a visual separation that the subjects can count to identify the floor on which they arrive (see Figure 12.7). Subjects are asked to keep track of the floor they are on (sustained attention and executive function); however, distractions occur during the entirety of the task. Preprogrammed sources of noise (e.g., telephone ringing; music) and questions (e.g., "What is your name?" "How many classes are you taking?") are presented during the task. The system measures how many errors occur during the task.

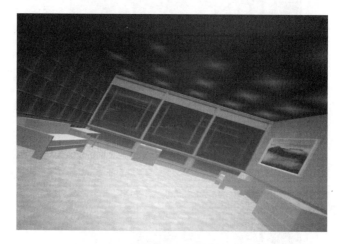

Figure 12.6. The reaction time scenario during a left–right (medial–lateral) movement. Copyright 2018 by HeadRehab, Inc.

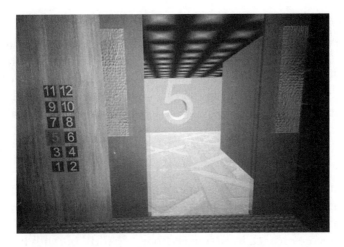

Figure 12.7. Visual representation of the virtual elevator scenario. Copyright 2018 by HeadRehab, Inc.

Recognition "A" Task

This task tests the subjects' visual recognition by asking them to remember and recall various objects as they are taken along a pathway. The computer leads the subjects (passively) through a hallway (see Figure 12.8) with seven different objects displayed along the way. Subjects are asked to remember the objects (both color and type are important) because they will be tested on them later. After completing the hallway, the subject is shown 14 objects and is given 120 s to select only the 7 objects they saw in the hallway (see Figure 12.9). The system measures number of errors and total time to complete the task.

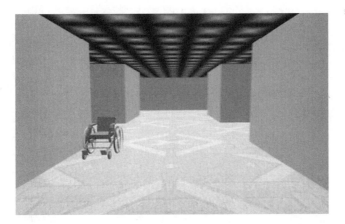

Figure 12.8. Visual representation of the hallway presented to the subject with an example object subjects are asked to memorize. Copyright 2018 by HeadRehab, Inc.

Recognition "B" Task

The subject is shown seven different objects to memorize, which slowly rotate for 70 s. After the 70 s, subjects are passively led through the hallway and asked to identify the objects they saw earlier. Each object is encased in a clear bubble and, using the trigger of a joystick, the subject will select the object, turning the bubble red. The system measures the number of errors that occur.

Scoring

While the participant is interacting with the virtual world, the system measures movements and responses to the environment. Using various mathematical algorithms, the SideLine Version 10.1 Test Oculus reporting module produces a score on a scale that ranges from 0.00 to 10.00, with higher scores representing better performance (Oculus VR, LLC, Menlo Park, CA; see Figure 12.10). This score quantifies each area of cognitive function during testing that is used for analysis.

SENSITIVITY AND SPECIFICITY OF VIRTUAL REALITY TASKS

Determining the sensitivity and specificity of a VR tool is currently a crucial part of its development in research. With recent developments in technology, proving its ability to be both sensitive and specific to cognitive changes in an individual is important, as is its ability to provide a distinction between a concussed and non-concussed individual. Although computer-based

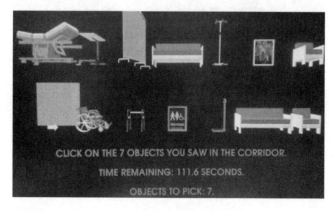

Figure 12.9. Display of the 14 choices. Subjects have to pick the correct 7 images they were presented in the hallway in 120 seconds. Copyright 2018 by HeadRehab, Inc.

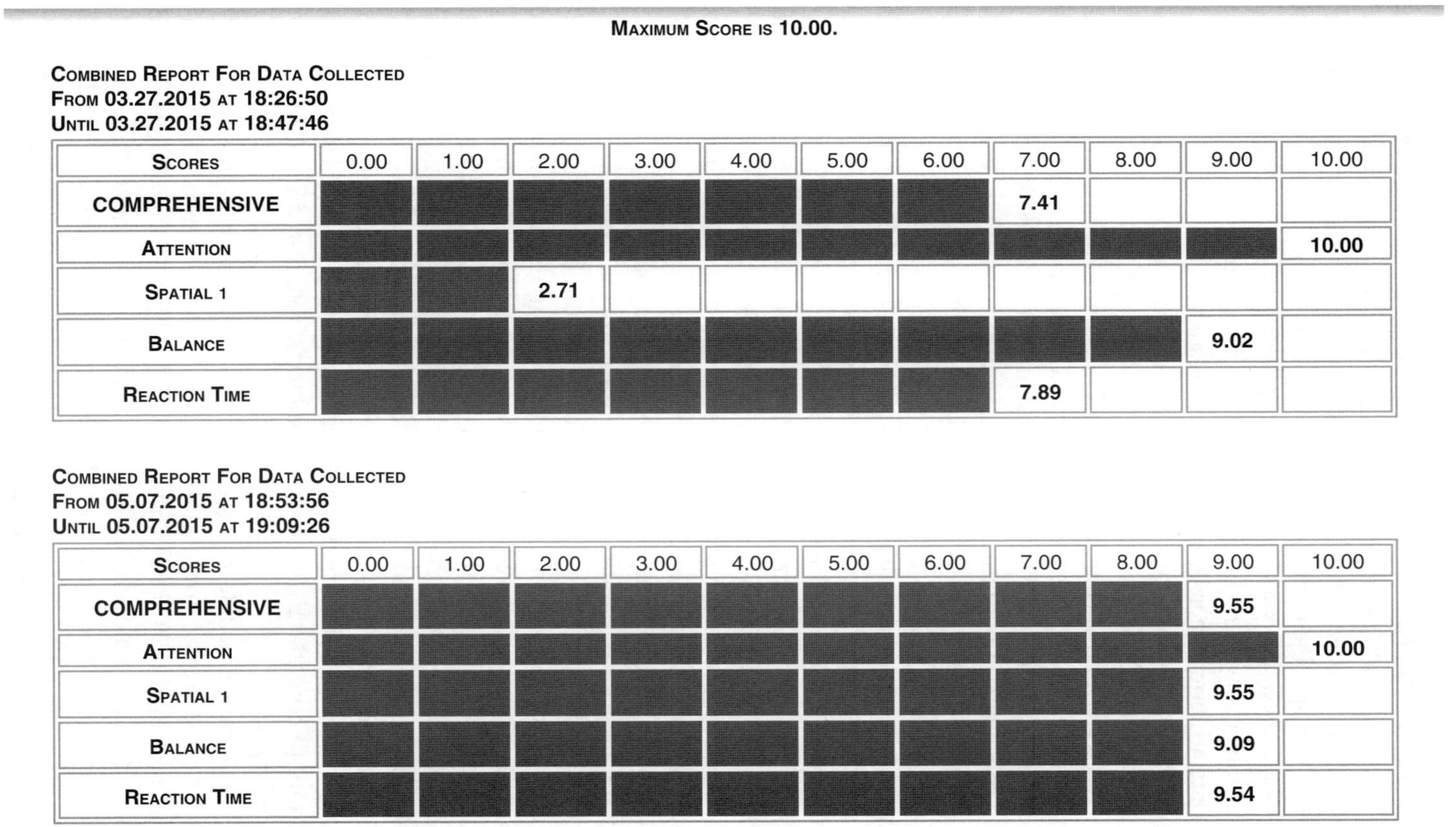

Maximum Score is 10.00.
Combined Report For Data Collected
From 03.27.2015 at 18:26:50
Until 03.27.2015 at 18:47:46
Scores
0.00
1.00
2.00
3.00
4.00
5.00
6.00
7.00
8.00
9.00
10.00
COMPREHENSIVE
7.41
Attention
10.00
Spatial 1
2.71
Balance
9.02
Reaction Time
7.89
Combined Report For Data Collected
From 05.07.2015 at 18:53:56
Until 05.07.2015 at 19:09:26
Scores
0.00
1.00
2.00
3.00
4.00
5.00
6.00
7.00
8.00
9.00
10.00
COMPREHENSIVE
9.55
Attention
10.00
Spatial 1
9.55
Balance
9.09
Reaction Time
9.54

Figure 12.10. Sample output report for virtual reality testing. Copyright 2018 by HeadRehab, Inc.

neuropsychological testing is widely used and can be an effective clinical tool, there is still an ongoing debate over its lack of ecological validity. Therefore, a retrospective study examined VR data (Teel, Gay, Johnson, & Slobounov, 2016) in nonconcussed ($n = 128$) and concussed ($n = 24$) subjects to examine the data's specificity and sensitivity. Because of the immersive nature of VR, concussed subjects were tested 7 to 10 days after the injury, whereas the control subjects, with no history of concussion, were tested once during their collegiate athletic career. All subjects were tested on VR modules, including balance, reaction time, attention, and spatial memory. The findings included that the individual modules of spatial navigation and reaction time produced high sensitivity and specificity when determining performance-based variability between concussed and nonconcussed subjects. In addition, when all modules were combined for a comprehensive score, there was high sensitivity to and specificity of performance-based cognitive variability when comparisons of concussed and non-concussed subjects were made. These two findings demonstrate that VR can be used to detect cognitive changes after a concussive injury. The specificity (96.1%) and sensitivity (95.8%) values for the combined score were also comparable to previously reported values in traditional neuropsychological testing, ranging from 81.95% to 96.6% for sensitivity (Erlanger, Feldman, et al., 2003; Erlanger, Saliba, et al., 2001) and 69.7% to 97.3% for specificity (Iverson, 2006; Louey et al., 2014).

The balance module was specifically examined for sensitivity in comparison with commonly used clinical balance tests (Teel, Gay, Arnett, & Slobounov, 2016). Balance problems are common following concussion and often are due to the inability of the brain to process and integrate vestibular, visual, and somatosensory information. A retrospective study focused on non-concussed ($n = 94$) and concussed ($n = 27$) individuals on the balance module. Ten trials were used, with the first trial taking place in a stationary room. Analyses revealed that this VR balance module had better overall sensitivity and specificity than typical clinically accepted balance measures; specifically, the VR module was able to discriminate 85.7% of concussed subjects, whereas the balance error scoring system could differentiate only 60% and sensory organization test differentiated only 61.9%. However, it is important to note that these concussed subjects were tested 7 to 10 days after their injury.

The balance module also was validated with center-of-pressure (COP) data obtained from a force platform (Teel & Slobounov, 2015). Non-concussed controls ($n = 60$) and concussed subjects ($n = 21$) were tested on the VR balance module and standard balance assessments (force plate). On the force plate, subjects were tested under two 1-minute conditions: (a) eyes open and (b) eyes closed. Additional subjects were included who completed only the VR balance module, bringing the total to 94 controls and

28 concussed subjects. The analysis showed that final VR yaw, pitch, and roll scores were significantly and negatively correlated with the area of the COP in both eyes closed and eyes open. VR final score correlations with COP data met or exceeded the established clinical validity measures. This suggests that the VR balance module validly measures postural stability and the nature of the test is able to detect postinjury deficits.

VIRTUAL REALITY AND ELECTROENCEPHALOGRAPHY

VR and EEG have successfully been used together, as both are valuable clinical tools for the assessment of concussion. VR has been proven to have a more immersive experience that requires the allocation of more brain and sensory resources for tasks (evaluated by EEG) than a two-dimensional (2D) environment (Slobounov, Ray, Johnson, Slobounov, & Newell, 2015). In this experiment, 12 subjects with no history of concussion participated in VR module 2D and 3D spatial navigation (spaced by 2 hours) while simultaneously undergoing an EEG recording. In the 3D scenario, subjects reported a significantly higher sense of presence as compared to the 2D scenario. In addition, an EEG analysis revealed an increase of frontal–midline theta during the encoding phases in both 2D and 3D, but the 3D frontal–midline theta power was significantly higher than the 2D scenario. Also, both visually and significantly, there was an increase of theta power in the right parietal region during the 3D retrieval phase and a significant increase of theta power in the left occipital region.

Because the 3D scenario has shown to be more effective with EEG, studies have also examined various stages of concussive injury. Teel, Ray, Geronimo, and Slobounov (2014) looked at clinically asymptomatic concussed subjects. The control group ($n = 12$) and recently concussed group ($n = 7$) underwent a 128-channel EEG under four conditions: (a) sitting with eyes closed, (b) sitting with eyes open, (c) standing with eyes closed, and (d) standing with eyes open. They then took the Immediate Post-Concussion Assessment and Cognitive Testing (ImPACT; Schatz, Pardini, Lovell, Collins, & Podell, 2006) while still undergoing EEG recordings. After the ImPACT, subjects completed the balance and spatial navigation VR modules, again while undergoing EEG recordings. ImPACT scores revealed no significant differences between the concussed and non-concussed groups. VR revealed that the concussed group had significantly lower scores than the control group. EEG revealed significantly decreased power during all three protocols; specifically, there was whole-brain reduction in the concussed group in theta and beta (EEG baseline), in frontal and posterior theta and posterior alpha (ImPACT), and in posterior delta (VR). Teel et al.'s (2014) study revealed that in ImPACT and VR modules (except balance), the asymptomatic concussed group performed as well as the non-concussed group. However, the EEG data revealed that the concussed group appeared to be recruiting additional brain resources that may have made up for the lack of power they had during tasks.

VIRTUAL REALITY AND MAGNETIC RESONANCE IMAGING

Virtual reality also has the ability to be used in conjunction with MRI. In one study, functional MRI (fMRI) was combined with VR to examine residual functional deficits in recently concussed but asymptomatic subjects (Slobounov et al., 2010). This study used an fMRI sequence that incorporated spatial tasks within a virtual environment. Fifteen controls (no history of concussion) and 15 recently diagnosed asymptomatic concussed athlete subjects were used. Subjects were placed in a supine position in the scanner and were asked to use their right thumb to navigate a joystick. The spatial navigation module, in which the subject is shown a route to and from a door (encoding stage), then immediately asked to navigate the same route using the joystick, was used. Also, subjects were asked to navigate randomly around the hallway and to trace a cross image using the joystick. Both groups reported a high sense of presence and performed similarly in the VR environment. These behavioral findings allowed the fMRI data to be viewed as a representing a cognitive process without significant confounding variables.

The fMRI data revealed significant increases during the encoding stage in several brain regions in both the non-concussed and concussed subjects. Concussed subjects, however, had significantly greater activation in the right dorsolateral–prefrontal cortex and the left parietal cortex. There was also additional activation of the cerebellum and left dorsolateral–prefrontal cortex that was not seen in non-concussed controls. In concussed subjects there was also a significantly larger cluster size around shared regions of activation during encoding (parietal cortex, right dorsolateral–prefrontal cortex) despite similar performance by both groups in VR. These findings suggest a task-related navigation network that can be interrupted by a concussive blow.

PRECLINICAL STUDIES USING VIRTUAL REALITY

The following two studies were completed with different companies: ENZO Nutraceuticals Ltd. (Enzogenol) and Spartan Medical Inc. (brain/neck cooling). These data are unpublished at this time.

Enzogenol

This study examined the feasibility of Enzogenol, a pine bark extract, as a potential treatment for concussed individuals with residual symptoms in the chronic phase of injury. Forty-two student athletes with a history of sport-related concussion were enrolled in a double-blind randomized clinical trial for a 6-week supplementation comparing Enzogenol versus a placebo. Subjects were tested before supplementation (baseline) and 6 weeks after taking either a placebo or Enzogenol by using VR and EEG in conjunction with a conventional neuropsychological testing battery.

For VR, subjects were tested on balance, spatial memory, reaction time, and attention modules. After 6 weeks, there were nonsignificant differences in scores compared with baseline for both placebo and Enzogenol groups. However, spatial navigation, balance, and reaction time modules (see Figure 12.11) for the Enzogenol group all had improved scores after 6 weeks that approached significance ($p \sim .10$).

Brain Cooling

The influence of hypothermia on traumatic brain injury has been well studied and is shown to have positive outcomes; however, there is limited evidence regarding selective brain cooling of the head and neck, especially in a concussed population. One study aimed to examine the effects of selective

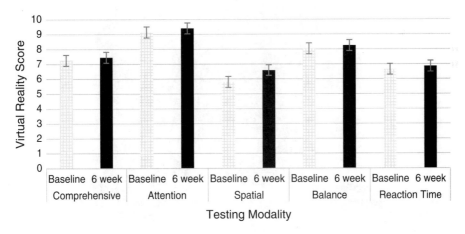

Figure 12.11. Mean virtual reality test scores for the Enzogenol group before and after supplementation. No significant differences were seen after 6 weeks, however, attention, spatial navigation, and balance modules all approached significance ($p \sim .10$). Copyright 2018 by HeadRehab, Inc.

brain cooling on clinical symptoms and biological functions of the brain after a concussive injury. The researchers hypothesized that cooling of the brain would modulate clinical symptom resolution that would be correlated with changes in neural and metabolic underpinnings.

Using VR, we expected to see positive changes in symptom resolution after a 30-min cooling period using the Spartan cooling system (see Figure 12.12) in athletes in the acute phase of concussive injury. The HeadRehab VR system (HeadRehab Inc., Sarasota, Florida) was used to collect data from nonconcussed controls ($n = 12$) and concussed athletes ($n = 12$) who also participated in an EEG. VR testing (and EEG) was done before and after a 30-min cooling period using the modules of balance, reaction time, and spatial navigation. However, most concussed athletes were unable to tolerate VR testing because of the recurrence of concussive symptoms while in the VR environment and the presence of motion sickness. Nonconcussed controls had no significant differences ($p > .05$) between their pre- and postcooling scores; however, scores did slightly increase after cooling. In the concussed group (see Figure 12.13), in those who could tolerate it, there were no significant differences in scores for balance ($p > .05$), but the spatial navigation and reaction time modules approached significance ($p \sim .09, p \sim .07$).

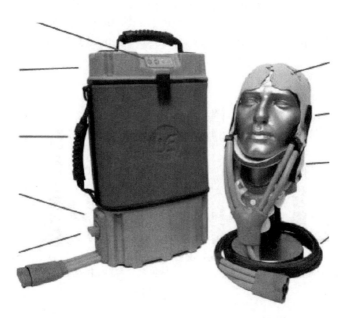

Figure 12.12. Spartan cooling device used in this study. Copyright 2018 by HeadRehab, Inc.

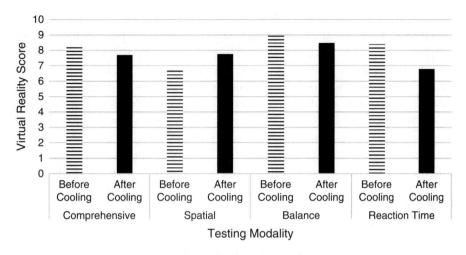

Figure 12.13. Average VR scores in concussed subjects before and after brain cooling. Average mean value for each virtual reality module before and after cooling in the concussed population (those who could tolerate it). Copyright 2018 by HeadRehab, Inc.

CASE STUDY

As discussed, most athletes are cleared and return to full play within 10 days of their injury. However, some subjects still exhibit decreased VR scores when compared with the baseline weeks after their concussive injury. The following is an example of an athlete who showed decreased VR scores after being cleared for return to play. Some of the original details of this case have been changed to protect the confidentiality of the individual tested.

The athlete is a 20-year-old male soccer player who was injured during a soccer scrimmage. He was going up for a head ball and was headed in the nose, which resulted in blood. Within minutes following the hit, he experienced blurry vision and slight fogginess. He reported no memory loss, and he stayed in the game and kept playing. He did not report his symptoms to anyone and finished the scrimmage, then played in another after lunch. Later, he experienced difficulty concentrating, headache, nausea, and mood changes. He sat out for one week after his first concussion and then he was cleared to return to play.

He had completed baseline testing before the start of the season and had normal VR score reports: 9.33 on comprehensive, 9.45 on balance, 9.80 on spatial memory, and 8.75 on reaction time. After receiving his concussive injury, he came back for more VR testing on postinjury Day 5. He appeared normal on his neuropsychological evaluation (31 seconds for Trail Making [Reynolds, 2002] and 71 boxes on the Symbol Digit Modalities Test [Smith, 1991]). However, his VR scores had significantly decreased from his baseline scores. On Day 5, he scored a 4.97 on comprehensive, 4.56 on balance, 2.76 on spatial, and 7.60 on reaction time. He was cleared for play on Day 10 and came back for VR testing on Day 15. His scores had improved from Day 5 but were still below his baseline scores (a 6.26 on comprehensive, 5.76 on balance, 4.82 on spatial, and 8.20 on reaction time). He was retested on Day 30 and still had scores well below his baseline values (a 6.69 on comprehensive, 6.37 on balance, 5.20 on spatial, and 8.50 on reaction time). During these appointments, he displayed clinical symptoms only during the Day 5 testing. On Days 10 and 30 he was clinically asymptomatic but his VR scores were still suffering. This case is just one example in which an athlete appears clinically asymptomatic after a concussion but still has lingering effects despite being cleared for full return to play.

CLINICAL TAKE-HOME POINTS

1. *Be mindful of the fact that the symptom resolution assessed by conventional tools (neuropsychological or neurological) used today may not mean that the concussive injury is fully resolved.*
2. *Be aware that a return to baseline of clinical symptoms may characterize a compensatory effect in the athletes rather than a true return to normal.*
3. *Work with scientists to develop more advanced technology that can help target these problems is critical.*

KEY QUESTIONS TO BE ANSWERED IN THE NEXT 5 YEARS

1. *A standard diagnostic treatment needs to be developed using precision medical tools with the goal of a standard for the assessment of concussion.*
2. *There needs to be clarification of an evidence-based definition of concussion, its severity, and the classification levels.*
3. *Researchers and clinicians should consider what treatment modalities can be used for concussion to speed up or facilitate the recovery of symptoms.*

CONCLUSION

Overall, VR has a unique ability to provide an interactive 3D environment, demonstrating both ecological validity and accurate and reliable results. Its high sensitivity and specificity in identifying symptoms and separating controls and concussed individuals makes it a worthwhile research and clinical tool for the assessment of concussion. Future research and development should be focused on the elaboration of a sport-specific VR scenario to further improve ecological validity; specifically, research could examine how changing the VR location and situation to a more gamelike situation would affect a person's performance on the various executive function tasks. Also, scholars could expand on current research to understand how a 3D environment affects a person's performance and how neural mechanisms are affected (using EEG) when exposed to a 2D versus 3D world.

REFERENCES

Abbas, K., Shenk, T. E., Poole, V. N., Breedlove, E. L., Leverenz, L. J., Nauman, E. A., . . . Robinson, M. E. (2015). Alteration of default mode network in high school football athletes due to repetitive subconcussive mild traumatic brain injury: A resting-state functional magnetic resonance imaging study. *Brain Connectivity, 5*, 91–101. http://dx.doi.org/10.1089/brain.2014.0279

Barkhoudarian, G., Hovda, D. A., & Giza, C. C. (2011). The molecular pathophysiology of concussive brain injury. *Clinics in Sports Medicine, 30*, 33–48. http://dx.doi.org/10.1016/j.csm.2010.09.001

Bartels, C., Wegrzyn, M., Wiedl, A., Ackermann, V., & Ehrenreich, H. (2010). Practice effects in healthy adults: A longitudinal study on frequent repetitive cognitive testing. *BMC Neuroscience, 11*, 118. http://dx.doi.org/10.1186/1471-2202-11-118

Barwick, F., Arnett, P., & Slobounov, S. (2012). EEG correlates of fatigue during administration of a neuropsychological test battery. *Clinical Neurophysiology, 123*, 278–284. http://dx.doi.org/10.1016/j.clinph.2011.06.027

Chang, T., Ramirez, A. M., Herbst, M., & Coris, E. E. (2009, April). *Detection of concussions in athletes combining CT, MRI, and PET neuroimaging: A community pilot study.* Paper presented at the 42nd Society of Teachers of Family Medicine (STFM) Annual Spring Conference, Denver, CO.

Chong, C. D., & Schwedt, T. J. (2015). White matter damage and brain network alterations in concussed patients: A review of recent diffusion tensor imaging and resting-state functional connectivity data. *Current Pain and Headache Reports, 19*, 485. http://dx.doi.org/10.1007/s11916-015-0485-0

Chun, I. Y., Mao, X., Breedlove, E. L., Leverenz, L. J., Nauman, E. A., & Talavage, T. M. (2015). DTI detection of longitudinal WM abnormalities due to accumulated head impacts. *Developmental Neuropsychology, 40*, 92–97. http://dx.doi.org/10.1080/87565641.2015.1020945

Erlanger, D., Feldman, D., Kutner, K., Kaushik, T., Kroger, H., Festa, J., . . . Broshek, D. (2003). Development and validation of a web-based neuropsychological test protocol for sports-related return-to-play decision-making.

Archives of Clinical Neuropsychology, 18, 293–316. http://dx.doi.org/10.1016/S0887-6177(02)00138-5

Erlanger, D., Saliba, E., Barth, J., Almquist, J., Webright, W., & Freeman, J. (2001). Monitoring resolution of postconcussion symptoms in athletes: Preliminary results of a web-based neuropsychological test protocol. *Journal of Athletic Training, 36,* 280–287.

Gardner, A., Iverson, G. L., & Stanwell, P. (2014). A systematic review of proton magnetic resonance spectroscopy findings in sport-related concussion. *Journal of Neurotrauma, 31,* 1–18. http://dx.doi.org/10.1089/neu.2013.3079

Gardner, A., Kay-Lambkin, F., Stanwell, P., Donnelly, J., Williams, W. H., Hiles, A., . . . Jones, D. K. (2012). A systematic review of diffusion tensor imaging findings in sports-related concussion. *Journal of Neurotrauma, 29,* 2521–2538. http://dx.doi.org/10.1089/neu.2012.2628

Gatson, J., & Diaz-Arrastia, R. (2014). Tau as a biomarker of concussion. *JAMA Neurology, 71,* 677–678. http://dx.doi.org/10.1001/jamaneurol.2014.443

Iverson, G. L. (2006). Sensitivity of computerized neuropsychological screening in depressed university students. *The Clinical Neuropsychologist, 20,* 695–701. http://dx.doi.org/10.1080/138540491005857

Keshner, E. A., & Kenyon, R. V. (2000). The influence of an immersive virtual environment on the segmental organization of postural stabilizing responses. *Journal of Vestibular Research: Equilibrium & Orientation, 10,* 207–219.

Kou, Z., Gattu, R., Kobeissy, F., Welch, R. D., O'Neil, B. J., Woodard, J. L., . . . Mondello, S. (2013). Combining biochemical and imaging markers to improve diagnosis and characterization of mild traumatic brain injury in the acute setting: Results from a pilot study. *PLoS One, 8*(11), e80296. Advance online publication. http://dx.doi.org/10.1371/journal.pone.0080296

Langlois, J. A., Rutland-Brown, W., & Wald, M. M. (2006). The epidemiology and impact of traumatic brain injury: A brief overview. *The Journal of Head Trauma Rehabilitation, 21,* 375–378. http://dx.doi.org/10.1097/00001199-200609000-00001

Louey, A. G., Cromer, J. A., Schembri, A. J., Darby, D. G., Maruff, P., Makdissi, M., & McCrory, P. (2014). Detecting cognitive impairment after concussion: Sensitivity of change from baseline and normative data methods using the CogSport/Axon cognitive test battery. *Archives of Clinical Neuropsychology, 29,* 432–441. http://dx.doi.org/10.1093/arclin/acu020

Lovell, M., Collins, M., & Bradley, J. (2004). Return to play following sports-related concussion. *Clinics in Sports Medicine, 23,* 421–441x. http://dx.doi.org/10.1016/j.csm.2004.04.001

Luther, N., Niogi, S., Kutner, K., Rodeo, S., Shetty, T., Warren, R., . . . Hartl, R. (2012). Diffusion tensor and susceptibility-weighted imaging in concussion assessment of National Football League players. *Neurosurgery, 71,* E558. http://dx.doi.org/10.1227/01.neu.0000417733.09300.04

McCrory, P., Meeuwisse, W., Dvorák, J., Aubry, M., Bailes, J., Broglio, S., . . . Vos, P. E. (2017). Consensus statement on concussion in sport—The 5th international conference on concussion in sport held in Berlin, October 2016. *British Journal of Sports Medicine, 51,* 838–847. http://dx.doi.org/10.1136/bjsports-2017-097699

McDevitt, J., Tierney, R., Phillips, J., Gaughan, J., Torg, J. S., & Krynetskiy, E. (2014). Supporting the concept of genetic predisposition to prolonged recovery following a concussion. *Orthopaedic Journal of Sports Medicine, 2*(7, Suppl. 2). http://dx.doi.org/10.1177/2325967114S00078

Meier, T. B., Bellgowan, P. S., Singh, R., Kuplicki, R., Polanski, D. W., & Mayer, A. R. (2015). Recovery of cerebral blood flow following sports-related concussion. *JAMA Neurology, 72,* 530–538. http://dx.doi.org/10.1001/jamaneurol.2014.4778

Merritt, V. C., & Arnett, P. A. (2016). Apolipoprotein E (APOE) ε4 allele is associated with increased symptom reporting following sports concussion. *Journal of the International Neuropsychological Society, 22,* 89–94. http://dx.doi.org/10.1017/S1355617715001022

Merritt, V. C., Ukueberuwa, D. M., & Arnett, P. A. (2016). Relationship between the apolipoprotein E gene and headache following sports-related concussion. *Journal of Clinical and Experimental Neuropsychology, 38,* 941–949. http://dx.doi.org/10.1080/13803395.2016.1177491

Nauman, E. A., Breedlove, K. M., Breedlove, E. L., Talavage, T. M., Robinson, M. E., & Leverenz, L. J. (2015). Post-season neurophysiological deficits assessed by ImPACT and fMRI in athletes competing in American football. *Developmental Neuropsychology, 40,* 85–91. http://dx.doi.org/10.1080/87565641.2015.1016161

Papa, L., Silvestri, S., Brophy, G. M., Giordano, P., Falk, J. L., Braga, C. F., . . . Robertson, C. S. (2014). GFAP out-performs S100β in detecting traumatic intracranial lesions on computed tomography in trauma patients with mild traumatic brain injury and those with extracranial lesions. *Journal of Neurotrauma, 31,* 1815–1822. http://dx.doi.org/10.1089/neu.2013.3245

Poole, V. N., Abbas, K., Shenk, T. E., Breedlove, E. L., Breedlove, K. M., Robinson, M. E., . . . Dydak, U. (2014). MR spectroscopic evidence of brain injury in the non-diagnosed collision sport athlete. *Developmental Neuropsychology, 39,* 459–473. http://dx.doi.org/10.1080/87565641.2014.940619

Radanov, B. (2001). PET, SPECT and their reliability for diagnosis of concussion. *British Journal of Sports Medicine, 35,* 375.

Reynolds, C. R. (2002). *Comprehensive Trail-Making Test (CTMT).* Austin, TX: Pro-Ed.

Schatz, P., Pardini, J. E., Lovell, M. R., Collins, M. W., & Podell, K. (2006). Sensitivity and specificity of the ImPACT Test Battery for concussion in athletics. *Archives of Clinical Neuropsychology, 21,* 91–9.

Schulte, S., Podlog, L. W., Hamson-Utley, J. J., Strathmann, F. G., & Strüder, H. K. (2014). A systematic review of the biomarker S100B: Implications for sport-related concussion management. *Journal of Athletic Training, 49*, 830–850. http://dx.doi.org/10.4085/1062-6050-49.3.33

Slobounov, S. M., Gay, M., Zhang, K., Johnson, B., Pennell, D., Sebastianelli, W., . . . Hallett, M. (2011). Alteration of brain functional network at rest and in response to YMCA physical stress test in concussed athletes: RsFMRI study. *NeuroImage, 55*, 1716–1727. http://dx.doi.org/10.1016/j.neuroimage.2011.01.024

Slobounov, S. M., Ray, W., Johnson, B., Slobounov, E., & Newell, K. M. (2015). Modulation of cortical activity in 2D versus 3D virtual reality environments: An EEG study. *International Journal of Psychophysiology, 95*, 254–260. http://dx.doi.org/10.1016/j.ijpsycho.2014.11.003

Slobounov, S., Sebastianelli, W., & Newell, K. (2011). Incorporating virtual reality graphics with brain imaging for assessment of sport-related concussions. *2011 Annual International Conference of the IEEE Engineering in Medicine and Biology Society, 2011*, 1383–1386. http://dx.doi.org/10.1109/IEMBS.2011.6090325

Slobounov, S., Slobounov, E., & Newell, K. (2006). Application of virtual reality graphics in assessment of concussion. *CyberPsychology & Behavior, 9*, 188–191. http://dx.doi.org/10.1089/cpb.2006.9.188

Slobounov, S. M., Zhang, K., Pennell, D., Ray, W., Johnson, B., & Sebastianelli, W. (2010). Functional abnormalities in normally appearing athletes following mild traumatic brain injury: A functional MRI study. *Experimental Brain Research, 202*, 341–354. http://dx.doi.org/10.1007/s00221-009-2141-6

Smith, A. (1991). *Symbol Digit Modalities Test.* Los Angeles, CA: Western Psychological Services.

Svaldi, D. O., Joshi, C., Robinson, M. E., Shenk, T. E., Abbas, K., Nauman, E. A., . . . Talavage, T. M. (2015). Cerebrovascular reactivity alterations in asymptomatic high school football players. *Developmental Neuropsychology, 40*, 80–84. http://dx.doi.org/10.1080/87565641.2014.973959

Talavage, T. M., Nauman, E. A., Breedlove, E. L., Yoruk, U., Dye, A. E., Morigaki, K. E., . . . Leverenz, L. J. (2014). Functionally-detected cognitive impairment in high school football players without clinically-diagnosed concussion. *Journal of Neurotrauma, 31*, 327–338. http://dx.doi.org/10.1089/neu.2010.1512

Teel, E. F., Gay, M. R., Arnett, P. A., & Slobounov, S. M. (2016). Differential sensitivity between a virtual reality balance module and clinically used concussion balance modalities. *Clinical Journal of Sport Medicine, 26*, 162–166. http://dx.doi.org/10.1097/JSM.0000000000000210

Teel, E. F., Gay, M. R., Johnson, B. A., & Slobounov, S. M. (2016). Determining sensitivity/specificity of virtual reality-based neuropsychological tool for detecting residual abnormalities following sport-related concussion. *Neuropsychology, 30*, 474–483. http://dx.doi.org/10.1037/neu0000261

Teel, E. F., Ray, W. J., Geronimo, A. M., & Slobounov, S. M. (2014). Residual alterations of brain electrical activity in clinically asymptomatic concussed individuals: An EEG study. *Clinical Neurophysiology, 125*, 703–707. http://dx.doi.org/10.1016/j.clinph.2013.08.027

Teel, E. F., & Slobounov, S. M. (2015). Validation of a virtual reality balance module for use in clinical concussion assessment and management. *Clinical Journal of Sport Medicine, 25,* 144–148. http://dx.doi.org/10.1097/JSM.0000000000000109

Terrell, T. R., Bostick, R., Rogers, G. L., Langston, M. A., Barth, J., Bennett, E., & Mihelic, F. M. (2014, May). *Association of APOE and other genetic polymorphisms with prospective concussion risk in a prospective cohort study of college athletes.* Paper presented at the 5th Annual Meeting of the Oak Ridge National Laboratory Biomedical Sciences Group. http://dx.doi.org/10.1109/BSEC.2014.6867745

Thompson, J., Sebastianelli, W., & Slobounov, S. (2005). EEG and postural correlates of mild traumatic brain injury in athletes. *Neuroscience Letters, 377,* 158–163. http://dx.doi.org/10.1016/j.neulet.2004.11.090

Trotter, W. (1924). On certain minor injuries of the brain. Being the annual oration, medical society of London. *The British Medical Journal, 1,* 816–819.

Wang, Y., Nelson, L. D., LaRoche, A. A., Pfaller, A. Y., Nencka, A. S., Koch, K. M., & McCrea, M. A. (2015). Cerebral blood flow alterations in acute sport-related concussion. *Journal of Neurotrauma.* Advance online publication.

13

NEUROPSYCHOLOGICAL ASSESSMENT OF CONCUSSION IN PEDIATRIC POPULATIONS

FRANK M. WEBBE AND DENISE S. VAGT

Assessment of sport-related concussion (SRC) in a pediatric context provides challenges that are not found in adult populations. Not surprisingly, age represents a wild card factor for at least three reasons. First, neuropsychological tests often used in older populations for assessing concussion in the sports context may not be appropriate for younger children, and the availability of comparable tests developed and normed for young children may be limited. Second, chronological age may not (and frequently does not) correspond to mental and emotional age. Two 9-year-olds may differ radically in their cognitive development, so norms listed for 9-year-olds may predict erroneously the level of actual performance in a given child. Third, developmental age invariably interacts with brain trauma but in unpredictable ways. Brain injuries that might lead to permanent functional loss in adults may have negligible long-term effects in children, but the reverse may also be true: Damage that occurs in childhood before specific nervous system growth has occurred may forever impair an individual.

http://dx.doi.org/10.1037/0000114-014
Neuropsychology of Sports-Related Concussion, P. A. Arnett (Editor)

In reviewing many studies with pediatric samples, we found that the accumulation of empirical data related positively to age. Thus, the bulk of the extant literature describes SRC in high school–age adolescents, and the smallest literature covers young children of primary school age.

In this chapter, we develop these topics and provide a guide for understanding the how, what, why, and when of sport concussion in children. Because the use of the terms *pediatric, child,* and *children* often extends over a range of ages from 5 to 18, sometimes with little regard for the obvious physical and cognitive developmental differences, for our own conclusions we will adhere to the following definitions: *young* child or children = ages 5 to 8, child or children = ages 9 to 12, and adolescents = ages 13 to 18. In reviewing data gathered from studies we will attempt to follow that convention where possible, or the convention of *primary school, middle school,* and *high school,* in an attempt to clarify age-based differences in outcome. If we cite a study that used participants who varied across the entire young child through adolescent range without parsing out age effects, we will so note.

Because the literature is replete with characterizations that show so many differences in considering SRC in pediatric versus adult populations, there will be instances of overlap in this chapter with the specific topics of other chapters. For example, validity of symptom report, methods of evaluation, persisting symptoms, and levels of evidence supporting particular aspects of management all differ between some or all pediatric versus adult populations. Overlap and repetition are kept to a minimum.

EPIDEMIOLOGY AND STATISTICS

Although SRC is a health concern for active persons of all ages, the high incidence of it in pediatric populations is particularly alarming given the potential ramifications of injury to the growing brain (Tator, 2013). Approximately 44,000,000 youth ages 6 to 18 years in the United States participate in organized youth sports annually, a number that has increased steadily over the past 20 years (National Council of Youth Sports, 2008). In 2010, 54% of Canadians ages 15 to 19 years reported regularly practicing a sport, but 75% of children ages 5 to 14 years had parental reports that they regularly practiced a sport (Canadian Heritage, 2013). High school sports in the United States alone attract more than 7,800,000 participants annually (National Federation of State High School Associations, 2015).

However, injuries in sport are also common. In the United States annually there are more than 3.5 million sport injuries in children age 14 and younger that were significant enough to cause loss of participation. Almost one third of all childhood injuries are due to sport participation or play, and sport-related injury is responsible for an estimated 21% of traumatic brain injuries in children. This number increases to 50% when recreational sport activities such as bicycling and skating are included (Stanford Children's Health, 2016). There are approximately 130,000 emergency room visits annually for SRC in individuals between ages 5 and 18 years (Centers for Disease Control and Prevention, 2006). However, this figure does not include the SRCs that are not treated in a hospital emergency department or urgent care center. The estimation of such unreported or uncharted injuries suggests no fewer than 400,000 annual SRCs for United States high school athletes (Yard & Comstock, 2009) and perhaps 5 to 10 times that many annual SRCs for all United States athletes under age 18 years.

Although the risk varies greatly by sport, an examination of 12 common youth sports indicated that the overall incidence of SRC per 1,000 pediatric athletes is estimated at 0.23 (95% confidence interval [0.19, 0.28]; Pfister, Pfister, Hagel, Ghali, & Ronksley, 2016). When examining high school sports alone, concussions represent over 13% of sports-related injuries, with an incidence of between 2.4 and 2.5 concussions per 10,000 athletic exposures (AEs), with an AE defined as one student participating in one game or practice. Further study of variation in concussions per 10,000 AEs demonstrates the much greater concussion risk in boys' football (approximate incidence of 6.4 concussions per 10,000 AEs) as compared with sports such as girls' and boys' track and field (approximate incidence of 0.2 concussions per 10,000 AEs) and girls' and boys' swimming (approximate incidence of 0.2–0.1 concussions per 10,000 AEs). Pediatric SRCs are more likely to occur during a game than during practice and are more commonly caused by player-to-player contact rather than player-to-playing surface contact (Marar, McIlvain, Fields, & Comstock, 2012).

Younger players demonstrate perhaps an even greater risk for concussion in some high contact sports, in particular during games. The incidence risk for concussion in football players age 8 to 12 years was estimated at 6.16 per 1,000 AEs during games and 0.24 per 1,000 AEs during practice. These practice rates are similar to high school and college concussion risk per AE but show approximately two times a greater risk during games (Kontos et al., 2013). Similarly, an investigation of concussion incidence in female youth soccer (ages 11–14 years) found the overall incidence rate to be 1.2 concussions per 1,000 AE hours, with 86% of the concussions occurring during a game (O'Kane et al., 2014). See Figure 13.1 for a summary of incidence risk across various studies.

These rates have been steadily increasing over the past two decades, most likely because of a combination of increased education and reporting, as well as more athletes participating in sports with full physical contact (Guerriero, Proctor, Mannix, & Meehan, 2012). In addition, individual-specific factors

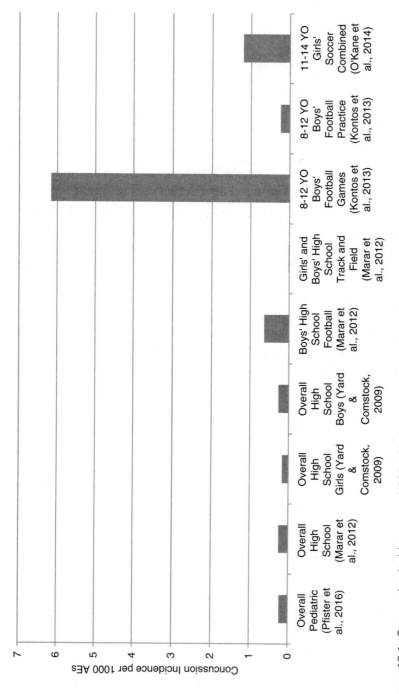

Figure 13.1. Concussion incidence per 1,000 athletic exposures across various ages and sports. AEs = Athletic Exposures; YO = years old.

may increase risk further for SRC in pediatric populations. For example, in a self-report measure of concussion and psychiatric history, 10.6% of high school and college athletes who reported a history of three of more concussions also reported a diagnosis of attention-deficit/hyperactivity disorder (ADHD), whereas only 3.6% of the group who denied any concussion history reported an ADHD diagnosis (Nelson et al., 2016).

Salinas and colleagues (2016) reported similarly that for 256 adolescents, ranging in age from 12 to 18, a history of ADHD was 2 times more likely to predict a previous concussion. Males are more likely to sustain a head-related injury during sport play compared with females; however, males are also more likely to participate in team sports in which player-to-player contact or collision is often seen, such as football or hockey (Stracciolini et al., 2014). When gender-comparable sports (e.g., soccer or basketball) are analyzed individually, female high school athletes are more likely than male counterparts to receive a SRC diagnosis; however, the influence of cultural and disparate reporting factors may bias these data, as concussions with loss of consciousness are similar between the two groups, possibly indicating that concussions occur with similar frequency, but "mild" concussions are less likely to be reported in male high school athletes (Yard & Comstock, 2009).

SYMPTOMS

Evaluation of initial baseline symptom reporting is helpful for accurate assessment of posttrauma symptom report across all ages, but it is less useful with young children, for whom symptom report is typically integrated with parental report and monitoring. Iverson et al. (2015) found, in a large sample of high school athletes, that the majority of athletes endorsed at least some symptoms during baseline assessment, and 19% of males and 28% of females reported baseline symptoms that are consistent with a diagnosis of post-concussion syndrome according to the *International Classification of Functioning, Disability and Health* (10th ed.; World Health Organization, 2001). These rates increase to as high as 72% in populations with certain previous or concurrent reported conditions, such as prior psychiatric diagnosis or treatment, history of migraines, substance abuse diagnosis, or ADHD. Interestingly, Iverson et al. (2015) found that a history of previous concussion was the weakest predictor of high symptom reporting consistent with post-concussion syndrome, as compared to the previous noted factors.

After sustaining a concussion, symptoms reported in pediatric populations are similar to those reported in adult populations. Physical symptoms often reported include headache, nausea, vomiting, balance or vision problems, fatigue, and sensitivity to light and noise. A second domain, cognitive symptoms, are commonly endorsed as well. These include feeling "slowed down" or "in a fog," difficulty concentrating and/or remembering, and general confusion. A sometimes-overlooked yet significant cluster of symptoms includes emotional symptoms of irritability, sadness, lability, and anxiousness. Finally, sleep problems are reported in the days and weeks after a concussion, including sleeping more or less than normal, difficulty falling asleep, and drowsiness (Halstead, Walter, & the Council on Sports Medicine and Fitness, 2010).

Headache is generally the most commonly reported symptom, with 53% of adolescent female soccer players reporting headache immediately after an injury (O'Kane et al., 2014), and 40% of male (48% of female) high school athletes reporting headache as their primary concussion symptom (Frommer et al., 2011). An increase in depression symptoms during the recovery period of a concussion has been documented in high school athletes (Kontos, Covassin, Elbin, & Parker, 2012). Although the severity of the symptoms does not cross the threshold of clinical significance on average, individual students may face function-limiting depression symptoms due to the injury, a lack of activity, removal from the team and the social support it provides, and anxiety regarding return to play or position.

The relationship between injury of any kind and increased risk for emotional difficulties is well documented, both in the athletic world and with nonathletes. However, the unknown and often-unexpected duration of concussion symptom recovery can exacerbate depression and anxiety in adolescent athletes. When faced with this uncertainty, combined with removal of an often-used stress reduction tool (exercise), depression symptoms can worsen, cycling into a positive feedback loop (Putukian, 2016).

This subgroup of student athletes who experience emotional symptoms, such as sadness or anxiety, is of particular note because of the impact these symptoms may have not only on intra- and interpersonal functioning but also, potentially, on academic performance. In a pediatric sample, those who reported depressive symptoms after a concussion demonstrated poorer school functioning than similarly concussed individuals who did not report an increase in negative emotional symptoms (O'Connor et al., 2012). It is clear that the evaluation, monitoring, and treatment provision options for emotional symptoms is a necessary part of managing concussions in pediatric samples of student athletes.

The time interval between appearance of symptoms and complete cessation of symptoms is typically within 2 weeks in pediatric groups; however, those (individuals ages 11–22 who presented to an emergency department) with a previous history of concussion had a longer duration of symptoms (M = 24 days) as compared to those without a previous concussion history (M = 12 days). In addition, individuals who reported more than one previous concussion had an even longer mean symptom duration (M = 35 days; Eisenberg, Andrea, Meehan, & Mannix, 2013). Evidence suggests that high school and college athletes who self-report memory problems in a post-trauma evaluation approximately 2 days after a concussion are more at risk for longer symptom duration than their counterparts who do not report memory impairment (Erlanger et al., 2003).

This timeline is generally consistent with the information gleaned from animal-model studies of the neurometabolic cascade of concussion, which demonstrates an initial period of acute chemical change within the brain as well as longer lasting neurotransmitter and glucose insufficiency and neuro-nal depression (Giza & Hovda, 2014). Because these changes mostly do not include significant cell death for the majority of concussions, full recovery is expected (and typically seen). The cellular energy crisis observed during the acute phase of a concussion places the brain at increased vulnerability for additional damage, in particular during already at-risk phases of brain development. A common reaction, therefore, is to drastically limit all physi-cal or mental activity of the individual during recovery. Although it initially seems protective, this approach can backfire, in particular with adolescents, because a moderate level of physical and mental stimulation is needed to facilitate recovery and limit risk for depression or anxiety symptom exacerba-tion (Choe, Babikian, DiFiori, Hovda, & Giza, 2012).

However, the average recovery timeline in pediatric populations is longer than what is typically observed in older individuals. Most college-age student athletes who sustain an SRC have a mean recovery time within 7 days (McCrea et al., 2013), and older adults playing professional sports have an even shorter recovery time (Pellman, Lovell, Viano, & Casson, 2006). However, evidence suggests that high school students are more likely to continue to expe-rience memory impairment 1 week or more after the injury (Field, Collins, Lovell, & Maroon, 2003) and can take an average of 10 to14 days to completely recover from a concussion. Younger children are likely to take even longer than 1 to 2 weeks, emphasizing the need for evaluators and medical providers working with this population to have pediatric-specific knowledge regarding expected concussion timelines across ages (Davis & Purcell, 2014).

DETECTION

As discussed later in this chapter, detection of SRC in pediatric samples is often initially started through alert from the child that he or she does not feel "right." McCrea, Hammeke, Olsen, Leo, and Guskiewicz (2004) provided the following definition of *concussion* to athletes:

> A blow to the head followed by a variety of symptoms that may include
> any of the following: headache, dizziness, loss of balance, blurred vision,

'seeing stars,' feeling in a fog or slowed down, memory problems, poor concentration, nausea, or throwing up. Getting 'knocked out' or being unconscious does not always occur with a concussion. (p. 14)

When provided with this definition, 47.3% of a sample of high school football players reported experiencing these symptoms, but decided not to report the injury and complete further evaluation. Common reasons given for not reporting a concussion included believing the injury was not serious enough, not wanting to leave the game, not knowing the symptoms experienced could be caused by a concussion, and not wanting to let teammates down.

There is evidence, however, that this trend of underreporting may be reduced through education. In a small sample of high school soccer players, those with reported concussion education, training, or both, were more likely to report that they would always notify a coach or trainers of concussion symptoms, compared with those who reported not receiving education or training (Bramley, Patrick, Lehman, & Silvis, 2012). Although this is encouraging, other research with high school student athletes shows that knowledge gained after receiving concussion education dissipates over the course of a playing season, and receiving concussion education does not influence the number of athletes who return to play before full resolution of symptoms (Kurowski, Pomerantz, Schaiper, Ho, & Gittelman, 2015).

Overall, research on concussion education points to possible improvement in reporting and detection through the use of didactic education for players and coaches; however, the magnitude of the effect is generally demonstrated to be small, and lack of standardization in the education provided limits meta-analysis of studies. In addition, some researchers use didactic education with quizzes or learning assessment incorporated, whereas others simply provide education with no knowledge checks. Finally, education effectiveness research is mostly limited to adolescent players and coaches; little is known about the usefulness of education in young child and child populations.

Even when concussion symptoms are recognized as such, reported to a coach, trainer, or parent, and deemed appropriate for follow-up medical care, pediatric emergency department or urgent care providers may not have the necessary tools and training to properly diagnose and treat concussion (Zonfrillo et al., 2012). Although courses such as those offered by *Heads Up* (e.g., "Concussion in Sports: What You Need to Know") are beginning to provide standardized concussion education with a demonstrated increase in concussion knowledge after course completion (Parker, Gilchrist, Schuster, Lee, & Sarmiento, 2015), the long-term increase in concussion knowledge, improvement in research-based clinical decision making, and overall decrease in mismanagement of concussion in pediatric samples is unknown.

Once the athlete has been flagged for further evaluation, many symptom scales are available for use, occasionally including symptom reports from parents or teachers, in particular when assessing younger children; however, few symptom scales for young children and adolescents have a solidly demonstrated foundation of reliability and validity (Gioia, Schneider, Vaughan, & Isquith, 2009). The gold standard for assessment of symptom report after a suspected pediatric concussion continues to be a clinical interview conducted by a trained provider. Many athletics systems have adopted management protocols that allow for standardized pathways of assessment and return to play and, ideally, minimize error in the process.

MANAGEMENT

Management of a concussion often implies different activities to different researchers and practitioners. For the purposes of this chapter, we define *concussion management* as the structured protocols that includes the following:

- education of athletes, their parents, and coaches about the signs, symptoms, and risks for concussion;
- identification of athletes who may have suffered a concussion and who are referred for evaluation;
- an outline of the steps taken to arrive at a diagnosis;
- implementation of interventions that are put into place after a diagnosis;
- follow-up examinations that track recovery progress;
- hard guidelines that result in the decision to return the athlete to their sport—and in the present case with children; and
- steps to take to help them return to their normal educational and social milieu.

In a perfect world, each stage of a concussion management plan would have empirical verification of its utility and the effectiveness of its procedures. However, the world of pediatric concussion management is far from perfect. Some procedures and the decisions that stem from their use do have empirical validation; many do not. For this latter category, the aim is to follow best practice guidelines. Such practice guidelines stem both from a professional consensus and from the outcome of studies that fall short of randomized control trial standards (Gioia, 2015).

An obvious and pervasive thread in discussing concussion management is the consideration of the child's age. In terms of physical and cognitive developmental milestones, we know that ages 5 to 11 are very different from 12 to 18. As Kirkwood and colleagues wrote so eloquently, "Children are not 'little adults'" (Kirkwood, Yeates, & Wilson, 2006, p. 1360). We could reduce the cohort range farther and describe significant cognitive developmental differences among 5- to 8-year-old, 9- to 13-year-old, and 14- to 18-year-old children. Whichever we choose, one obvious finding is that most of the data on management reside with the older adolescent cohort—typically, high schoolers—and the least with the youngest cohort (Halstead et al., 2010). Although this correlation of data quantity and quality with age makes sense given epidemiology that shows many more concussions in older children (Yue et al., 2016), it still leaves practitioners grasping for empirically valid diagnostic methods and interventions when their patient is a young child. One good example relates to cognitive and physical rest after a diagnosis. Practice guidelines have historically mandated days, weeks, or months of rest (Moser, Glatts, & Schatz, 2012; Valovich McLeod & Gioia, 2010). More recently, a group comparison study of older adolescents and young adults showed that minimal periods of rest were associated with faster recovery than longer periods (Buckley, Munkasy, & Clouse, 2016). This developing guideline still requires empirical support for true pediatric samples.

In pediatric populations, as in adults, a structured protocol for concussion management ensures that every athlete receives care and attention regardless of personal attributes or opinions held by the athlete or the treating professional. Although various organizations and leagues will establish idiosyncratic protocols, some characteristics are common. These include education, sideline evaluation, diagnostic assessment, a return-to-play decision tree, intervention for persisting symptoms, and retirement from play. Because many of these categories are discussed at length in other chapters of this book, we comment here only on ones that are particularly critical in pediatric settings.

Education

Education of athletes and coaches is mandated in U.S. intercollegiate play by the sanctioning bodies, frequently in structured programs (NCAA Sport Science Institute, 2017). With their HEADS UP Resource Center, the Centers for Disease Control and Prevention aggressively have promoted education about concussion for youth athletes, their parents, and coaches (see https://www.cdc.gov/headsup/resources/). The adoption by the State of Washington of the Zackery Lystedt Law in 2009 (H.R. 1824) stimulated all other states to legislate some aspect of concussion education and management. The implementation of programs has varied widely, ranging from pro forma adoptions to empirically researched efforts (Williamson et al., 2014). The bottom line is that decent (some validated) education programs for children and adolescents—and parents and coaches—are available for the asking (Sady, Vaughan, & Gioia, 2011). With pediatrics, the onus of education rests firmly on parents and coaches, because children may have limited insight into the term *concussion* and its meaning. Gioia, Vaughan, and Sady (2012) noted also that, with young children, conceptual disconnects with their parents occurs also in symptom recognition and identification.

Sideline Evaluation

Professional and college leagues, including the National Football League, the National Hockey League, and the National Collegiate Athletic Association Division I football, now have paid professionals on the sideline or in the press box who are tasked with identifying players who are involved in incidents that warrant sideline evaluation for concussion. The actual tests that will be performed there or in the locker room vary by league, and sometimes by team, but they have the potential for identifying athletes who need to be withheld from further play pending a more complete evaluation. Thoroughness of sideline evaluations may range from the basic questions of the Maddocks Scale (e.g., "Where are you?" "What's the Score?" "What's your name?"; Maddocks, Dicker, & Saling, 1995); to visual scanning tests, such as the King–Devick (Galetta et al., 2011); balance tests, such as the BESS (Guskiewicz, 2001); to a complete SCAT5 (McCrory et al., 2017). If that scenario is considered day, then the situation in youth sports is the darkest night. At best, a single, overworked athletic trainer may be observing a practice or game for some high schools. Most often, however, the task of singling out a child or adolescent who may be concussed is left to coaches and parents. The effectiveness of such monitoring can be decent if the coach or parent has attended (and attended to) education classes and has learned what to be on the lookout for. This best case is probably rare. Parents may not even be present, and coaches—in particular, youth sport coaches—are one-person shows and must multitask at practices and games. If the child reports feeling "off," and such a report garners attention then, depending on the geographic location, the sport, and the coach, some rudimentary assessment may be conducted. The availability of professionals capable of assessing on the sideline is very low, so at best the child will be kept out the rest of the session and the parents will be notified that an examination may be in order. Some youth football and hockey leagues have adopted rudimentary accelerometer-based helmet or mouth guard alert systems that announce when a blow exceeding a preset threshold has occurred (Straus, 2017). Although the use of such devices may be better than rudimentary monitoring by parents, it also runs the risk of being accepted as the only bellwether of concussion, and children who should be removed and evaluated may be permitted to continue playing simply because a sensor has not sounded an alert. Although empirical demonstration of the effectiveness of such systems in identifying and reducing the number of concussions has not been reported, there certainly can be a role for novel detection devices in comprehensive concussion prevention and diagnostic programs (McCrory et al., 2017; Mihalik, Lynall, Wasserman, Guskiewicz, & Marshall, 2017).

Diagnostic Evaluation

The actual assessment of children and adolescents who have been observed, referred, or self-reported to have suffered a traumatic event that may have produced a concussion is the meatiest section of management in this chapter. Issue No. 1 is the model used or, to paraphrase Shakespeare, "To baseline or not to baseline, that is the question." Irrespective of the age of the athlete, there is ongoing empirical investigation into whether baseline procedures should continue to be considered the gold standard in concussion management programs. The issue arose partly in considering the level of confidence clinicians may have in their posttrauma assessment outcomes when baseline data are not available (Echemendia et al., 2012; Schmidt, Register-Mihalik, Mihalik, Kerr, & Guskiewicz, 2012). Given that the field of clinical neuropsychology was built on comparing test outcomes with valid group norms, this framing of baseline versus normative comparison is somewhat hollow. Indeed, the few studies available have found that, statistically, clinicians make similar decisions independent of the mode of comparison (Haran et al., 2016). The original rationale for the baseline approach, as Barth and colleagues (Barth, Harvey, Freeman, & Broshek, 2011) later described it, was to eliminate sources of variability that are due to the individual. The importance of eliminating errors in diagnostics remains very important, as it does in research, and, although statistical appraisals of the baseline-versus normative-comparison methods may not favor either protocol, individual clinical decision making likely is facilitated when a major source of variance is eliminated (Webbe & Zimmer, 2015). What is not so clear is whether the baseline procedure as employed in many concussion management programs actually uses procedures that allow baseline advantages to shine forth (Moser, Schatz, & Lichtenstein, 2015; Moser, Schatz, Neidzwski, & Ott, 2011). As Moser and colleagues have noted, whatever advantage in reducing error that occurs theoretically in prospective baseline procedures may be lost or worse if environmental conditions are not well controlled during testing.

When we now focus directly on the pediatric context, the virtue of baseline as a longitudinally replicable snapshot of normal functioning has severe conceptual limitations (Kirkwood, Randolph, & Yeates, 2009). With young children, cognitive developmental change occurs very rapidly, and the use of annual baselines—the most common approach—might, and probably would, result in many false negative outcomes. In other words, the level of cognitive development in one year might or would be great enough so that impairment due to mild brain trauma would be obscured by improved performance. Although reliable change indices are seen as mandatory in the baseline approach because of the necessary repeat testing, it would be difficult to conceptualize a reliable change statistical model that could adapt to the cognitive changes in young children that are not due to head trauma. Unfortunately, the situation with age-based group norms also carries considerably greater inherent variability than is seen with older adolescents and adults (Baron, 2008); that is, two 9-year-olds may be at different levels of intellectual development: Both are normal but have very different developmental slopes, both have possibly suffered a concussion. The slower developing child might appear impaired on testing and yet be normal, whereas the quicker developing child may appear normal or better and yet be impaired compared with his or her premorbid functioning. As Baron (2008) commented about the more general pediatric setting, "whether a measured change in function over time is genuine and inherent to a child's changing neurocognitive status, or a misleading or skewed change that does not accurately reflect true progress or decline over time" (pp. 96–97) demands great skill and knowledge on the part of the clinician. A case certainly can be made that concussion management in children is considerably more complicated than in adults, and more demanding of a pediatric sports neuropsychologist to interpret the meaning of test outcomes and integrate them with other aspects of the clinical examination, review of records, and social and educational history (Gioia, 2015).

Computerized neuropsychological batteries, in which significant numbers of athletes receive baseline testing as part of precompetition medical examinations, have become the staple of most concussion management programs (Webbe & Zimmer, 2015). As mentioned earlier, the reliability and validity of baseline performance on these instruments depend directly on the strict control of ecological variables. Several computerized tests are available to use with adults and adolescents over 12. As of this writing, only the ImPACT and the Pediatric ImPACT (Newman, Reesman, Vaughan, & Gioia, 2013) have been approved by the U.S. Food and Drug Administration (FDA) as a medical device for assessment of cognitive functioning following head trauma in children (FDA, 2016). The family of ImPACT tests are thus the first that have passed this hurdle, which was recommended as critical in the joint position paper of the National Academy of Neuropsychology and the American Academy of Clinical Neuropsychology (Bauer et al., 2012). Although such approval does not equate to an endorsement of effectiveness, it does ensure that certain standards of care and analysis have been taken in test development, quality testing, and independent review of use outcomes. Other tests are used routinely with older children and adults, with levels of reliability and validity reasonably equivalent to ImPACT (Nelson et al., 2016).

Given that the one normative study of performance on ImPACT with 10- to 12-year-old children (Reynolds, Fazio, Sandel, Schatz, & Henry, 2016) showed many significant differences in subtest and domain performance across the single age groups, the development of Pediatric ImPACT has been an important addition to tests designed for younger children. Pediatric ImPACT provides for 5- to 12-year-olds a computerized battery that measures attention, memory, reaction time, and cognitive speed. Pediatric ImPACT is a significant departure from the adult version of ImPACT, with the subtests geared toward children's more limited abstract abilities, fluency, and experience. Gioia and colleagues (2012) reported age-related differences in reaction time and memory, with younger children slower to react and more challenged on the memory tasks, as one would expect (Newman et al., 2013). These early reports suggest that children interact with the subtests of Pediatric ImPACT in a manner that is encouraging of understanding rules and responding as directions demand. Given the earlier cautions about using baseline approaches with young children, considerably more empirical data on clinical outcomes with ImPACT in a baseline protocol is desirable, as is the collection of normative performance for the young child population. In the meantime, conservative practice would suggest relying on ImPACT more as a posttrauma measure in combination with standard neuropsychological tests and batteries.

Generally speaking, normative data for youth who sustain a concussion are sparse, and relying on psychometrically sound neuropsychological measures may produce more accurate results. At a minimum, test selection should include measures of attention and concentration, executive functioning, visual and verbal memory, visuomotor ability, processing speed, verbal fluency, and sensorimotor skills. Moreover, tests or structured observations of emotional behavior and mood should be used. Tests that appear reasonably robust or that have child norms are listed in Table 13.1.

Return to Play

It is now the case that youth leagues and high schools are governed, however loosely, by state regulations that require certification by a health care professional before a concussed child is returned to play (Centers for Disease Control and Prevention, 2015; Harvey, 2013). Regrettably, the definition of *health care professional*, as well as the stringency of procedures required, extends from disappointing to good. We recommend that coaches and parents emphasize the importance of safe play and should err on the side of caution concerning a child's return to athletic practice and play. The recommendations of the 5th International Conference on Concussion in Sports, as

TABLE 13.1
Standard Neuropsychological Tests That Have Been Used
in the Management of Pediatric Concussion

Domain	Test
Auditory/verbal learning and memory	California Verbal Learning Test, Children's Version (Horton et al., 1996); Rey Auditory Verbal Learning Test (Schmidt, 1996)
Visual/spatial learning and memory	Brief Visuospatial Memory Test—Revised (Benedict et al., 1996), WRAML–II Picture Memory, WRAML–II Design Memory, TVPS Visual Memory, TVPS Sequential Memory, Rey–Osterreith Complex Figure Test (Meyer & Meyers, 1995)
Processing speed	Symbol Digit Modalities Test; Children's Trail Making Test, Parts A and B (Allen et al., 2011); WISC–IV Symbol Search; WISC–IV Digit Symbol Coding
Executive function	Tower of London–Drexel (Culbertson & Zillmer, 1998), NEPSY–II Inhibition
Attention	WISC–IV Digit Span
Word fluency	NEPSY–II Word Generation, COWAT; NEPSY–II Speeded Naming

Note. WRAML = Wide Range Assessment of Memory and Learning (Sheslow & Adams, 1990); TVPS = Test of Visual–Perceptual Skills, Non-Motor (Gardner, 1982); WISC–IV = Wechsler Intelligence Scale for Children—Fourth Edition (Wechsler, 2004); NEPSY–2 = A Developmental NEuroPSYchological Assessment, Second Edition (Korkman, Kirk, & Kemp, 2007); COWAT = Controlled Oral Word Association Test (Benton, 1969).

well as other bodies, including the National Athletic Trainers' Association, the American Academy of Neurology, and the National Academy of Neuropsychology, all advocate that athletes should not return to play if they continue to be symptomatic after a concussion, either at rest or under physical or cognitive exertion (Broglio et al., 2014; Giza et al., 2013; McCrory et al., 2017; Moser et al., 2007).

Because the consequences of concussion for young athletes are still not fully understood, there are two reasons why it is important to be conservative when making return-to-play decisions in child athletes. First, children apparently take longer to reach the point of symptom resolution, thus extending the time when their vulnerability to additional injury is high (Crowe et al., 2016). Second, an emphasis on the safety of young athletes may support continued athletic participation into college and beyond, and at the same time promote brain health for a lifetime.

CASE STUDY

Some of the original details of this case have been changed to protect the confidentiality of the individual tested.

Nick, an 11-year-old boy, has been playing football in a community league for 3 years. His parents like how active the sport keeps him and the commitment he shows to his teammates. During Nick's Friday night game he was running with the ball when he was tackled from behind. His coach and teammates were pleased his hard work in practice had paid off, given that he tucked the ball in when falling instead of dropping it and trying to catch himself with his hands. Nick struck the ground hard with his right shoulder, but quickly and easily got back up. His adrenaline was pumping, he was exhausted and hot, but he was elated he had kept the ball! His coach checked in with him briefly, but Nick denied any injury to his shoulder. He felt dazed and a little "off," but this was not an unfamiliar feeling for him during a long, hot game and he didn't want to leave his team to get checked out. He went back into play but did not accomplish much during the remaining 30 seconds of the game.

Nick thought once he had taken a shower, cooled down, and eased back from the adrenaline of the game he would feel more like himself. However, he had a hard time keeping up with his teammates as they bantered about the game in the locker room. He noticed a steady increase in the headache he had developed during the end of the game, and he suddenly just really wanted to go to bed. His parents were surprised by his request to go straight home, but they figured he was likely just tired from a long week of school, practices, and an evening game. Nick slept for 11 hours that night but still felt foggy and not like himself the next day. His headache continued, and his parents wondered if he was getting sick. He mostly slept and watched TV the rest of the weekend because his headache got worse when he attempted to do his favorite hobbies of playing video games or riding his bike.

Nick had a test in math class on Monday, but he wasn't worried about it because it was his best subject. He reviewed a little on Sunday but had a hard time focusing. About 20 minutes into the test, he began panicking—he couldn't keep his mind focused enough to complete the longer equations, and he was only two questions into the 15-question exam. Nick became more agitated as the remaining exam time ticked away, and he felt miserable when his teacher collected the half-completed paper at the end of the class. He asked to go to the nurse's office to be evaluated and possibly sent home.

Nick sat with the nurse, Ms. Chelsea, and described his current symptoms of headache, difficulty focusing, agitation, fatigue, and general sense of not feeling "right." Ms. Chelsea had recently attended a concussion educational presentation through the school's athletic department and recognized Nick's symptoms as possible indications of a concussion. She questioned him further about the game and eventually learned about the hard hit Nick took toward the end of the game. While describing the tackle, Nick again focused on hitting the ground with his shoulder, but he also remembered that the right side of his head hit the ground as well when he bounced from the impact. Ms. Chelsea recognized how Nick's likely concussion would interfere with his ability to focus on his exam or other classes. She also knew an increase in rest during the acute recovery period of concussion was recommended. She called Nick's parents and recommended Nick go home and not engage in any strenuous activity but to take a short walk a few times a day and to do some brief reading, as long as it did not increase his headache.

Nick stayed home for the next two days, mostly engaged in restful activity but taking a few short walks a day and doing some reading for school in brief 20-minute sessions. His headache slowly subsided, and by the second day home he was no longer feeling fatigued or foggy. Because Ms. Chelsea provided an explanation of Nick's symptoms to his math teacher, he was permitted to retake the exam the following week. He had to sit out of practice for the rest of the week, but he kept up with the team by reading the playbook and sitting on the sidelines of practice from Wednesday onward.

Ms. Chelsea also recommended the community football league have an athletic trainer or other qualified professional who could evaluate Nick to determine when he was fully recovered from his concussion and could return to play. The athletic trainer who was present for some of the team's games was surprised to learn Nick likely had a concussion and felt guilty he did not see the tackle or suspect Nick had sustained a concussion during Friday's game. He was diligent in working with Nick to monitor his symptoms. He also used brief tests to monitor Nick's memory, processing speed, and balance. Eleven days after the hit, Nick met with the athletic trainer for the third time and reported that he had not experienced any symptoms in the past two days. The athletic trainer had Nick complete some brief drills, tested his memory and balance, and was satisfied he had recovered from his concussion when Nick denied any breakthrough symptoms during the exercises and seemed back to his typical self. The athletic trainer kept a close eye on Nick during the next several practices.

CLINICAL TAKE-HOME POINTS

1. *Children are not "little adults."* Their mental and cognitive frame is qualitatively different, their emotional responses will be less predictable and possibly more florid, than those of adults, and thus the methods for assessing symptom exacerbation and of neuropsychological testing differ in kind from adults'.
2. *Awareness of the impact of the injury on the child's social functioning, academic work, and continued integration with his or her*

teammates is necessary. Because of these differences there is a greater onus on the clinician in conducting concussion evaluations, and the knowledge and skill base of the practitioner must be oriented toward these idiosyncrasies.

KEY QUESTIONS FOR FUTURE RESEARCH

1. *What are the long-term outcomes for children who sustain a concussion during young childhood, childhood, or adolescence? Does the age at first concussion have an impact on long-term memory and processing speed performance?*
2. *To what extent do the severity and duration of symptoms after a pediatric concussion predict greater morbidity after brain trauma later in development?*
3. *Can baseline procedures be perfected so as to be a useful protocol in concussion management with young children?*

REFERENCES

Allen, D., Thaler, N., Ringdahl, E., Vogel, S., & Mayfield, J. (2011). Comprehensive Trail Making Test performance in children and adolescents with traumatic brain injury. *Psychological Assessment, 24,* 556–564.

Baron, I. S. (2008). Growth and development of pediatric neuropsychology. In J. E. Morgan & J. H. Ricker (Eds.), *Textbook of clinical neuropsychology* (pp. 91–104). New York, NY: Taylor & Francis.

Barth, J. T., Harvey, D. J., Freeman, J. R., & Broshek, D. K. (2011). Sport as a laboratory assessment model. In F. M. Webbe (Ed.), *Handbook of sport neuropsychology* (pp. 75–89). New York, NY: Springer.

Bauer, R. M., Iverson, G. L., Cernich, A. N., Binder, L. M., Ruff, R. M., & Naugle, R. I. (2012). Computerized neuropsychological assessment devices: Joint position paper of the American Academy of Clinical Neuropsychology and the National Academy of Neuropsychology. *The Clinical Neuropsychologist, 26,* 177–196. http://dx.doi.org/10.1080/13854046.2012.663001

Benedict, R. H. B., Schretlen, D., Groninger, L., Dobraski, M., & Shpritz, B. (1996). Revision of the Brief Visuospatial Memory Test: Studies of normal performance, reliability, and validity. *Psychological Assessment, 8,* 145–153.

Benton, A. L. (1969). Development of a multilingual aphasia battery: Progress and problems. *Journal of the Neurological Sciences, 9,* 39–48.

Bramley, H., Patrick, K., Lehman, E., & Silvis, M. (2012). High school soccer players with concussion education are more likely to notify their coach of a suspected concussion. *Clinical Pediatrics, 51*, 332–336. http://dx.doi.org/10.1177/0009922811425233

Broglio, S. P., Cantu, R. C., Gioia, G. A., Guskiewicz, K. M., Kutcher, J., Palm, M., . . . National Athletic Trainer's Association. (2014). National Athletic Trainers' Association position statement: Management of sport concussion. *Journal of Athletic Training, 49*, 245–265. http://dx.doi.org/10.4085/1062-6050-49.1.07

Buckley, T. A., Munkasy, B. A., & Clouse, B. P. (2016). Acute cognitive and physical rest may not improve concussion recovery time. *The Journal of Head Trauma Rehabilitation, 31*, 233–241. http://dx.doi.org/10.1097/HTR.0000000000000165

Canadian Heritage. (2013). *Sport participation 2010* [Research paper]. Gatineau, Quebec, Canada: Author.

Centers for Disease Control and Prevention. (2006). *Nonfatal traumatic brain injuries from sports and recreation activities*. Atlanta, GA: Author.

Centers for Disease Control and Prevention. (2015). *Sports concussion policies and laws*. Retrieved from https://www.cdc.gov/headsup/policy/index.html

Choe, M. C., Babikian, T., DiFiori, J., Hovda, D. A., & Giza, C. C. (2012). A pediatric perspective on concussion pathophysiology. *Current Opinion in Pediatrics, 24*, 689–695. http://dx.doi.org/10.1097/MOP.0b013e32835a1a44

Crowe, L., Collie, A., Hearps, S., Dooley, J., Clausen, H., Maddocks, D., . . . Anderson, V. (2016). Cognitive and physical symptoms of concussive injury in children: A detailed longitudinal recovery study. *British Journal of Sports Medicine, 50*, 311–316.

Culbertson, W. C., & Zillmer, E. A. (1998). The Tower of London[DX]: A standardized approach to assessing executive functioning in children. *Archives of Clinical Neuropsychology, 13*, 285–301.

Davis, G. A., & Purcell, L. K. (2014). The evaluation and management of acute concussion differs in young children. *British Journal of Sports Medicine, 48*, 98–101. http://dx.doi.org/10.1136/bjsports-2012-092132

Echemendia, R. J., Bruce, J. M., Bailey, C. M., Sanders, J. F., Arnett, P., & Vargas, G. (2012). The utility of post-concussion neuropsychological data in identifying cognitive change following sports-related MTBI in the absence of baseline data. *The Clinical Neuropsychologist, 26*, 1077–1091. http://dx.doi.org/10.1080/13854046.2012.721006

Eisenberg, M. A., Andrea, J., Meehan, W., & Mannix, R. (2013). Time interval between concussions and symptom duration. *Pediatrics, 132*, 8–17. http://dx.doi.org/10.1542/peds.2013-0432

Erlanger, D., Kaushik, T., Cantu, R., Barth, J. T., Broshek, D. K., Freeman, J. R., & Webbe, F. M. (2003). Symptom-based assessment of the severity of a concussion. *Journal of Neurosurgery, 98*, 477–484. http://dx.doi.org/10.3171/jns.2003.98.3.0477

Field, M., Collins, M. W., Lovell, M. R., & Maroon, J. (2003). Does age play a role in recovery from sports-related concussion? A comparison of high school and

collegiate athletes. *The Journal of Pediatrics, 142,* 546–553. http://dx.doi.org/
10.1067/mpd.2003.190

Frommer, L. J., Gurka, K. K., Cross, K. M., Ingersoll, C. D., Comstock, R. D., &
Saliba, S. A. (2011). Sex differences in concussion symptoms of high school
athletes. *Journal of Athletic Training, 46,* 76–84. http://dx.doi.org/10.4085/
1062-6050-46.1.76

Galetta, K. M., Barrett, J., Allen, M., Madda, F., Delicata, D., Tennant, A. T., . . .
Balcer, L. J. (2011). The King–Devick test as a determinant of head trauma
and concussion in boxers and MMA fighters. *Neurology, 76,* 1456–1462. http://
dx.doi.org/10.1212/WNL.0b013e31821184c9

Gardner, M. F. (1982). *Test of Visual–Perceptual Skills (Non-Motor).* Seattle, WA:
Special Child.

Gioia, G. A. (2015). Multimodal evaluation and management of children with
concussion: Using our heads and available evidence. *Brain Injury, 29,* 195–206.
http://dx.doi.org/10.3109/02699052.2014.965210

Gioia, G. A., Schneider, J. C., Vaughan, C. G., & Isquith, P. K. (2009). Which
symptom assessments and approaches are uniquely appropriate for paediatric
concussion? *British Journal of Sports Medicine, 43*(Suppl. 1), i13–i22. http://
dx.doi.org/10.1136/bjsm.2009.058255

Gioia, G. A., Vaughan, C. G., & Sady, M. D. S. (2012). Developmental considerations in pediatric concussion evaluation and management. In J. N. Apps
& K. D. Walter (Eds.), *Pediatric and adolescent concussion: Diagnosis, management and outcome* (pp. 151–176). New York, NY: Springer. http://dx.doi.org/
10.1007/978-0-387-89545-1_12

Giza, C. C., & Hovda, D. A. (2014). The new neurometabolic cascade of
concussion. *Neurosurgery, 75*(4, Suppl. 4), S24–S33. http://dx.doi.org/10.1227/
NEU.0000000000000505

Giza, C. C., Kutcher, J. S., Ashwal, S., Barth, J., Getchius, T. S., Gioia, G. A., . . .
Zafonte, R. (2013). Summary of evidence-based guideline update: Evaluation
and management of concussion in sports. *Neurology, 80,* 2250–2257. http://
dx.doi.org/10.1212/WNL.0b013e31828d57dd

Guerriero, R. M., Proctor, M. R., Mannix, R., & Meehan, W. P., III. (2012). Epidemiology, trends, assessment and management of sport-related concussion in
United States high schools. *Current Opinion in Pediatrics, 24,* 696–701. http://
dx.doi.org/10.1097/MOP.0b013e3283595175

Guskiewicz, K. M. (2001). Postural stability assessment following concussion: One
piece of the puzzle. *Clinical Journal of Sport Medicine, 11,* 182–189.

Halstead, M. E., Walter, K. D., & the Council on Sports Medicine and Fitness.
(2010). Clinical report—Sport-related concussion in children and adolescents.
Pediatrics, 126, 597–615. http://dx.doi.org/10.1542/peds.2010-2005

Haran, F. J., Dretsch, M. N., Slaboda, J. C., Johnson, D. E., Adam, O. R., & Tsao,
J. W. (2016). Comparison of baseline-referenced versus norm-referenced

analytical approaches for in-theatre assessment of mild traumatic brain injury neurocognitive impairment. *Brain Injury, 30*, 280–286. http://dx.doi.org/10.3109/02699052.2015.1118766

Harvey, H. H. (2013). Reducing traumatic brain injuries in youth sports: Youth sports traumatic brain injury state laws, January 2009–December 2012. *American Journal of Public Health, 103*, 1249–1254. http://dx.doi.org/10.2105/AJPH.2012.301107

Horton, A. M., Russo, A. A., & Bigler, E. D. (1996). The California Verbal Learning Test—Children's Version (CVLT–C). *Archives of Clinical Neuropsychology, 11*, 171. http://dx.doi.org/10.1093/arclin/11.2.171

Iverson, G. L., Silverberg, N. D., Mannix, R., Maxwell, B. A., Atkins, J. E., Zafonte, R., & Berkner, P. D. (2015). Factors associated with concussion-like symptom reporting in high school athletes. *JAMA Pediatrics, 169*, 1132–1140. http://dx.doi.org/10.1001/jamapediatrics.2015.2374

Kirkwood, M. W., Randolph, C., & Yeates, K. O. (2009). Returning pediatric athletes to play after concussion: The evidence (or lack thereof) behind baseline neuropsychological testing. *Acta Paediatrica, 98*, 1409–1411. http://dx.doi.org/10.1111/j.1651-2227.2009.01448.x

Kirkwood, M. W., Yeates, K. O., & Wilson, P. E. (2006). Pediatric sport-related concussion: A review of the clinical management of an oft-neglected population. *Pediatrics, 117*, 1359–1371. http://dx.doi.org/10.1542/peds.2005-0994

Kontos, A. P., Covassin, T., Elbin, R. J., & Parker, T. (2012). Depression and neurocognitive performance after concussion among male and female high school and collegiate athletes. *Archives of Physical Medicine and Rehabilitation, 93*, 1751–1756. http://dx.doi.org/10.1016/j.apmr.2012.03.032

Kontos, A. P., Elbin, R. J., Fazio-Sumrock, V. C., Burkhart, S., Swindell, H., Maroon, J., & Collins, M. W. (2013). Incidence of sports-related concussion among youth football players aged 8–12 years. *The Journal of Pediatrics, 163*, 717–720. http://dx.doi.org/10.1016/j.jpeds.2013.04.011

Korkman, M., Kirk, U., & Kemp, S. L. (2007). *NEPSY II: Administrative manual.* San Antonio, TX: Psychological Corporation.

Kurowski, B. G., Pomerantz, W. J., Schaiper, C., Ho, M., & Gittelman, M. A. (2015). Impact of preseason concussion education on knowledge, attitudes, and behaviors of high school athletes. *The Journal of Trauma and Acute Care Surgery, 79*(3, Suppl. 1), S21–S28. http://dx.doi.org/10.1097/TA.0000000000000675

Maddocks, D. L., Dicker, G. D., & Saling, M. M. (1995). The assessment of orientation following concussion in athletes. *Clinical Journal of Sport Medicine, 5*, 32–35.

Marar, M., McIlvain, N. M., Fields, S. K., & Comstock, R. D. (2012). Epidemiology of concussions among United States high school athletes in 20 sports. *The American Journal of Sports Medicine, 40*, 747–755. http://dx.doi.org/10.1177/0363546511435626

McCrea, M., Guskiewicz, K., Randolph, C., Barr, W. B., Hammeke, T. A., Marshall, S. W., . . . Kelly, J. P. (2013). Incidence, clinical course, and predictors of prolonged recovery time following sport-related concussion in high school and college athletes. *Journal of the International Neuropsychological Society, 19,* 22–33. http://dx.doi.org/10.1017/S1355617712000872

McCrea, M., Hammeke, T., Olsen, G., Leo, P., & Guskiewicz, K. (2004). Unreported concussion in high school football players: Implications for prevention. *Clinical Journal of Sport Medicine, 14,* 13–17. http://dx.doi.org/10.1097/00042752-200401000-00003

McCrory, P., Meeuwisse, W., Dvořák, J., Aubry, M., Bailes, J., Broglio, S., . . . Vos, P. E. (2017). Consensus statement on concussion in sport—The 5th International Conference on Concussion in Sport held in Berlin, October 2016. *British Journal of Sports Medicine, 51,* 838–847.

Meyer, J. E., & Meyers, K. R. (1995). *Rey Complex Figure Test and Recognition Trial Professional Manual.* Odessa, FL: Psychological Assessment Resources.

Mihalik, J. P., Lynall, R. C., Wasserman, E. B., Guskiewicz, K. M., & Marshall, S. W. (2017). Evaluating the "threshold theory": Can head impact indicators help? *Medicine and Science in Sports and Exercise, 49,* 247–253. http://dx.doi.org/10.1249/MSS.0000000000001089

Moser, R. S., Glatts, C., & Schatz, P. (2012). Efficacy of immediate and delayed cognitive and physical rest for treatment of sports-related concussion. *The Journal of Pediatrics, 161,* 922–926. http://dx.doi.org/10.1016/j.jpeds.2012.04.012

Moser, R. S., Iverson, G. L., Echemendia, R., Lovell, M., Schatz, P., Webbe, F. M., . . . Barth, J. T. (2007). Neuropsychological testing in the diagnosis and management of sports-related concussion. *Archives of Clinical Neuropsychology, 22,* 909–916.

Moser, R. S., Schatz, P., & Lichtenstein, J. D. (2015). The importance of proper administration and interpretation of neuropsychological baseline and postconcussion computerized testing. *Applied Neuropsychology: Child, 4,* 41–48. http://dx.doi.org/10.1080/21622965.2013.791825

Moser, R. S., Schatz, P., Neidzwski, K., & Ott, S. D. (2011). Group versus individual administration affects baseline neurocognitive test performance. *The American Journal of Sports Medicine, 39,* 2325–2330. http://dx.doi.org/10.1177/0363546511417114

National Council of Youth Sports. (2008). *Market research report: NCYS membership survey.* Stuart, FL: Author.

National Federation of State High School Associations. (2015). *2014–2015 High school athletics participation survey.* Indianapolis, IN: Author.

NCAA Sport Science Institute. (2017). Concussion Safety Protocol Checklist. Retrieved from https://www.ncaa.org/sites/default/files/2017SSI_ConcussionSafetyProtocolChecklist_20170322.pdf

Nelson, L. D., Guskiewicz, K. M., Marshall, S. W., Hammeke, T., Barr, W., Randolph, C., & McCrea, M. A. (2016). Multiple self-reported concussions are more prevalent in athletes with ADHD and learning disability. *Clinical Journal of Sport Medicine, 26,* 120–127. http://dx.doi.org/10.1097/JSM.0000000000000207

Newman, J. B., Reesman, J. H., Vaughan, C. G., & Gioia, G. A. (2013). Assessment of processing speed in children with mild TBI: A "first look" at the validity of pediatric ImPACT. *The Clinical Neuropsychologist, 27,* 779–793. http://dx.doi.org/10.1080/13854046.2013.789552

O'Connor, S. S., Zatzick, D. F., Wang, J., Temkin, N., Koepsell, T. D., Jaffe, K. M., . . . Rivara, F. P. (2012). Association between posttraumatic stress, depression, and functional impairments in adolescents 24 months after traumatic brain injury. *Journal of Traumatic Stress, 25,* 264–271. http://dx.doi.org/10.1002/jts.21704

O'Kane, J. W., Spieker, A., Levy, M. R., Neradilek, M., Polissar, N. L., & Schiff, M. A. (2014). Concussion among female middle-school soccer players. *JAMA Pediatrics, 168,* 258–264. http://dx.doi.org/10.1001/jamapediatrics.2013.4518

Parker, E. M., Gilchrist, J., Schuster, D., Lee, R., & Sarmiento, K. (2015). Reach and knowledge change among coaches and other participants of the online course: "Concussion in Sports: What You Need to Know." *The Journal of Head Trauma Rehabilitation, 30,* 198–206. http://dx.doi.org/10.1097/HTR.0000000000000097

Pellman, E. J., Lovell, M. R., Viano, D. C., & Casson, I. R. (2006). Concussion in professional football: Recovery of NFL and high school athletes assessed by computerized neuropsychological testing—Part 12. *Neurosurgery, 58,* 263–274. http://dx.doi.org/10.1227/01.NEU.0000200272.56192.62

Pfister, T., Pfister, K., Hagel, B., Ghali, W. A., & Ronksley, P. E. (2016). The incidence of concussion in youth sports: A systematic review and meta-analysis. *British Journal of Sports Medicine, 50,* 292–297. http://dx.doi.org/10.1136/bjsports-2015-094978

Putukian, M. (2016). The psychological response to injury in student athletes: A narrative review with a focus on mental health. *British Journal of Sports Medicine, 50,* 145–148. http://dx.doi.org/10.1136/bjsports-2015-095586

Reynolds, E., Fazio, V. C., Sandel, N., Schatz, P., & Henry, L. C. (2016). Cognitive development and the Immediate Postconcussion Assessment and Cognitive Testing: A case for separate norms in preadolescents. *Applied Neuropsychology: Child, 5,* 283–293. http://dx.doi.org/10.1080/21622965.2015.1057637

Sady, M., Vaughan, C. G., & Gioia, G. A. (2011). School and the concussed youth: Recommendations for concussion education and management. *Physical Medicine and Rehabilitation Clinics of North America, 22,* 701–719. http://dx.doi.org/10.1016/j.pmr.2011.08.008

Salinas, C. M., Dean, P., LoGalbo, A., Dougherty, M., Field, M., & Webbe, F. M. (2016). Attention-deficit hyperactivity disorder status and baseline neuro-

cognitive performance in high school athletes. *Applied Neuropsychology: Child,*
5, 264–272. http://dx.doi.org/10.1080/21622965.2015.1052814

Schmidt, J. D., Register-Mihalik, J. K., Mihalik, J. P., Kerr, Z. Y., & Guskiewicz, K. M.
(2012). Identifying impairments after concussion: Normative data versus individualized baselines. *Medicine and Science in Sports and Exercise, 44,* 1621–1628.
http://dx.doi.org/10.1249/MSS.0b013e318258a9fb

Schmidt, M. (1996). *Rey Auditory and Verbal Learning Test: A handbook.* Los Angeles,
CA: Western Psychological Association.

Sheslow, D., & Adams, W. (1990). *Wide range assessment of memory and learning.*
Wilmington, DE: Wide Range.

Stanford Children's Health. (2016). *Sports injury statistics.* Retrieved from http://
www.stanfordchildrens.org/en/topic/default?id=sports-injury-statistics-90-P02787

Stracciolini, A., Casciano, R., Levey Friedman, H., Stein, C. J., Meehan, W. P., III,
& Micheli, L. J. (2014). Pediatric sports injuries: A comparison of males versus
females. *The American Journal of Sports Medicine, 42,* 965–972. http://dx.doi.org/
10.1177/0363546514522393

Straus, L. B. (2017). *Concussion hit count and impact sensor product guide.* Retrieved
from http://www.momsteam.com/health-safety/sports-concussion-safety/
impact-sensors/hit-count-impact-sensors-buying-guide

Tator, C. H. (2013). Concussions and their consequences: Current diagnosis, management and prevention. *Canadian Medical Association Journal, 185,* 975–979.
http://dx.doi.org/10.1503/cmaj.120039

U.S. Food and Drug Administration. (2016, August 22). *FDA allows marketing*
of first-of-kind computerized cognitive tests to help assess cognitive skills after a
head injury [News release]. Retrieved from https://www.fda.gov/newsevents/
newsroom/pressannouncements/ucm517526.htm

Valovich McLeod, T. C., & Gioia, G. A. (2010). Cognitive rest—The often
neglected aspect of concussion management. *Athletic Therapy Today, 15,* 1–3.
http://dx.doi.org/10.1123/att.15.2.1

Webbe, F. M., & Zimmer, A. (2015). History of neuropsychological study of sport-
related concussion. *Brain Injury, 29,* 129–138. http://dx.doi.org/10.3109/
02699052.2014.937746

Wechsler, D. (2004). *Wechsler Intelligence Scale for Children—Fourth Edition.* London,
England: Pearson Assessments.

Williamson, R. W., Gerhardstein, D., Cardenas, J., Michael, D. B., Theodore, N., &
Rosseau, N. (2014). Concussion 101: The current state of concussion education
programs. *Neurosurgery, 75*(Suppl. 4), S131–S135. http://dx.doi.org/10.1227/
NEU.0000000000000482

World Health Organization. (2001). *International classification of functioning, disability*
and health. Geneva, Switzerland: Author.

Yard, E. E., & Comstock, R. D. (2009). Compliance with return to play guidelines following concussion in U.S. high school athletes, 2005–2008. *Brain Injury, 23,* 888–898. http://dx.doi.org/10.1080/02699050903283171

Yue, J. K., Winkler, E. A., Burke, J. F., Chan, A. K., Dhall, S. S., Berger, M. S., . . . Tarapore, P. E. (2016). Pediatric sports-related traumatic brain injury in United States trauma centers. *Neurosurgical Focus, 40,* e3. http://dx.doi.org/10.3171/2016.1.FOCUS15612

Zackery Lystedt Law of 2009, H.R. 1824, 61 Wa. § 475, 2009.

Zonfrillo, M. R., Master, C. L., Grady, M. F., Winston, F. K., Callahan, J. M., & Arbogast, K. B. (2012). Pediatric providers' self-reported knowledge, practices, and attitudes about concussion. *Pediatrics, 130,* 1120–1125. http://dx.doi.org/10.1542/peds.2012-1431

14

MANAGEMENT OF SPORTS-RELATED CONCUSSIONS IN AN ORTHOPAEDIC SETTING

NEHA GUPTA AND WAYNE J. SEBASTIANELLI

On any given Sunday during the season, millions of fans gather in stadiums and around their televisions, eagerly anticipating the thundering clash of helmets, the exhilarating roar of the crowd, and the thrill of a hard-won touchdown, as players battle over the prized pigskin. This is football—arguably America's most popular sport. However, over the past decade, a darker side of football has surfaced. This side reveals the startling connection between football and long-term brain damage caused by repetitive mild traumatic brain injuries, which are an inherent risk of the game.

A *concussion* is a type of traumatic brain injury (TBI) caused by a blow to the head or the body that forces the brain to slam against the skull, temporarily impeding its function. Once regarded as benign and even downright exciting in the context of a football game, concussions have recently been proven to have life-altering implications. Before the surge in concussion research, blows to the head were considered trivial. The mind-set toward concussions in

http://dx.doi.org/10.1037/0000114-015
Neuropsychology of Sports-Related Concussion, P. A. Arnett (Editor)

the sports world was well summarized by Dan Bernstein, cohost of the sports radio program *Boers and Bernstein*, as "You got dinged; you got your bell rung; you had cobwebs; you were seeing stars—there was every euphemism to say, 'You're OK'" (Cole, 2012). As long as a player did not lose consciousness, he was expected to "tough it out" and charge back on the field. No one stopped to consider that these seemingly innocuous "dings" could have more than a transient effect.

There is now an understanding that repetitive concussions can cause chronic headaches and depression and may lead to long-term disorders such as dementia and irrational aggression, although these latter links are only speculative. A speculative relationship to the neurodegenerative disease chronic traumatic encephalopathy (CTE) is also of concern (McCrory et al., 2017). Unable to live with these debilitating conditions, several afflicted athletes, such as Andre Waters and Junior Seau, have resorted to suicide in the past 10 years, sending the sports world, the media, and the public into a frenzy. New research spawned by these high-profile suicides has brought to light an unquestionable correlation between football and TBIs, precipitating a paradigm shift in the understanding and treatment of concussions, suggesting that concussions are not merely transient ailments but can be lifelong, compounding TBIs (see Chapter 6, this volume, for a more detailed discussion of CTE).

It is not only in football that concussions occur. Approximately 5.3 million Americans live with disabilities caused by TBIs in the general population, which could result from vehicle accidents, falls, or sports (Centers for Disease Control and Prevention [CDC], 2016b). In the athletic population, 37% of all sport-related concussions occur in football, 16% occur in basketball, and 14% occur in soccer (CDC, 2016a). Specifically in the realm of football, 75% of players sustain a concussion during their career (CDC, 2016a). Athletes, coaches, trainers, and doctors must all join forces to ensure proper management of and prevention against concussions. This chapter highlights the biological impacts of concussions on the brain, the role of orthopedists in the diagnosis and management of sports-related injuries, a summary of numerous treatment options, steps for prevention, and a case study that ties all aspects of the chapter together.

ANATOMY OF A CONCUSSION

Because the brain is the most intricate part of the body and the controller of movement and translator of senses, injury to this structure leads to short- and long-term consequences. Despite being encased in a bony skull and surrounded by protective cerebrospinal fluid, the brain is susceptible to mechanical forces because of its soft and gelatinous consistency (Novack & Bushnik, 2016).

Composed of billions of nerve cells (neurons), the brain is responsible for creating electrical and chemical signals that control the body. One specific neuron consists of a cell body; a nerve fiber, called the *axon*; and body projections that help create connections with other cells called *dendrites* (Nucleus Medical Media, 2012).

When a rapid direct or indirect force is applied to the head, the differential movement of the skull and brain (produced by the difference in their densities) causes the brain to violently move back and forth or side to side, thus colliding with the hard skull that surrounds it. This jarring movement can result in a brain injury due to diffuse axonal shearing, bruising of brain tissue (clinically known as *contusion*) and/or tearing of blood vessels (Nucleus Medical Media, 2012).

When axons are damaged, they break down, and decreased communication occurs between neurons of the brain. In addition, cell injury creates leakage of ions and chemicals from the cells, impairing nerve cell function and membrane pump physiology. Severely injured fibers can permanently lose their ability to communicate with other brain cells. When this occurs, the neurons will die. The tearing of the axon and its surrounding myelin sheath releases neurotransmitters into extracellular spaces, which also causes inflammation and additional injury, extending the zone of damage produced by the initial mechanical force trauma (Nucleus Medical Media, 2012).

Even with sophisticated imaging (computed tomography [CT], magnetic resonance imaging [MRI] scan), most concussions cannot be viewed. Routine scanning techniques reveal only significant contusion, edema, or hemorrhage. When it comes to sport-related mild TBI, imaging is virtually negative, with damage being assessed only by changes in brain function as determined by behavior and cognition (CDC, 2016c).

The majority of people recover within a few days or weeks from a concussion. In a small proportion of individuals, symptoms can extend beyond several weeks. When symptoms occur beyond 3 months, postconcussion syndrome (PCS) must be entertained. Because these symptoms can include fogginess and balance dysfunction, athletic performance will suffer. It is therefore imperative to ensure proper return-to-play protocols, including appropriate rest and management after injury.

SYMPTOMS

It is important to note that every individual's experience with a concussion is different. No two cases are the same. Common symptoms are listed in Exhibit 14.1 (CDC, 2016b).

EXHIBIT 14.1
Common Symptoms of Concussions

Headaches or pressure in the head
Nausea and vomiting
Balance issues and dizziness
Intolerance to bright lights and loud sounds
Ocular issues
Feeling of fogginess, sluggishness, or grogginess
Confusion or concentration issues
Ringing in the ears
Difficulty with memory
Cognitive changes
Emotional changes: irritability, sadness, anxiety, depression, personality shifts
Sleep disturbances
In some cases, loss of consciousness

Cognitive dysfunction in concussion is primarily associated with injury to functioning of the frontal and temporal lobes (U.S. Department of Health and Human Services, n.d.). Headache varieties include migraines, tension, cervicogenic, and rebound headaches. These headaches can be accompanied by nausea, vomiting, and sensitivity to light and noise. Occipital or C2 neuralgia can cause headaches that emanate from the base of the skull and radiate across the scalp ("Occipital Neuralgia," 2016; see Chapter 2, this volume, for more detailed discussion of postconcussion headaches).

Damage to the vestibular system (consisting of the utricle, saccule, and three semicircular canals) can cause the transmission of asymmetrical impulses to the brain. These in turn lead to a dysfunction in head–eye movement and stable gaze, accompanied by vertigo, dizziness, and nausea. Injury to the cerebellum and other parts of the brain can result in impaired balance and posture (National Institute on Deafness and Other Communication Disorders, 2015).

Ocular dysfunction includes difficulties with eye teaming, leading to convergence or divergence excess, saccadic or eye tracking deficiency, focusing or accommodative insufficiency, visual motor integration deficits, and visual vertigo syndrome. These manifest as blurred vision, double vision, headaches, and sensitivity to light. This dysfunction is primarily associated with occipital lobe injury ("Occipital Neuralgia," 2016).

Psychological disorders, such as anxiety, depression, irritability, sadness, and overall personality changes are common after brain injuries (U.S. Department of Health and Human Services, n.d.). Diffuse axonal injury in the frontal lobes and limbic system often disrupt the transmission of endorphins such as serotonin and dopamine, contributing to these mood disorders (Schwarzbold et al., 2008; see Chapter 3, this volume, for more on depression and anxiety in sports-related concussion). Sleep disturbances are also common symptoms after a mild TBI (U.S. Department of Health and Human Services, n.d.).

Along with concussions, other injuries to the body can occur. A spinal cord injury can occur from an axial load to the head, inappropriate tackling technique, twisting of the body, or falling from a height. Whiplash is also common, causing neck pain and stiffness (Jagannathan, Dumont, Prevedello, Shaffrey, & Jane, 2006).

THE ROLE OF ORTHOPAEDIC SURGEONS

Orthopedists focus on injuries and diseases of the body's musculoskeletal system. This system includes bones, joints, ligaments, tendons, muscles, and nerves. Orthopedists are involved in diagnosis, treatment (with medication, exercise, or surgery), rehabilitation (using exercise and physical therapy), and prevention (with future treatment plans) of injuries.

Orthopedists actively work athletic events and must remain alert to a potential injury. Mild TBI must be properly diagnosed to prevent prolonged disability and brain damage. Some athletic programs incorporate telemetry technology that records every head impact the player experiences. An impact above a predetermined threshold can alert sideline personnel to have that athlete removed for assessment.

It is imperative that an individual suffering from a concussion seek medical attention. A thorough and systematic assessment of the injury and its manifestations by a trained medical practitioner is vital in ensuring a rapid and full recovery. To facilitate a speedy and full recovery, it is also critical for physicians to develop individualized management plans.

The first step in treatment should be rest. When a concussion has occurred, the brain is very sensitive to further damage, and continued brain activity can hinder recovery. School, sports, TV, computers, cell phones, and crowded places should be avoided. Analyzing screens is very challenging for the first few days after the injury. Flickerings of 30 Hz can prolong symptoms while the brain needs the most rest (Stone, 2013). Screen usage should be completely avoided during the first 24 hours and should also be limited during the recovery to avoid headaches and excess eyestrain. Concussed athletes should also not return to play or engage in high-risk activities (e.g., exercise) until cleared by a doctor trained in concussion management. Cognitive exertions that involve concentration for reading or writing should be limited during the initial recovery stages. On the basis of present research efforts, what the actual length of time of relative rest should be remains unclear. Close monitoring of symptoms and their resolution can allow activity to be restored relatively quickly. Within the first 24 hours, a patient should be watched closely to see if symptoms escalate, indicating bleeding or swelling in the brain and mandating referral to a neurologist/emergency care provider. High-level imaging (CT, MRI) is not frequently indicated but should be considered in scenarios with symptom progression over time.

Immediate Post-Concussion Assessment and Cognitive Testing (ImPACT; https://www.impacttest.com/products/?ImPACT-Workplace-27), the Standardized Assessment of Concussion—2 test (SAC–2; Graham, Rivara, Ford, & Spicer, 2014), and the Acute Concussion Evaluation (Gioia, Collins, & Isquith, 2008) assess the neurocognitive consequences and severity of concussion. Professionals can also measure progress and determine whether the individual can return to school or sports.

ImPACT evaluates current symptoms, verbal and visual memory, processing speed, and reaction time to 1/100th of a second. With this test, athletes often display concussion symptoms because it is based on test performance compared with baseline data. (See Chapter 10, this volume, for a more detailed exploration of the complex issues involved in neuropsychological assessment in sports-related concussion.)

The SAC–2 is a very useful tool for immediate sideline examination of athletes. Several impairments can be found, including disruptions in orientation, memory, and concentration, that can determine an athlete's mental state.

The Acute Concussion Evaluation characterizes an injury, identifies the type and severity of symptoms, and shows the individualized risk factors that could impede recovery.

An athlete should return to play when cleared by a doctor. The Pennsylvania State University's return-to-play protocol (National Collegiate Athletic Association, 2015) is given in Exhibit 14.2.

EXHIBIT 14.2
Pennsylvania State University's Return-to-Play Protocol

Step 1: No activity, complete rest
Step 2: Light aerobic exercise (walking, stationary cycling keeping intensity < 70% mph); no resistance training
Step 3: Sport-specific exercise (skating in hockey, running in soccer); no head impact activities
Step 4: Noncontact training drills; progression to more complex training drills (passing drills in football and ice hockey). May start progressive resistance exercise.
Step 5: Full contact training
Step 6: Game play—full clearance

Note. Athletes cannot pass two steps in 1 day.

Physical therapy/athletic training for injuries to the body that occur simultaneously with concussion, such as neck and spine injuries, should be initiated. Rehabilitation of associated injuries decreases pain and swelling and increases strength, range of motion, flexibility, coordination, and endurance.

The high velocity applied to the head during whiplash can cause a concussion, and vice versa. Whiplash includes spraining of the neck ligaments and straining of neck muscles, resulting in pain, stiffness, vertigo, shoulder and back pain, and headaches (Wellmont Health System, 2016). Therefore, not only the symptoms of the concussion but also those of whiplash must be addressed.

Some patients experience poor cognitive performance, sleep disturbances, anxiety, depression, or posttraumatic migraines. Medications can alleviate some of these symptoms when cognitive and physical rest or mechanical treatments do not improve PCS symptoms. These medications include nonsteroidal anti-inflammatory drugs, amitriptyline, topiramates, gabapentins, beta blockers, calcium channel blockers, valproic acid, triptans, sertraline, and dihydroergotamine (Meehan, 2011). Medications that affect platelet formation or clotting should be avoided in the acute phase of treatment (nonsteroidal anti-inflammatory drugs, aspirin).

OTHER OPTIONS THAT MAY ALLEVIATE SYMPTOMS OF POSTCONCUSSION SYNDROME

Those treating concussions and those being treated should be aware of the various treatment options that may alleviate symptoms caused by concussions. The recommended treatment plan depends on the patient's symptoms. Many treatment options are still experimental, so we recommend that you first speak with a medical professional and a professional trained in the treatment specialty before initiating any treatment. Further evidence-based research should investigate the efficacy of symptom management options.

PREPARING STUDENT ATHLETES TO PREVENT CONCUSSIONS

When resources are available, baseline assessments such as impact, the SAC–2, or virtual reality programs can be helpful (McCrory et al., 2017; see also Exhibit 14.3). These instruments can then be readministered after a concussion to see what deficits are present. The results can also be used to assess recovery and guide return to play.

EXHIBIT 14.3
Various Options That Might Alleviate Postconcussion Symptoms

Vision therapy works on correcting visual–motor and perceptual–cognitive deficiencies. Activities are done to enhance the brain's ability to control eye alignment, eye teaming, eye focusing, eye movements, and visual processing (Gallaway, Scheiman, & Mitchell, 2017; U.S. Department of Health and Human Services, n.d.).

Acupuncture is an ancient Chinese healing technique. Research is being conducted to test the efficacy of acupuncture in relieving post-concussion symptoms such as headaches, anxiety, depression, insomnia, and cognitive deficits. Although measuring the cause and effect of acupuncture is difficult, several studies have indicated that further research of well designed, adequately powered studies is warranted (Pilkington, Kirkwood, Rampes, Cummings, & Richardson, 2007).

Active Release Techniques alleviate pain and other symptoms associated with scar tissue buildup. This patented method involves precisely directed manual tension with very specific muscle-lengthening movements. It restores the motion and function of the soft tissue. Entrapped nerves and blood vessels are also released in the process. This may help with chronic neck pain associated with post-concussion syndrome (Kim, Lee, & Park, 2015; "What Is Active Release Techniques (ART) to individuals, athletes, and patients?", n.d.).

Vestibular rehabilitation therapy is a specialized exercise-based program that aims to alleviate vestibular disorders such as vertigo and dizziness, gaze instability and imbalance. Vestibular rehabilitation therapy also reduces secondary vestibular problems such as nausea and/or vomiting and fatigue (Alsalaheen et al., 2010; Vestibular Disorders Association, 2016).

Neurofeedback involves the direct training of brain function, enabling it to function more efficiently. Electrodes placed on the scalp read brainwave frequencies, a process known as *electroencephalography*. Electroencephalography is often sensitive to the impacts on the brain after a concussion. Through beeps and video game–like settings, the brain is taught to self-regulate: Some brain frequencies are promoted, whereas others are diminished. Experiments have tested the efficacy of neurofeedback in reducing a variety of psychiatric disorders, migraines, anxiety, memory dysfunctions, and other effects of a concussion. This is experimental, and further research is being conducted (Esty & Shifflett, 2014).

Atlas Readjustment Mobilizations (C1), or "Atlas," can affect alignment of the spine. The head is tilted and the spine shifts to support the head, causing postural strains and nerve dysfunctions. The atlas is gently and noninvasively manipulated using X rays and a specified machine. The intended outcome is to generate proper nerve flow. Research is still being conducted to test efficacy for migraine and neck pain patients (Atlas Orthogonal Chiropractic, 2016).

Occipital Nerve Block Injection is an injection of a steroid or medication around the greater or lesser occipital nerves at the back of the head. This reduces the inflammation around the nerves and can lead to a reduction in tension and migraine headaches (Ashkenazi & Young, 2005).

Proper fitting of equipment is crucial for player safety. Football helmets should fit properly to ensure maximum protection. Coaches and trainers should learn the procedures to measure head size and adjust the fit of helmets with inflation tools. Coaching can influence injury risk, such as heading a ball in soccer and tackling in football. Strengthening the neck is crucial in sports in which blows to the head are common. A strong neck dampens the force applied to the head. A strong neck lessens the severity of concussions. People with a smaller mean neck circumference and weaker neck strength should be targeted for concussion prevention programs that focus on neck strengthening (Collins et al., 2014).

The Pennsylvania Amended Early Intervention Services System Act (Pub. L. 1372) set standards for managing concussions and TBIs to student athletes. There are penalties if these requirements are not followed. These strict guidelines should be replicated in every state.

The shift in society's perception of concussions has fostered better research and, consequently, a superior understanding of these injuries. It is important for athletes to report a potential concussion and for parents, coaches, or teammates to report an athlete suspected of having a concussion. This culture of reporting needs to be spearheaded by the health care team. If individuals become more open to seeking treatment and preventing injury, the paradigm will likely continue to shift and allow for a deeper understanding of the brain's rehabilitative abilities.

CASE STUDY

Some of the original details of this case have been changed to protect the confidentiality of the individual tested

An 18-year-old female college basketball freshman fell onto the court, from a height of 3 feet, landing on the back of her head. She did not lose consciousness, and denied any immediate changes in vision, chest pain, shortness of breath, or vomiting. She did note a headache. Several hours later she started to vomit. She was taken to the emergency room. A CT scan showed no evidence of skull fracture, hemorrhage, or contusion. Intravenous Zofran was administered.

After she was discharged, fatigue and reduced appetite persisted. Reports of balance and sleep disturbances continued. Hypersensitivity to sound and light led her to leave school. After 5 weeks of relative rest, symptoms continued. She was referred for additional treatment programs, including vestibular therapy, physical therapy, vision therapy, the atlas procedure, acupuncture, and occipital nerve block injections.

A physical assessment revealed the following:

- Convergence excess: She was unable to use both eyes together.
- Accommodative insufficiency: She was unable to track a moving target and switch fixation from one target to another, which hindered her ability to read or take notes in class.
- Saccadic eye movement deficiency: She had trouble with shifting attention from one distance to another with instantaneous clarity.
- Visual motor integration deficits: She had some trouble with eye–hand coordination.
- Visual vertigo syndrome: She exhibited signs of postconcussive balance disorder, visual contexts (including movement of two- or three-dimensional objects), words on a page, and navigating supermarkets), which aggravated her symptoms.

Vestibular therapy escalated her nausea. Acupuncture was initiated and was successful in improved tolerance to sound and light and decreased her headache intensity. Atlas therapy also decreased her headache severity. Six months after her injury, symptoms continued as she returned to school. All therapies continued, and additional treatments were started, including occipital blocks and medications (amitriptyline, propranolol, prednisone, dihydroergotamine, metoclopramide, nabumetone, sumatriptan, divalproex sodium, topiramate, gabapentin, and frovatriptan). Despite marked improvement 18 months later, her symptoms persist, and the athlete is functional but not competitive. Day-to-day symptoms can be managed by medications and antiemetics when necessary.

This case highlights the poor correlation between the apparent initial severity and recovery from a "mild" TBI or concussion. It illustrates how an individualized model of care is crucial in treating a concussion effectively in an orthopaedic setting and ensuring that symptoms are comprehensively treated.

CLINICAL TAKE-HOME POINTS

1. *There are several treatments and therapies that should be considered.* This chapter includes a comprehensive list of therapies, but the therapies must be tailored to the individual.
2. *Concussion severity is not dictated by loss of consciousness.*
3. *Physical exercise progression needs to be monitored for symptom escalation.*
4. *Cognitive rest is just as important as physical rest.*
5. *Symptom resolution may not mean injury resolution.*

KEY QUESTIONS TO BE ADDRESSED IN THE NEXT 5 YEARS

1. *What is the role of biomarkers in determining level or severity of a concussion?* Do elevated nerve biomarkers in the saliva or blood correlate with TBI?
2. *What rule changes for contact sports will be necessary to reduce the risk of concussions?* How can we change the play of the game to minimize head injury risk?
3. *Do multiple subconcussive blows lead to CTE?* What level of frequency and severity of concussion leads to CTE?

REFERENCES

Alsalaheen, B. A., Mucha, A., Morris, L. O., Whitney, S. L., Furman, J. M., Camiolo-Reddy, C. E., . . . Sparto, P. J. (2010). Vestibular rehabilitation for dizziness and balance disorders after concussion. *Journal of Neurologic Physical Therapy, 34*, 87–93. http://dx.doi.org/10.1097/NPT.0b013e3181dde568

Amended Early Intervention Services System Act, H.R. 20 (Penn.), Pub. L. 1372 (2017).

Ashkenazi, A., & Young, W. B. (2005). The effects of greater occipital nerve block and trigger point injection on brush allodynia and pain in migraine. *Headache, 45*, 350–354. http://dx.doi.org/10.1111/j.1526-4610.2005.05073.x

Atlas Orthogonal Chiropractic. (2016). *Our techniques.* Retrieved from http://www.atlasorthogonalchiro.com/About-Us/Our-Techniques.aspx

Centers for Disease Control and Prevention. (2016a). *Concussion awareness* [Digital image]. Retrieved from https://www.cdc.gov/headsup/resources/graphics.html

Centers for Disease Control and Prevention. (2016b). *Severe TBI.* Retrieved from http://www.cdc.gov/traumaticbraininjury/severe.html

Centers for Disease Control and Prevention. (2016c). *TBI: Get the facts.* Retrieved from http://www.cdc.gov/traumaticbraininjury/get_the_facts.html

Cole, C. (2012). *Uncovering concussions: How they're changing our brains and the game.* Retrieved from http://chicagohealthonline.com/uncovering-concussions/

Collins, C. L., Fletcher, E. N., Fields, S. K., Kluchurosky, L., Rohrkemper, M. K., Comstock, R. D., & Cantu, R. C. (2014). Neck strength: A protective factor reducing risk for concussion in high school sports. *The Journal of Primary Prevention, 35*, 309–319. http://dx.doi.org/10.1007/s10935-014-0355-2

Esty, M. L., & Shifflett, C. M. (2014). *Conquering concussions: Healing TBI symptoms with neurofeedback and without drugs.* Sewickley, PA: Round Earth.

Gallaway, M., Scheiman, M., & Mitchell, G. L. (2017). Vision therapy for post-concussion vision disorders. *Optometry and Vision Science, 94*, 68–73. http://dx.doi.org/10.1097/OPX.0000000000000935

Gioia, G. A., Collins, M., & Isquith, P. K. (2008). Improving identification and diagnosis of mild traumatic brain injury with evidence: Psychometric support for the Acute Concussion Evaluation. *The Journal of Head Trauma Rehabilitation, 23,* 230–242. http://dx.doi.org/10.1097/01.HTR.0000327255.38881.ca

Graham, R., Rivara, F. P., Ford, M. A., & Spicer, C. M. (2014). *Sports-related concussions in youth: Improving the science, changing the culture.* Washington, DC: National Academies Press.

Jagannathan, J., Dumont, A. S., Prevedello, D. M., Shaffrey, C. I., & Jane, J. A., Jr. (2006). Cervical spine injuries in pediatric athletes: Mechanisms and management. *Neurosurgical Focus, 21*(4), 1–5. http://dx.doi.org/10.3171/foc.2006.21.4.7

Kim, J. H., Lee, H. S., & Park, S. W. (2015). Effects of the active release technique on pain and range of motion of patients with chronic neck pain. *Journal of Physical Therapy Science, 27,* 2461–2464. http://dx.doi.org/10.1589/jpts.27.2461

McCrory, P., Meeuwisse, W., Dvořák, J., Aubry, M., Bailes, J., Broglio, S., & Vos, P. E. (2017). Consensus statement on concussion in sport—The 5th international conference on concussion in sport held in Berlin, October 2016. *British Journal of Sports Medicine, 51,* 838–847. http://dx.doi.org/10.1136/bjsports-2017-097699

Meehan, W. P., III. (2011). Medical therapies for concussions. *Clinical Sports Medicine, 30,* 115–124. http://dx.doi.org/10.1016/j.csm.2010.08.003

National Collegiate Athletic Association. (2015). *The Pennsylvania State University sports medicine concussion management policy.* Retrieved from https://www.ncaa.org/sites/default/files/2017-18CProto65_PennStateU_Protocol_20170803.pdf

National Institute on Deafness and Other Communication Disorders. (2015). *Balance disorders.* Retrieved from https://www.nidcd.nih.gov/health/balance-disorders

Novack, T., & Bushnik, T. (2016). *Understanding TBI: Part 1. What happens to the brain during injury and the early stages of recovery from TBI?* Retrieved from http://www.msktc.org/tbi/factsheets/Understanding-TBI/What-Happens-During-Injury-And-In-Early-Stages-Of-Recovery

Nucleus Medical Media. (2012, March 14). *Concussion/traumatic brain injury* [Online video]. Retrieved from https://www.youtube.com/watch?v=55u5Ivx31og

Occipital neuralgia. (2016). Retrieved from http://www.webmd.com/migraines-headaches/occipital-neuralgia-symptoms-causes-treatments

Pilkington, K., Kirkwood, G., Rampes, H., Cummings, M., & Richardson, J. (2007). Acupuncture for anxiety and anxiety disorders—A systematic literature review. *Acupuncture in Medicine, 25,* 1–10. http://dx.doi.org/10.1136/aim.25.1-2.1

Schwarzbold, M., Diaz, A., Martins, E. T., Rufino, A., Amante, L. N., Thais, M. E., . . . Walz, R. (2008). Psychiatric disorders and traumatic brain injury. *Neuropsychiatric Disease and Treatment, 4,* 797–816.

Stone, P. (2013). *How is your TV making your concussion symptoms worse?* Retrieved from http://www.traumaticbraininjury.net/how-is-your-tv-making-your-concussion-symptoms-worse/

U.S. Department of Health and Human Services. (n.d.). *Facts for physicians about mild traumatic brain injury (MTBI)*. Retrieved from http://www.brainlinemilitary.org/concussion_course/course_content/pdfs/mtbi.pdf

Vestibular Disorders Association. (2016). *Vestibular rehabilitation therapy (VRT)*. Retrieved from http://vestibular.org/understanding-vestibular-disorder/treatment/treatment-detail-page

Wellmont Health System. (2016). *Whiplash*. Retrieved from http://www.wellmont.org/Our-Services/Orthopedics/Conditions-and-diseases/Spine-and-neck/Whiplash/

What is Active Release Techniques® (ART) to individuals, athletes, and patients? (n.d.). Retrieved from http://www.activerelease.com/ART-for-Patients.asp

15

WHERE ARE WE NOW, AND WHERE DO WE GO FROM HERE?

PETER A. ARNETT

I hope you have enjoyed this book and have expanded your knowledge on sports-related concussions. With the knowledge from this cast of esteemed researchers and clinicians, you should be able to improve your clinical care of athletes who suffer from concussions and have a much better understanding of the directions that research will take us in the next few years. In this final chapter, I am going to highlight some of the key take-home points from this book.

PREMORBID FACTORS ARE IMPORTANT PREDICTORS OF OUTCOME

Preexisting psychiatric symptomatology, premorbid problems with headache, and having the ε4 allele of the apolipoprotein (APOE) gene are risk factors for poor outcome after sports-related concussion. As such, knowing about these factors in individual athletes could help guide post-concussion

http://dx.doi.org/10.1037/0000114-016
Neuropsychology of Sports-Related Concussion, P. A. Arnett (Editor)

treatment and management. More work is needed, however, in terms of exactly how this information could be used in clinical management.

Regarding the ε4 allele of the *APOE* gene, for example, assuming future work replicates the initial findings of risk for poor outcome outlined in the chapter in this book by Victoria C. Merritt and me, how can this information be used? Should athletes be informed of their *APOE* allele status before engaging in sports in which the risk of head trauma is high? If so, who should convey this information? In addition, how early on should such information be gathered? When athletes begin playing at very young ages? Before embarking in contact sports as late adolescents or young adults? Also, to what extent might genetic risk factors for recovery (e.g., the *APOE* ε4 allele) be integrated with genetic vulnerabilities that might also underlie the development of posttraumatic headache and migraine, as articulated so convincingly by Womble, Henley, Fedor, and Collins in their chapter in this volume? Ultimately, there are ethical issues at play here with which future researchers and clinicians will have to grapple if more research supports genetic risk factors for poor outcome after concussion.

In terms of psychiatric symptomatology and premorbid problems with headache as risk factors for poor outcome, how should this information be used? Should such potential problems be evaluated at baseline and then athletes who experience these problems be treated even before they experience any type of concussion related injury? A case could be made for this, in that successful treatment of these problems before any injury occurs might lessen the likelihood of a poor outcome should such an athlete ever experience a concussion. An alternative approach could be to have those involved in concussion management simply be aware of these risk factors more generally, and then treat these problems aggressively should the athlete experience a concussion to reduce the risk of poor outcome at that point in the process. However, again, the optimal timing of such interventions is not known. As Erin Guty, Megan Bradson, and I outline in our chapter herein, the implications of these kinds of risk findings need to be further considered in terms of how they might inform clinical management. Ideally, treatment outcome studies could examine the relative efficacy of interventions at different time points in the process.

BIOMARKERS OF CONCUSSION AND OUTCOME NEED FURTHER EXPLORATION

As Grossner, Mayer, and Hillary, outline in their chapter on neuroimaging methods in this book, brain imaging approaches have become increasingly sophisticated in recent years and have helped characterize functional brain changes that commonly occur after a sports-related concussion.

However, at present there is still no clear functional brain change signature that can be used as a postconcussion biomarker. Continued work in this realm is needed in terms of short-term functional brain changes that can serve as biomarkers. Related to these issues, as Echemendia, Bruce, and Glusman note in their chapter, more work is needed to determine the extent to which physiological recovery extends beyond clinical recovery and whether patterns of physiological recovery have implications for physical or cognitive functioning.

Beyond their examination during the relatively acute post-concussion period, biomarkers that may be evident later on in life that may serve as biomarkers of the presence of chronic traumatic encephalopathy (CTE) should also be investigated further. As Alosco, Healy, and Stern note in their fine chapter on CTE, it is not possible to diagnose CTE during an athlete's life, and even the clinical presentation of CTE is not well characterized. In addition to in vivo functional biomarkers from brain imaging, structural biomarkers (e.g., using diffusion tensor imaging indices) might be useful as predictors and correlates of CTE during life. Finally, as Echemendia and colleagues clearly lay out in their chapter, whether or not a particular number of concussions warrants retirement from play is unclear. In addition to considering the sheer number of concussions, the characteristics of concussions, including their severity and temporal sequencing, may be important. Some integration of these issues with work on CTE and genetic work would help clarify risk profiles for CTE. More research clearly is needed to explore some of these possibilities.

AN AWARENESS OF SEX AND DEVELOPMENTAL DIFFERENCES IN CONCUSSION PRESENTATION AND RECOVERY SHOULD INFORM CARE

There is now substantial evidence showing that females report more concussions than males in comparable sports. Knowing this, treatment providers will very likely see more females than males clinically, and they should generally expect that females will report more symptoms and take longer to recover than males. In addition, given their report of more symptoms, females will very likely need more treatment options than males. Covassin, Bretzin, and Fox's outstanding chapter details some of these issues in a compelling way, but more work on sex differences in concussion by a broader range of investigators is clearly needed.

Regarding potential negative long-term outcomes, the vast majority of work on CTE to date has focused on male athletes. More work is also needed to assess the extent to which female athletes involved in sports where repeated head injuries occur are at elevated risk for CTE and other negative long-term outcomes compared with males.

Analogous to the work on sex differences, Webbe and Vagt's chapter on pediatric concussion is noteworthy. As they note, children are not "little adults," and their symptom profile and recovery patterns differ in ways that appear to be less predictable than those of adults. More attention is often needed regarding the impact of concussion on a child's social and academic functioning in a way that is less salient for adults. Also, more work is needed regarding the severity and timing of pediatric concussion in terms of predicting long-term outcomes. This is difficult work to do, because it requires long-term follow-up, but it is necessary for us to gain a full understanding of the potentially different character and risk profile associated with pediatric concussions relative to concussions that occur in late adolescence and adulthood.

MORE WORK ON THE TIMING OF POSTCONCUSSION PHYSICAL AND COGNITIVE EXERTION IS NEEDED

As detailed so cogently in McCrea and colleagues' chapter on persistent postconcussion symptoms, and discussed by Gupta and Sebastianelli in their chapter, one counterintuitive finding that has emerged in recent years is that completely eliminating cognitive and physical exertion after an injury can prolong negative outcomes. Before these recent findings, the standard of clinical care was generally complete cognitive and physical rest prior to symptom resolution. Now, it does appear that engaging in at least some light cognitive and physical activity before complete symptom resolution is beneficial to most concussed athletes' recovery. As yet, however, the ideal timing of when athletes in recovery should start to engage in such exertion is not known. Additional outcome studies on this topic are clearly needed. Some integration of such research with biomarkers of recovery would be especially appealing. For example, if functional brain imaging signatures that indicate different stages of recovery can be identified, such markers could be timed with the onset of the beginning of postinjury physical and cognitive exertion. Also, some investigation of sex differences in such brain imaging signatures and their timing with recovery would be optimal, given the somewhat different postinjury symptom presentations characteristic of females versus males.

MORE WORK IS NEEDED THAT COMPARES COMPUTERIZED WITH TRADITIONAL NEUROPSYCHOLOGICAL MEASURES

The chapter by Jessica Meyer and me in this volume shows that traditional paper-and-pencil neuropsychological measures are more sensitive to the neurocognitive effects of concussion than computerized measures like

Immediate Post-Concussion Assessment and Cognitive Testing (ImPACT). However, this is only one study, and there were limitations of this research in terms of subject selection and the timing of testing after the injury. In addition, the logistical challenges to widespread use of more traditional measures that require fact-to-face testing are not trivial. More work is clearly needed on this topic to see whether these types of results will be replicated. Also, if replication studies confirm the initial finding of less sensitivity of computerized measures, then this could stimulate more work on how computerized measures could be made more sensitive such that they are comparable to traditional measures. If our results are replicated, then there are serious issues that need to be addressed in terms of the widespread use of computerized tests given that such an approach could likely result in an uncomfortably high number of false negatives and put concussed athletes back to play before they are fully recovered.

The sports-concussion literature has moved along at a geometrically increasing pace over the past 10 to 15 years. However, as this book has demonstrated, even though we know much more about risk factors and outcome and recovery patterns, sports concussion research is still in its infancy. I hope that the research and clinical issues detailed in this book will help push the field forward in ways that will enhance our understanding of sports concussion and result in better clinical care and long-term outcomes.

INDEX

ABOUT THE EDITOR

Peter A. Arnett, PhD, received his doctorate in clinical psychology from the University of Wisconsin–Madison and completed a postdoctoral fellowship in clinical neuropsychology at the Medical College of Wisconsin. He is currently a psychology professor and director of the Neuropsychology of Sports Concussion and Multiple Sclerosis (MS) Programs at Pennsylvania State University (Penn State). Dr. Arnett's research has focused on clinical neuropsychology, with an emphasis on understanding cognitive and emotional functioning in those who have suffered from sports-related concussion or MS. He is a fellow of the National Academy of Neuropsychology (NAN), a past winner of NAN's Nelson Butters Award for Research Contributions to Clinical Neuropsychology, and is President-Elect of NAN. He is the author of more than 130 research articles and book chapters and has edited another book, *Secondary Influences on Neuropsychological Test Performance*. Dr. Arnett has given numerous national and international talks on sports-related concussion and on MS, and he has worked clinically with hundreds of people who have experienced sports-related concussions. Dr. Arnett has served as the program chair of the International Neuropsychological Society (INS) meeting, editor of the *NAN Bulletin*, a board member of the INS, and the director of clinical training at Penn State. He is an editorial board member of several journals and has received grant funding from the National Institutes of Health, National Institute of Mental Health, and National Multiple Sclerosis Society.